Family Carers in Palliative Care

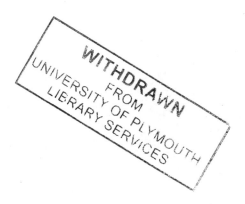

Family Carers in Palliative Care

A Guide for Health and Social Care Professionals

Edited by

Peter Hudson

Associate Professor and Director,
Centre for Palliative Care Education and Research,
St Vincent's Hospital and The University of Melbourne,
Victoria, Australia

Sheila Payne

Professor,
Help the Hospices Chair in Hospice Studies,
International Observatory on End of Life Care,
Lancaster University,
Lancaster, UK

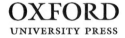

OXFORD
UNIVERSITY PRESS

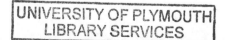

2013 → Plymouth

OXFORD
UNIVERSITY PRESS

Great Clarendon Street, Oxford OX2 6DP

Oxford University Press is a department of the University of Oxford.
It furthers the University's objective of excellence in research, scholarship,
and education by publishing worldwide in

Oxford New York

Auckland Cape Town Dar es Salaam Hong Kong Karachi
Kuala Lumpur Madrid Melbourne Mexico City Nairobi
New Delhi Shanghai Taipei Toronto

With offices in

Argentina Austria Brazil Chile Czech Republic France Greece
Guatemala Hungary Italy Japan Poland Portugal Singapore
South Korea Switzerland Thailand Turkey Ukraine Vietnam

Oxford is a registered trade mark of Oxford University Press
in the UK and in certain other countries

Published in the United States
by Oxford University Press Inc., New York

© Oxford University Press 2009

The moral rights of the authors have been asserted
Database right Oxford University Press (maker)

First published 2009

British Library Cataloguing in Publication Data
Data available

Library of Congress Cataloging-in-Publication Data
Family carers in palliative care: a guide for health and social care professionals / edited by Peter
Hudson, Sheila Payne.
   p. ;cm.
Includes bibliographical references and index.
ISBN 978–0–19–921690–1
1. Palliative treatment. 2. Terminally ill—Home care. 3. Terminally ill—Family relationships.
4. Caregivers. I. Hudson, Peter, 1965- II. Payne, Sheila, 1954-[DNLM: 1. Palliative Care—
methods. 2. Family Relations. WB 310 F1982 2008]
R726.8.F353 2008
616'.209—dc22
2008031671

Typeset by Cepha Imaging Private Ltd., Bangalore, India
Printed in Great Britain
on acid-free paper
by Biddles Ltd., King's Lynn, UK
ISBN 978–0–19–921690–1

1 3 5 7 9 10 8 6 4 2

Whilst every effort has been made to ensure that the contents of this book are as complete,
accurate and up-to-date as possible at the date of writing, Oxford University Press is not
able to give any guarantee or assurance that such is the case. Readers are urged to take
appropriately qualified medical advice in all cases. The information in this book is
intended to be useful to the general reader, but should not be used as a means of
self-diagnosis or for the prescription of medication.

Foreword

Peter Hudson and Sheila Payne's book provides a valuable overview of key issues related to the challenges faced by family carers of individuals receiving palliative care. The breadth and depth of topics covered in this volume serve as a helpful guide to those endeavouring to understand better the experiences of these families.

Barbara Monroe and David Oliviere's engaging opening chapter cautions us about the risk of romanticizing families and presuming how they ought to respond. The authors anchor their analysis in systems theory, reinforcing the usefulness of both a health and social approach to care. This novel analysis challenges service providers to work across traditional boundaries to offer the range of supports that families require. The authors reinforce the notion of potential cultural variations in communication and encourage health professionals to quarantine assumptions that may create barriers.

Allan Kellehear provides a cogent argument for the necessity of a public health approach to palliative care, offering a more holistic framework for constructing health family caregiving. He reminds us that the notion of caring within families is interactive; and that patients also care for and support families, as they work through the emotions, tasks and adjustments associated with a terminal illness. Kellehear cautions the reader to beware of superficial stereotypes related to cultural beliefs and hidden assumptions about what may be best (for example, the notion that a home death is the ideal).

The spiritual needs of family carers is a topic that has, to date, been poorly researched. Rosalie Hudson provides a comprehensive summary of relevant literature and poses useful questions about how to sensitively attend to matters relating to spiritual well-being. The importance of communication skills is reinforced in this chapter and the call to reflective practice is particularly pertinent. The world of palliative care can attract individuals who are open to conversations about meaning, spirituality, and religious inquiry. There is also a risk that boundaries related to these topics are crossed and Hudson alerts the reader to this possibility. The notion of a team approach, the importance of training related to spiritual support and the need for transparency related to this aspect of palliative practice, are essential.

Hilary Arksey and Anne Corden provide a valuable chapter related to policy initiatives for family carers, through their analysis and comparison of policies in England, Canada, Australia and European states. The social policies related to caregiving provide the architecture that shapes service provision. Therefore, it is essential that palliative care providers contribute to social policies relevant to palliative care practice. Although some countries have adopted polices that recognize, to some extent, the role of family caregiving, the economic, psychological and practical impacts of family caregiving are generally not well resourced and consequently much invisible, unpaid family caregiving occurs in most countries, subsidizing the paid palliative care workforce.

Jennifer Hunt's account of the issues faced by family carers in resource-poor countries is extremely informative and points to the need to look beyond usual social and geographic boundaries. The difficulties of providing family support in countries ravaged by years of HIV/AIDS are particularly sobering, stressing the inter-generational legacy of a terminal illness on struggling nations. The need for fundamental public health infrastructure is evident in Hunt's analysis and she emphasizes the importance of a primary care approach to community based palliative care that educates and empowers volunteers, families and the wider community.

Ethical and legal issues related to family caregiving are thoughtfully addressed by Michael Ashby and Danuta Mendelson. Their chapter reinforces the earlier notion of death as a community experience and the importance of a health-promoting approach to death and dying. Their conclusions regarding the significance of communication and the process of ethical consultation are valuable when considering how best to support families through decisions. The tables summarizing information about how to conduct family meetings and tips about how to work with families who are reluctant to discuss a poor prognosis offer sound, practical information that will be helpful to clinicians.

Kevin Brazil provides a summary of family carer satisfaction literature, highlighting the measurement complications associated with this construct. However, the importance of a family member's views of care is not something to be dismissed, and conceptual clarity and trustworthy assessment of the care experience through the eyes of the family are essential if we are to understand their experiences and better meet their needs. A number of instruments to measure family care satisfaction have been tested over the years and have demonstrated sound psychometric properties, being translated into different languages. The theoretical and clinical links between family care satisfaction and other critical care indicators have also been demonstrated. For example, family carers who report lower levels of care satisfaction are less likely to have their needs met and cope more poorly in the bereavement period following the patient's death (1). The 'so what factor' related to family care satisfaction is the potential for families to feel guilty and experience more despair during the patient's illness and after the patient's death because they believed that they should have been a better advocate for the patient. It is essential that we continue to index the perceptions of families in relation to the care received so that we might align our support more appropriately.

The editors of this book also recognize that family carers' needs may differ according to care setting. Betty Ferrell, Tami Borneman and Chan Thai have contributed a reflective chapter with useful case illustrations focusing on the challenges of family caregiving in hospitals and in-patient palliative care units. They remind us that in many instances, a hospital setting may be the setting of choice and may be the most appropriate choice. However, in these settings the role of the family as carer may be more complex and the legitimacy of the family as a recipient of care poorly recognized. As well, a less familiar care setting may prompt families to retreat from the care experience. They may be less confident about expressing their own needs for support. If family members withdraw or feel side-lined by the routine and busy-ness of hospital life, they may suffer from a lack of information and subsequent anxiety and uncertainty about how to participate. The importance of communication, family conferences and engagement with the family in care decisions are critical strategies for family support in these care settings.

Kelli Stajduhar and Robin Cohen offer a coherent analysis of the needs of families providing care at home. The suggested questions to help assess needs of families and the role(s) they wish to play are particularly helpful. The strategies outlined to support home-based palliative carers provide a useful framework for structuring focused intervention studies and clinical choices.

Mike Nolan and Rosalie Hudson provide a careful synthesis of relevant literature related to family care in the context of palliative aged care. The importance of communication, engagement with the family and the value of a care partnership are particularly relevant in mapping a framework for family support in this context.

The needs of family carers of children confronting life-threatening illnesses are comprehensively summarized by Sharon De Graves and Jenny Hynson. It is evident that less research has been undertaken with the paediatric palliative care population and their families and that further research is needed to identify interventions that are most helpful.

Donna Milne and Karen Quinn document the importance of targeted and tailored care interventions for families of individuals with advanced cancer. The authors identify the challenges of helping families to acknowledge and attend to their own needs for support during a progressive, and sometimes fast-moving downward, illness trajectory.

The inclusion of chapters related to family carers of individuals with non-malignant diseases is important given expected trends in palliative care service provision. Janice Brown and Julia Addington-Hall provide a valuable summary of relevant empirical findings related to the needs of families of individuals with organ failure and neurodegenerative conditions. The unique features of these illness trajectories merit targeted intervention studies aimed at evaluating the most appropriate approaches to support family carers in these circumstances.

Sheila Payne and Liz Roll's chapter on 'Support for bereaved family carers' navigates a vast and complex body of literature constructively. This dimension of palliative care is encumbered by a number of assumptions and a lack of sound evidence to guide practice decisions and service provision. The correct 'dose' of bereavement support is not known. The notion of who is 'at risk' for a 'complicated grief response' is also poorly understood. It is unclear when normal grief and the process of grieving warrants intervention. And again, our approach to supporting grieving individuals is shaped, and likely hampered by, the lack of community education about how to respond and support individuals during their grieving. The need for further research to address these questions is evident.

Peter Hudson and Sheila Payne's final chapter underscores the point that there is a notable gap between the rhetoric of family centred palliative care and actual practice, with the clear conclusion that family centred social policy, further research and improved service delivery is warranted. The number of family members of individuals with progressive disease will continue to increase as we are faced with the caregiving requirements of an ageing population (2). Notwithstanding the demands of caregiving, family carers report benefits and rewards from the caring role (3). There is also evidence that family carers may feel a strong sense of duty to provide good quality care to their relative. Helping family members to assume the caregiving role in a way that is sustainable and fulfilling should be the aim. Healthcare providers who view the family as the unit of care are better able to assess and identify supports for those in need of assistance. Attention to families in a palliative phase of illness who may be psychologically vulnerable, lack resources or have concomitant health issues and concerns, constitutes good preventive family care.

This book makes a significant contribution to our understanding of family carers in palliative care and will be a valuable resource. This comprehensive and thoughtful summary of the empirical evidence related to this population will be frequently cited by researchers, students and clinicians who are endeavouring to know how to use these findings to guide their work.

Professor Linda Kristjanson
Deputy Vice-Chancellor, Research and Development
Curtin University of Technology
Australia

References

1. Kristjanson LJ, Sloan JA, Dudgeon DJ and Adaskin E (1996). Family members' perceptions of palliative cancer care: predictors of family functioning and family members' health. *Journal of Palliative Care* **12**(4): 10–20.

2. Kristjanson LJ (1999). Families of palliative care patients: a model for care. In: Aranda S and O'Connor M (ed.). *Palliative Care for Nursing: A Guide to Practice*. Richmond, VIC: Ausmed Publications, 279–293.

3. Hudson P (2004). Positive aspects and challenges associated with caring for a dying relative at home. *International Journal of Palliative Nursing* **10**: 58–65.

Preface

Dying is a family affair, its impact ripples out to affect close friends, neighbours and the wider social network. When a person is diagnosed with a life-threatening illness, the impact of this event extends to the entire family and close friends. The quality of life of the person confronting the end stages of their life may be severely compromised without the support of family carers. Indeed, most people requiring palliative care would not be able to be cared for at home or to realize their preferences, such as for dying at home, without significant family carer input. Furthermore, healthcare services acknowledge that, without the involvement of family carers and/or close friends, healthcare costs would substantially increase.

Remarkably, most families and friends respond to these challenges by mobilizing their social networks, sharing resources, skills and knowledge to provide compassionate care. While the role of family carers varies with each situation, it is not uncommon for carers to provide symptom management, hygiene and practical care, together with emotional and spiritual support for their relative or friend. This responsibility can be extremely demanding; some carers suffer financially and socially as a consequence of their role, and others are overwhelmed by the psychological and physical issues confronting them. It must be emphasized, however, that some carers will also derive positive outcomes from the experience.

Since its inception, the modern hospice/palliative care movement has recognizd the role family carers play in end-of-life care. As a consequence, health and social care professionals are obliged to support the family alongside the person diagnosed with a life-threatening illness. In short, palliative care is supposed to be family centred. We acknowledge, however, the considerable challenges impacting upon health and social care workers' capacity to deliver family centred palliative care. Meeting the needs of family members is not simple, considering, for example, the increasingly complex patterns of relationships in contemporary families. Friends, neighbours and other social networks are often crucial to caring directly for people with advanced disease or indirectly in supplying support to family carers.

It is easy to highlight shortcomings and challenges. Our aim in preparing this book was not only to acknowledge the issues related to family carers but, most importantly, to provide readers with suggested strategies and resources (based on available evidence) in order to improve the care available to families. In so doing, we invited experts from several continents and a variety of multidisciplinary backgrounds to contribute to this book. We have endeavoured to cover a broad range of topics related to family carers, including social policy and public health, communication, ethico-legal, research, cultural and spiritual dimensions, and exploration of caregiver roles across a broad spectrum of disease states and care delivery settings. We also outline a revised scope for the interface between palliative care and family carer support and highlight the priorities for the future.

Our passion for preparing this book stems from our own backgrounds as (a) providers of palliative care (clinicians), (b) observers of palliative care (researchers) and (c) our interest in the social aspects of palliative care (policy informers). At the 'coal face' of palliative care we have witnessed exemplary support for some family carers, while observing that overall attention to families and friends is highly variable. We have identified an increasing number of family carer research projects, while noting also the lack of comprehensive intervention studies. We are also conscious of some new social policy and public health initiatives but also mindful of the lack of resources to match these and ongoing issues of access and availability of support services. Moreover, quality service delivery for families needs to be complemented by strong social policy, appropriate resources and robust research. We believe these areas need to be strengthened significantly.

In summary, we are concerned about the current level of quality of support offered to family carers, despite the emphasis over four decades of 'modern' hospice/palliative care. We hope that health and social care workers, palliative care specialists, academics and policy makers who read this book will be inspired to have greater respect for, and understanding of, the experiences of family carers, and to work with them to plan and deliver care that is inclusive of their needs and concerns. We believe there is a gap between the description of 'family centred care' in palliative care and its application in practice. This book attempts to bridge that gap.

Peter Hudson
Sheila Payne
2008

Contents

Contributors

Julia Addington-Hall
Professor in End of Life Care,
Co-Director of the NCRI-funded
Cancer Experiences Supportive and
Palliative Care Research
Collaborative (CECo),
School of Nursing and Midwifery
University of Southampton,
Southampton, UK

Hilary Arksey
Senior Research Fellow,
Social Policy Research Unit,
University of York,
York, UK

Michael Ashby
Director of Palliative Care,
Royal Hobart Hospital, and
Professor of Palliative Care,
School of Medicine,
Faculty of Health Science,
University of Tasmania,
Tasmania, Australia

Tami Borneman
Senior Research Specialist,
Department of Nursing Research
and Education,
City of Hope,
California, USA

Kevin Brazil
Associate Professor,
Department of Clinical
Epidemiology and Biostatistics,
Division of Palliative Care,
Family Medicine Faculty of Health
Science, McMaster University and
Director, St Joseph's Health System
Research Network,
Ontario, Canada

Janice Brown
Senior Lecturer,
Cancer, Palliative Care and
End of Life Research Group,
School of Nursing & Midwifery,
University of Southampton,
Southampton, UK

Robin Cohen
Research Director and Associate,
Professor, Division of Palliative Care,
Departments of Oncology and
Medicine, McGill University,
Quebec, Canada

Anne Corden
Senior Research Fellow,
Social Policy Research Unit,
University of York,
York, UK

Sharon De Graves
Clinical Nurse Educator,
Children's Cancer Centre,
Royal Children's Hospital, Melbourne,
Victoria, Australia

Betty Ferrell
Research Scientist,
Department of Nursing Research
and Education,
City of Hope,
California, USA

Peter Hudson
Associate Professor and Director,
Centre for Palliative Care Education
and Research, St Vincent's Hospital
and The University of Melbourne,
Victoria, Australia

Rosalie Hudson
Palliative and Aged Care Consultant
and Associate Professor and
Honorary Senior Fellow,
School of Nursing,
The University of Melbourne,
Victoria, Australia

Jennifer Hunt
Social Work Consultant
Harare, Zimbabwe

Jenny Hynson
Consultant Paediatrician,
Victorian Paediatric Palliative
Care Program,
Royal Children's Hospital,
Melbourne,
Victoria, Australia

Allan Kellehear
Professor of Sociology and
Head of Department,
Department of Social & Policy Sciences
University of Bath,
Bath, UK

Danuta Mendelson
Professor, School of Law,
Deakin University,
Victoria, Australia

Donna Milne
Clinician Researcher,
Nursing and PhD candidate
(The University of Melbourne),
Department of Nursing and

Supportive Care Research,
Peter MacCallum Cancer Centre,
Victoria, Australia

Barbara Monroe
Chief Executive,
St Christopher's Hospice,
London, UK

Mike Nolan
Professor of Gerontological Nursing,
Sheffield Institute for Studies
on Ageing,
University of Sheffield,
Sheffield, UK

David Oliviere
Director of Education and Training,
St Christopher's Hospice,
London, UK

Sheila Payne
Professor, Help the Hospices Chair in
Hospice Studies, and Co-Director of
the NCRI-funded Cancer
Experiences Supportive and
Palliative Care Research
Collaborative (CECo),
International Observatory on
End of Life Care, Institute for
Health Research,
Lancaster University,
Lancaster, UK

Karen Quinn
Research Fellow,
Centre for Palliative Care,
Education & Research,
St Vincent's Hospital and
The University of Melbourne,
Victoria, Australia

Liz Rolls
Senior Research Associate and
Honorary Research Fellow,
University of Gloucestershire
International Observatory on End of
Life Care, Institute for Health
Research, Lancaster University,
Lancaster, UK

Kelli Stajduhar
Assistant Professor,
School of Nursing and
Centre on Aging

University of Victoria,
British Columbia,
Canada

Chan Thai
Coordinator,
Department of Nursing Research,
and Education,
City of Hope,
California, USA

Chapter 1

Communicating with family carers

Barbara Monroe and David Oliviere

Families are not fairytales whose last line is 'and they all lived happily ever after'. They are places of conflict and stress. But they are also places where we learn to resolve them by honest communication, mutual understanding and forgiveness. The family is where we learn the grammar of emotional intelligence by not giving up when the going gets tough. It's our ongoing seminar on the meaning of loyalty.

Rabbi Jonathan Sacks (1)

Families are made up of ordinary people. As a result of illness, death and bereavement, they react, respond, adjust and achieve. It is an indication of the resilience of families that they can do these things (2). The medium for families is communication. It is the job of health and social care professionals to facilitate these processes, not try and do it for them. We cannot give families what they ultimately wish: to take away the illness, keep the person alive or bring back their family member following bereavement. Some families struggle to care, communicate, collaborate or cohere. We need to give special attention to these families.

This chapter focuses on the family in terms of a social care and family 'systems' approach. It considers the family as a group with the patient as an integral part, rather than addressing the needs of family carers as a separate entity, and outlines some of the communication issues and challenges in family work in palliative care. In terms of 'who' the 'family' is, we recommend the Kissane and Bloch (3) definition: 'the family is who the patient says it is'. This can include a whole range of relationships of blood, care, commitments, duty, friendship and of love.

Families can be seen as both 'patient' and 'staff': recipients of care and providers of care. One of the ambiguities for palliative care professionals is that family carers are separate from, and yet the same as, the patient. They are second-order 'patients', but sometimes also 'colleagues' in the care of the patient. They have identified needs of their own (4) but are heavily influenced by, and have an influence on, the patient's needs. We cannot assume that family members are also carers. Family members may move in and out of caring tasks during the illness trajectory and non-biological members of the patient's network may emerge as significant contributors to care.

The family as a 'system'

Events have a history and a future. Illness, death and bereavement are events and processes. The family lives in a web of relationships from the past, in the present and into the future. Families function within a social, cultural, economic and environmental context. All these factors considered together create a meaning system, a lens through which the family views the world and other people.

One way of understanding families and family carers, and of gaining insights into the dynamics at play in palliative care, is through a systems approach to working with families. The family is a set of relationships— functional and dysfunctional—a set of dynamic and changing bonds. Family relationships and attitudes are interacting, interconnected and interdependent. In everyday living, family members are mutually dependent, taking on different roles and tasks. They develop their own idiosyncratic patterns of communication and norms of behaviour. There is a 'system' or 'pattern' that gives the family unit meaning and equilibrium in coping with the ups and downs of living. Change in one part of the system will have a corresponding effect on another part of the system, rather like a 'see-saw' effect. For example, deterioration in the health of one family member will impact psychologically on another; the daughter's depression following diagnosis of her father's stroke results in increased guilt in the patient. The crucial function of the family system is to give balance and stability.

Health and social care approaches

There are varying perceptions between healthcare and social care professionals about the way work with families is identified, defined and approached. There are overlapping but differing skills and knowledge, professional values, tasks and working contexts, which can result in a divergence in defining the problem, causation and focus for intervention, as seen in Table 1.1.

Both perspectives are needed to meet holistically the complex needs of patient and family carer in modern palliative care. Traditional healthcare approaches to the family involve treating the patient as an individual whilst assessing family carers separately in terms of their set of needs. Although proper attention is now being demanded for the diverse and specific needs of

Table 1.1 Health and social care continuum

Health	Social
'Management' of situation	Facilitation of change at a personal and societal level
Focus on individuals	Focus on system/group
Individual's responsibility	Society's influence
Current circumstances	Context of past, present, future
Professional expertise	User/carer choice/empowerment

family carers in their own right (4, 5), from a social care and systems perspective it is also essential to perceive the family as a whole entity.

Carers' concerns may need to be discussed separately before attempts to integrate patient and family issues in a joint meeting. It often helps to legitimize separate meetings in initial assessments with patient and family. However, this should not be used as a justification for avoiding the offer of a powerful therapeutic opportunity to engage the patient and family in revealing concerns and problem-solving together. A typical scenario might be: 'Don't tell Jack I can't cope any longer. It would kill him.' A potential response might be: 'My experience is that most couples who have been together as long as you and Jack get pretty good at guessing one another's thoughts.' Left unspoken these hunches can loom much larger than they really are and cause even more fear and worry. An appropriate alternative might be: 'Would you be prepared to try talking to Jack if I were there to help and to keep things safe?' The Australian clinical practice guidelines for communicating prognosis and end-of-life issues contain many helpful suggestions for managing exchanges with the family, including those who wish to withhold information from the patient (6).

Translating the systems approach to healthcare

There has been long-standing interest in end-of-life care about the potential benefit of family therapy (7) and family-based approaches (8). Early interest coincided with more general observations that intractable grief in individuals was often reflected in family patterns. A few studies offered tentative indications that a systemic approach might offer benefits (9, 10). Nadeau's research (11) demonstrates the importance of 'family meaning making' in bereavement. Clinical experience over many years suggests that in most situations one or two family sessions, of whatever grouping is permitted by the patient and can be practically arranged, can facilitate coping. Griffith *et al.* (12) offers suggestions about improving family meetings with older people in a rehabilitation setting and provides some indication of their potential to contribute to outcomes. Walsh (13) reviews strengths-based approaches to working with families and promoting resilience. However, there is little significant research data on the outcomes of the family-meeting approach in palliative care. Kissane's work on 'Family Focused Grief Therapy' offers one methodology for a more specifically targeted and therapeutic approach, and has now demonstrated beneficial outcomes for those assessed to be 'at risk' by the model (14).

From a clinician's perspective, it is important to see the needs of individuals—patient and family carer(s)—but also to appreciate the sum of the parts: the whole, a set of relationships that act, react and interact. In family work, it is desirable to become attuned to the dynamics of the family, which give clues to the quality of their communication, cohesion and ability to resolve conflict (3). The belief is that focused interventions can trigger one or two changes in the family system, which, in turn, has the potential for a catalytic effect on producing more basic change in functioning—at least sufficient for family coping to improve. What is not attempted is the amelioration of long-term family issues or problems, although this is sometimes the outcome.

The family system resembles a series of interlocking parts, rather like a jigsaw puzzle. Indeed, 'puzzle' may be apt as the patterns of relationship and communication are often subtle, unique to the family and a mystery to outsiders. Sometimes one may wonder how the particular system functions and remains intact, as the relationships and communication in the family may be quite different from our own—unusual or harmful and hurtful as viewed by an outsider. The system can be compared to a 'dance' where the moves and style are characteristic of and known to the participants, as in the following scenario.

> Mrs S, 48 years old with advanced multiple sclerosis, complained to staff of her struggles to manage all the shopping, cleaning and cooking. It transpired that her two adult children were unemployed, yet did little to help. Staff in the multi-professional home care team became critical of the adult children and of their mother in 'allowing' this. Systems understanding threw light on the family behaviour of mother taking responsibility for doing all and the whole family feeding into this established pattern. Skilled help from the team confronted the inadequacy of their coping at a time when the patient's condition was deteriorating.

Impact of crisis on communication

The crisis of impending death is the ultimate threat to the family system. The system is thrown 'off balance'. Members hold on to the ill member, struggling to retain familiar coping patterns. How well the family communicates, shares, supports its members, operates as a team and tolerates difference of opinion, defines its functioning. In their research, Kissane and Bloch (3) demonstrated that family functioning has a striking impact on bereavement outcome. They concluded that cohesion, conflict and communication (expressiveness) were core components in assessing and working with families in palliative care to enhance family functioning.

No one model of intervention fits all families (13). What matters most are effective family processes and core to these is communication.

Common challenges

Some familiar family scenarios are summarized below. Various elements can be identified in each situation.

Collusions

Family members not wishing to address issues of the patient deteriorating and dying. A typical scenario is when the family carer insists, 'don't tell him, it'll kill him'; whilst the patient states, 'don't tell her, she cannot take it'. The two positions are held by the two parties colluding with each other in a 'game'.

Denial

Denial can exist on many levels and be more or less healthy, depending on how safe and useful a defence it is. If denial is too strong and key aspects of life are compromised, then denial serves a less useful purpose, as family function-ing is adversely affected; for example, the person who blocks any conversation related to the illness.

Isolation

When the patient or family carer gives signals that they want/need to express their feelings or elicit more information or discuss significant decisions—for example, future care of the children—and attempts are blocked by other family members, there can be profound isolation, leading to sadness, depres-sion and anxiety.

Scapegoating

Blaming another, projection or dividing into 'good' and 'bad' can be an attempt to leave the family intact whilst rallying against an 'enemy'. For example, seeing the nurse as 'good', whilst rejecting the doctor or social worker who discussed the possibility of a poor prognosis as 'bad'. A family must not be labelled as 'scapegoating' when there are real issues and inadequacies in services.

Withdrawn families

Families who exhibit clear signs of distress about what is happening to their patient but who are 'hard to reach' and display the signals to 'keep off'. Attempts to penetrate their 'system' are firmly rejected.

Family secrets

A variety of 'secrets' relating to the past (for example, how a grandparent died) or in the present (for example, father's affair) can impede family communication. The past often surfaces in time of illness and crisis. Previous life events can be actively present in the current situation, with feelings, thoughts and behaviours being acted out and accessible. Skilled work with the family can help them identify the issues and offer an opportunity to work through them.

Anger and conflict

Anger can often emerge, based on reality or fantasy, and directed against a range of people, God or things. It is sometimes directed towards the teams and professionals or volunteers working with the family. Families can present long-standing conflicts from their past; for example, non-communication between parties, or the surfacing of powerful feelings in terms of a father who has abused his children. This can result in acting out behaviour and conflict in the present.

Abusive families

Abuse does not have to take the form of extreme behaviours, bullying, or physical or psychological ill-treatment, although this can be a possibility. Subtle forms of abuse include exclusion from conversations or decision-making, depersonalizing the patient or neglectful physical care. The patient, too, can be abusive through insistent demands and verbal, sometimes physical, threats.

Multiple losses

It is common to see previous losses and the grief still attached to them, surface in the present crisis. The current bereavement can become mixed up with earlier ones and present an opportunity to revisit the pain, the issues involved and their meaning.

Cultural variations

All these family manifestations (listed above) can be affected by culture, another lens through which to see the world.

Culture fundamentally shapes how individuals and families make meaning out of illness and death. Nunez Olarte (15) describes how family attitudes, behaviours and patterns may be influenced by cultural variations. In traditional family systems—for example, in Southern Europe—the tendency is for the family to filter and control information regarding diagnosis and prognosis. In Northern Europe and North America, with the emphasis on patient autonomy and rights, the pattern is for the patients to be given priority to receive information regarding their condition.

There is a range of considerations required to meet varying cultural and religious needs (16). Gunaratnam warns against checklists and generalizations of cultural requirements, as they fail to 'reveal the complexity of the life history of individuals and their communities and the diversity of their human experience' (17). There are clearly a range of family patterns within each culture or religious group. Increasingly, sensitivity to inter-generational differences and understanding the complex mix of western/eastern influences will be important.

Cultural competence has been defined as a 'set of congruent behaviours, practices, attitudes and policies that come together in a system or agency, or among professionals, enabling effective work to be done in cross-cultural situations' (18). Effective culturally focused care needs to take into account:

- language and meaning of jargon, e.g. 'cancer', 'bereavement';
- interpreting and translation;
- record-keeping in terms of names, languages, forms of address;
- personal care requirements, e.g. modesty;
- environmental aspects, e.g. offensive images;
- empowerment of families, e.g. families screening information for patient;
- food and dietary requirements, e.g. sensitivity of fasting times, appropriate foods and handling of foods;
- respect for spiritual and religious practices and rituals, e.g. religious festivals;
- respect for roles, gender differences, beliefs and values, e.g. role of elders, male responsibilities; and
- norms of behaviour and expectations, e.g. children caring for parents, care of the body.

The most important question when working with families is to ask what is of cultural importance to them. It is essential to create a trusting relationship so that a useful conversation can emerge over what aspects of care need adapting to cultural or religious preferences and for the family to feel safe enough to ask for what they want without feeling that they are being made a 'special case'. An approach might include: 'We want to get this right for you. You might have to help us to understand your cultural needs. We want to look after your mum/dad, while respecting your religious requirements. If things are not going quite as you would like, please let us know.' Another approach is to check with the patient before making assumptions, as in the following scenario:

> Zara, 53, was dying in a hospice in-patient unit. The nursing staff were troubled with the huge number of visitors who kept calling and surrounding her bed as they felt she had no personal space. In a conversation with a key nurse, Zara was able to say how much she valued these visits, even when she was asleep.

Family assessment

The goals of family assessments are to provide a clear and adequate flow of information, with opportunities for shared questions and responses to increase mutual understanding; to support the development of shared and manageable priorities; to underpin and develop existing coping mechanisms; to acknowledge emotional pain and, where appropriate, to facilitate its expression and sharing; and to help family members to tolerate and understand differences. Individual and family assessments are inextricably intertwined. Assessments should be made early and often. Assessment is not a one-off process—circumstances alter and people change their minds. The aim is to create a partnership between the patient and their family, and the professional teams and organizations involved in their care. Consent must be obtained and checked regularly. 'Please tell us if there is something we ask that you would rather not discuss.' Confidentiality must be discussed and agreements made about those with whom information may be shared, both within professional teams and the patient's family and friendship network. It should also be recognized that information giving and gathering, assessment, planning, intervention and review are parts of a continuous and sometimes overlapping cycle.

Most assessments will have four main perspectives: the individual, the family, and their physical and social resources. The assessment will cover practical issues such as housing, finances, employment, unmet physical needs relating to caring, informal and formal caring resources. The effect of the illness on family roles and relationships and the personal histories of family members and any likely impact on caring capacity will need to be considered. Life cycle issues of family members, such as retirement or children leaving home, should be explored. It will be important to understand the history of any previous crises and their management and any additional concurrent crisis, such as job loss. The presence of other vulnerable individuals in the family, such as dependent elderly relatives, needs to be reviewed alongside attention paid to issues of culture, ethnicity and potential discrimination because of pre-existing vulnerabilities, such as learning disability or poverty.

Family and carer needs will emerge during assessment and may require differentiation. For example, it may become clear who is the lynch-pin of care and whether that person should be routinely involved in negotiations about care planning. Equally, a withdrawn or less obviously demanding family member may have masked needs for personal support, information or education.

Factors that may predispose the family to emotional risk include:

- close, dependent relationships or a carer with little perceived support;
- anger about delays in diagnosis or treatment, or lack of realism about prognosis;
- significant previous or current mental health problems or previous complicated losses;
- history of abuse or trauma, or evidence of dependency on drugs or alcohol;
- significant financial difficulties; and
- persistent family conflict or estranged family members (19).

Tools for intervention

These can include family trees/genograms and ecomaps (20), family meetings (either one-off or as a programme of sessions), and multi-professional and multi-agency work. Family care may be undertaken indirectly through others: advising or giving information to other health or social care professionals; mobilizing resources; co-ordinating agency efforts. A family focus can be maintained even when the whole family is not present. For example, carers may be asked in the absence of a semi-conscious patient, 'What do you imagine your mother would have wanted in these circumstances?'

A family tree is an assessment tool giving a snapshot of relationships and the availability of care, as well as a loss history to help in identifying those who may benefit from particular support (21). It is also a therapeutic tool that, when used with families, can encourage discussion and reveal concerns and issues to explore.

Family meetings

Brief, routine family sessions can be very valuable. The following guidelines are intended to describe the objectives and management of family meetings.

More structured therapeutic techniques, designed for interventions with families determined to be at serious risk, are detailed in the work of Kissane and Bloch (3).

Preparation

The team should discuss their objectives in advance. Any tensions between team members will emerge in the meeting, if not addressed beforehand. Goals may include: understanding patient and family views about prognosis and place of death, giving information about the illness and its management and care options, information about financial and other benefits, an assessment of carers' needs and family coping, and the identification of those at particular risk. It is important to consider who in the team will facilitate the meeting. It often helps to have a doctor or nurse joined by a team member with a psychological focus, so that both medical and broader psychosocial needs can be explored and the tasks of observing, offering information and time-keeping can be shared.

The patient's involvement and permission for such meetings should be obtained, even if they do not wish to be present. Where possible, patients should be asked who they would like to be present and whether they are comfortable with their illness, treatment and prognosis being discussed. Consideration should also be given on how to include people in the meeting who cannot be physically present.

There should be clear pre-planning about what will be said to the family about the purpose of the meeting. Family meetings offer a positive opportunity but often generate anxiety and so require focused, confident introductions. 'We want to talk about Jonathan's illness, your needs as a family and the support you may need as carers of Jonathan. We have found that it's useful to talk about these sorts of issues together.' Ensure that the environment is prepared with appropriate seating, and with televisions or bleeps turned off, where possible. Tensions can be high, so meetings should start on time.

Structure the session

- ♦ People feel safe with clear boundaries. Begin with proper introductions and set an expectation about the length of the meeting.
- ♦ Find out what the family would like to add to the team's agenda at the beginning of the meeting and attempt to create consensus about objectives.
- ♦ Adopt an open style with frequent checks on pace, comprehension and permission. 'Are we going too fast? Do we need to recap? Does this feel comfortable?'

- It helps if team members acknowledge uncertainty, where it exists. 'It's hard to know how to proceed with this.'
- Using simple feeling words such as 'sad, angry, frightened' can help people to say difficult things and to acknowledge painful emotions.
- Use questions to assess family functioning and promote open communication:
- How did each of you learn about/respond to the diagnosis?
  - Is there anyone significant who does not know?
  - How openly do you talk about the illness?
  - Who supports who at the moment?
  - How does your family handle disagreement?
  - Does your family share special beliefs?
  - What are the strengths of your family?
  - Is there anyone you are particularly worried about?
  - How are important decisions made in your family?

Normalize and anticipate problems and anxieties

- Conflicts of need should be openly acknowledged. 'You would like to go home to your daughter but you are anxious about the burden it might be for her.' 'You want to support your mother but you are worried about giving up your job.'
- Give information about how difficulties might be managed. For example, symptoms as death approaches, ways of managing financial problems.
- Recognize and permit differences. 'It is normal for illness to affect everyone differently and for there to be some areas of disagreement.'
- Use inclusive statements. 'A lot of people worry about… is this a concern for you?'
- Reinforce similarities and strengths. 'The important thing is that you all love your father and want to do your best to support him.'
- Confirm coping, remembering that caring can be a source of satisfaction and fulfilment, and that these positive attributes need reinforcement as well as the definition of any difficulties.

Encourage change

- Re-define problems in a positive form so that families can see things slightly differently rather than react defensively. 'You love your children and you want to protect them.'

- Help people to compromise. For example, where there is considerable denial it can help to say something like: 'It sounds as if you are unsure about how serious things are. It's important to hope for the best outcome but we also need to make plans in case things do not turn out as you hope'.

- Give clear information about the resources available and find out which of them the family would like to use. Families may need help to adjust expectations, to segment problems and to focus on one or two goals at a time.

- Help the family to concretize the steps needed to attain future objectives with questions like: 'How would we know that had changed? What would it look like?'

- Manage changes of direction. Use silence and touch. Challenge appropriately. 'We seem to be going round and round at the moment'. 'He just doesn't listen to me.' 'Then talk to him now.'

End in a safe place

- Give a warning shot. 'We've got about five minutes left. Is there anything else that is important for you to mention?'

- It is important that everyone feels that you understand their point of view, so summarize decisions in a way that reflects any family differences without showing a preference. The aim is to help them solve the problems they face in a way that they feel reasonably comfortable with, not to sort everything out for them. Agree who will action what and when.

- Offer the opportunity to rehearse concerns. 'Who are you most worried about telling? How do you think you might do it?'

- Acknowledge the emotional intensity of the meeting. 'We've talked about a lot of painful things today.'

- Validate the family's contribution to care and reinforce their confidence with specific examples of their coping strengths.

- Try to lower the emotional tone by moving on to more everyday topics, remembering that, if appropriate, body language such as shaking hands can be helpful in closing conversations.

- If a family makes it very difficult to end, take control. 'I am sorry but I think we have gone as far as we can at the moment, we will have to leave it there for now. There will be another opportunity to talk about this.'

- Be clear about the next opportunity to meet or follow-up contact.

Families with long-standing relationship difficulties

Using family meetings to achieve simple targets may be difficult or counter-productive in such families. Warning signs include families who frequently have hostile communications with professionals; family members who try to exclude others from meetings or care-giving; unrelenting hostility between family members, sometimes in the context of severe mental illness, substance abuse or physical or emotional abuse. In these circumstances it is important to maximize communication between service providers to avoid mixed messages, agree on modest targets in advance, and develop plans for managing violence or abusive behaviour or language (22).

Be explicit about ground rules at the beginning of meetings. 'Everyone will be asked to speak in turn. Abusive language or violent behaviour will not be tolerated.' A calm, firm tone helps. 'I understand that this is very important to you but shouting will not be allowed in this meeting.' Try to recognize over-protection or conflict. 'I think we need to let James talk for himself.' Bring unspoken feelings into play, 'You say you are unconcerned, but you look very tense.' Try to recognize and name anger: 'Something has happened to make you very angry'. Hypothesize about the possibility of other more painful feelings. 'It sounds very lonely too.' Recognize that sometimes working with the family together is an unrealistic goal and that team efforts may need to be focused on helping individuals to maintain their relationship with the patient in structured ways; for example, helping a divorced and a current wife to visit at separate times. Doka's work on disenfranchised grief (23) reminds us of the importance of recognizing and acknowledging the needs of hidden loss, such as that of secret lovers. It is also important to acknowledge the sometimes unrecognized significance of neighbour and friendship relationships and to validate their grief when families are excluding them.

Families and children

Many studies emphasize the potential of negative consequences if children are given inadequate support or involvement when facing the death of someone important to them (24, 25). Research confirms the importance of children's pre-death experiences in influencing and mediating the course and outcome of bereavement (26). Research findings also emphasize the particular importance of continued and competent parenting (27). Adult efforts to protect children often leave them confused and alone with their fears and fantasies, which may be much worse than the reality. Children always notice when something important is happening in their family: they are aware of adult anxieties, observe body language and practical changes, and often overhear adult conversations.

Children need simple, truthful, repeated information about what is happening and why and what might happen next; reassurance about practical concerns including their own care; to know that nothing they did or said made the illness happen; a chance to talk about feelings with adults prepared to share theirs; appropriate involvement in helping the patient; and help to manage changes.

Parents will often need support with their own emotional needs before they can contemplate the support of their children. The aim should be to help parents to talk to their children themselves and to give them the confidence and skills to begin to understand and meet their children's needs. Christ's research (24) underlines the value of giving parents information about their children's developmental needs. Many parents will also value rehearsal of possible questions from children and examples of appropriate responses (28). It can help to offer parents booklets to read for themselves about children's needs and books, or workbooks to read and complete with children. Including children in one-off family meetings can be a useful way of helping parents to develop the confidence to proceed for themselves.

Working with couples

In a recent survey on the emotional impact of cancer, 45 per cent of respondents said that the emotional aspects of the disease were more difficult to cope with than physical effects and 26 per cent reported significant difficulties in their relationship with their partner (29). People have a fundamental need to give and to receive love, to experience physical closeness and to feel some sense of ease with their bodies (30). Research indicates that sexual behaviour, self concepts and relationships are deeply affected in many adults with life-threatening disease (31, 32). Couples may collude to cope with the pressures of serious illness by blaming the outside world or by defending themselves against intimacy. Physical dependency needs created by the illness may disturb a well-established pattern of separation. Some partners find that physical changes in the patient, or a change of role—for example, from partner or spouse to carer—can alter their desire for intimacy. Addressing issues of sexuality and intimacy is part of professionals' responsibility towards couples. Professionals need to be able to initiate dialogue and discussion, and to offer first-line help, where appropriate (33). A study reports that when this was done, the majority of patients with advanced cancer actively wished to discuss issues of intimacy (34). Monroe (30) offers useful practice guidelines.

Families and teams

The palliative care literature offers considerable discussion and evidence about the effective working of recognized multi-professional teams internal to organizations (35). The importance of trust, clear formal systems of communication, coordination, and a mature, mutual understanding of, and respect for, differences in professional knowledge bases, codes of ethics, values, languages, cultures and goals, has been emphasized (36, 37). If these conditions are not met, the capacity of troubled families to divide and 'split' team members is apparent (20).

The current drive to deliver integrated 'seamless' support to patients and families across traditional health and social care divides makes the adherence to such professional behaviours even more important. We now see a wide variety of teams trying to coordinate a network of resources relevant to need, across complex boundaries, often with differing agency perceptions of who the 'real' client is (38). The different and jointly held identities of family as 'patient/client' and 'carer/support worker' can add to the confusion, as can different models of understanding; for example, a primarily 'physical health' or 'social' model of disability. Inter-agency tensions can be magnified by separate budgets and attendant financial pressures. In all circumstances, organizations and the teams and individuals within them, must take active steps to avoid mirroring the scapegoating that can emerge in family systems under stress.

Clear inter-agency protocols are essential and must include shared understandings about confidentiality. Recording must not become judgemental shorthand that promotes 'labelling'; for example, using the ubiquitous term 'problem family'. Equally important is effective signposting for patient and family about professional roles and areas of responsibility, if they are not to become disabled by bureaucratic overload. For example, a patient and family could be the focus for professional attention from a specialist palliative care team, the general practitioner and district nurse, social services, social security, housing, immigration services and community mental health services. Proposals for 'one-stop shop' environments and 'polyclinics' may provide more productive settings for coordination of support (39). The 'key worker' concept is rightly promoted. However, managing this level of continuity of personnel is often difficult to achieve in practice. Although expensive in terms of resources, case conferences where otherwise 'virtual teams' come together physically, can promote trust, achieve consensus about appropriate objectives and strategies, and deliver clarity about the allocation of tasks. Similarly, occasional debriefing meetings about deaths that have been complex to manage can be beneficial in terms of team-building and joint exploration of the need and mechanisms for changes in practice.

In complex inter-agency teams, the possibility is increased for family 'knowledge' and goals to become marginalizd (40). Family presence in meetings must be promoted actively so that the full potential of support and creative outcomes is achieved. Handled sensitively, inter-agency involvement can work positively to meet what patients and families want and need in complex circumstances. In an audit of adult protection work in a palliative care setting, Payne (41) reports that appropriate inter-agency assessments and interventions can support families and improve circumstances of abuse.

Family work matters

Care experiences can complicate or ameliorate individual and family experiences of bereavement and may influence the process and outcome of future difficult experiences (42, 3). In this sense, family work is proactive health promotion. All families find the experience of terminal illness challenging to normal patterns of communication and decision-making (43). The provision of clear information and support for family communication can help the family come together in its own way to collaborate and to support the patient. In addition there is substantial evidence for links between patient and family functioning (28). It is also clear that social support is a key factor in maintaining coping and in promoting adaptation in terminally ill patients (44). Since the quality of life of patients and families is intertwined, patient and family should be treated as the unit of care. However, in resource-constrained healthcare economies with increasing need and demand, there is a risk of a return to the privileging of a narrow medicalized model. A recent critique of the philosophy of palliative care suggests that 'the central aspect of palliative care is symptom control delivered humanely with adequate information. Undue emphasis on attending to families is demanding of resources which might be better devoted to a wider population of patients.' (45). Interestingly, the mantra of choice and the realities of constrained budgets may also be coming to the rescue of families with an assessment of the possible financial benefits of care provided at home. A systematic review of factors influencing home deaths emphasizes the importance of the role of prevention, public education, and family support and empowerment (46). It is apparent that home deaths are more likely in the presence of families that function well.

Conclusion

In the future there will simply not be enough professional carers to meet all end-of-life care needs. There must, therefore, be a focus on altering public attitudes and enhancing family and community resilience and capacity, so that families and communities themselves are resourced and enabled to respond sensitively and compassionately to the needs of the dying and the bereaved (47). Efforts to deliver public education and effective social marketing will become more important (48). Professionals must be realistic in the goals they set themselves in working with families. Loss hurts; we cannot make a family's experience something other than sad; but we can offer them support through a painful experience and help them to feel that they did what they could in caring. As Dame Cicely Saunders (49) said: 'We cannot take away the whole hard thing that is happening, but we can help bring the burden into manageable proportions.'

Key learning points

+ The family is defined by the patient and can include blood relatives, friends, neighbours and other significant relationships.
+ The family is an interdependent and interacting system.
+ The family exists in a social, cultural, economic and environmental context, which must be taken into account in assessment.
+ Facilitating family communication promotes health.
+ Good inter-professional and inter-agency communication is essential to effective family support.

Recommended reading and resources

Childhood Bereavement Network. Online directory and resources. www.childhoodbereavementnetwork.org.uk

Institute of Family Therapy, 24–32 Stephenson Way, London NW1 2HX. www.instituteoffamilytherapy.org.uk

King DA and Quill T (2006). Working with families in palliative care: one size does not fit all. *Journal of Palliative Medicine* 9(3): 704–715.

Kissane D and Bloch S (2002) *Family Focused Grief Therapy*. Oxford: Oxford University Press.

Monroe B (2004) Social work in palliative medicine. In: Doyle D, Hanks G, Cherny N and Calman K (3rd edn) *Oxford Textbook of Palliative Medicine*. Oxford: Oxford University Press.

Monroe B and Kraus F (ed.) (2005). *Brief Interventions with Bereaved Children*. Oxford: Oxford University Press.

Monroe B and Sheldon F (2004). Psychosocial dimensions of care. In: Sykes N, Edmonds P and Wiles J (ed.) *Management of Advanced Disease* (4th edn). London: Arnold.

Sheldon F (1997). *Psychosocial Palliative Care. Good Practice in the Care of the Dying and the Bereaved*. Cheltenham: Stanley Thornes.

Sheldon F and Oliviere D (2005). Family information and communication. *EJPC*, 12(6): 254–256.

Walsh F (2006) *Strengthening Family Resilience* (2nd edn) New York/London: Guilford Press.

References

1. Sacks J (2004). Credo. *The Times Newspaper*. International Day of Families, 15 May, p.49.

2. Stratton P (2005) *Report of the Evidence Base for Systematic Family Therapy*. Association for Family Therapy. London.

3. Kissane D and Bloch S (2002) *Family Focused Grief Therapy*. Oxford: Oxford University Press.

4. Payne S (2004) Carers and caregivers. In: Oliviere D and Monroe B (ed.) *Death, Dying and Social Differences*. Oxford: Oxford University Press, 181–198.

5. Payne S (2007) Resilient carers and caregivers. In: Monroe B and Oliviere D (ed.) *Resilience and Palliative Care. Achievement in Adversity*. Oxford: Oxford University Press, 83–98.

6. Clayton JM, Hancock KM, Butow PN, Tattersall MHN and Currow, DC (2007). Clinical practice guidelines for communicating prognosis and end-of-life issues with adults in the advanced stages of a life-limiting illness, and their caregivers. *Medical Journal of Australia* **186**(12): 18 June, S77–S108.

7. Walsh W and McGoldrick M (2004) (ed.). *Living Beyond Loss. Death in the Family* (2nd edn). New York: Norton.

8. Earnshaw-Smith E (1981). Dealing with dying patients and their relatives. *British Medical Journal* **282**: 1779.

9. Lieberman S (1978). Nineteen cases of morbid grief. *British Journal of Psychiatry* **132**: 159–163.

10. Rosenthal PA (1980). Short-term family therapy and pathological grief resolution with children and adolescents. *Family Process* **19**: 151–159.

11. Nadeau JW (1998). *Families Making Sense of Death*. London: Sage.

12. Griffith JC, Brosnan M, Lacey K, Keeling S and Wilkinson TJ (2004). Family meetings—a qualitative exploration of improving care planning with older people and their families. *Age and Ageing* **33**: 577–581.

13. Walsh F (2006). *Strengthening Family Resilience* (2nd edn). New York/London: Guilford Press.

14. Kissane DW, McKenzie M, Bloch S, Moskowitz C, Mckenzie DP and O'Neill I (2006). Family focused grief therapy: a randomized, controlled trial in palliative care and bereavement. *American Journal of Psychiatry* **163**(7): 1208–1218.

15. Nunez Olarte J (2003). Cultural difference and palliative care. In: Monroe B and Oliviere D (ed.). *Patient Participation in Palliative Care. A Voice for the Voiceless*. Oxford: Oxford University Press.

16. Oliviere D (2004) Cultural issues in palliative care. In: Sykes N, Edmonds P and Wiles J (ed.). *Management of Advanced Disease* (4th edn). London: Arnold, 438–449.

17. Gunaratnam Y (1997). Culture is not enough. A critique of multi-culturalism in palliative care. In: Field D, Hockey J and Small N (ed.). *Death, Gender and Ethnicity*. London: Routledge, 166–186.

18. Cross T, Bazron B, Dennis K and Isaacs MR (1989). *Towards a Culturally Competent System of Care*, Vol. 1. Washington, DC: Georgtown University Child Development Center: CASSP Technical Assistance Center.

19. Oliviere D, Hargreaves R and Monroe B (1998). Working with families. In: *Good Practices in Palliative Care: a Psychosocial Perspective*. Aldershot: Ashgate.

20. Sheldon F (1997). *Psychosocial Palliative Care. Good Practice in the Care of the Dying and the Bereaved*. Cheltenham: Stanley Thornes.

21. McGoldrick M and Gerson R (1985). *Genograms in Family Assessment*. New York: Stanley Thornes.

22. King DA and Quill T (2006). Working with families in palliative care: one size does not fit all. *Journal of Palliative Medicine* **9**(3): 704–715.

23. Doka L (2002) (ed). *Disenfranchised Grief: New Directions, Challenges and Strategies for Practice*. Champaign, IL: Research Press.

24. Christ GH (2000). *Healing Children's Grief: Surviving a Parent's Death from Cancer*. Oxford: Oxford University Press.

25. Silverman PR (2000). *Never too Young to Know. Death in Children's Lives*. Oxford: Oxford University Press.

26. Christ GH, Raveis VH, Siegal K, Karus D and Christ AE (2005). Evaluation of a preventive intervention for bereaved children. *Journal of Social Work in End-of-Life and Palliative Care* **1**(3): 57–81.

27. Worden WJ (1996). *Children and Grief. When a Parent Dies*. New York: Guilford Press.

28. Monroe B (2003). Psychological evaluation of patient and family. In: Sykes N, Fallon MT and Patt RB (ed.). *Cancer Pain*. London: Arnold, 73–85.

29. Cardy P, Corner J, Evans J, Jackson N, Shearn K and Sparham L (2006). *Worried Sick: the Emotional Impact of Cancer*. London: Macmillan Cancer Support.

30. Monroe B (1997). A sexual-sensitive approach to palliative care. In: Oliviere D, Hargreaves R and Monroe B (ed.). *Good Practices in Palliative Care: a Psychosocial Perspective*. Aldershot: Ashgate, 96–112.

31. Fallowfield L (1992). The quality of life: sexual function and body image following cancer therapy. *Cancer Topics* **9**: 20–21.

32. Schover LR (1998). Sexual dysfunction. In: Holland JC (ed.) *Psycho-oncology*. Oxford: Oxford University Press, 494–499.

33. Cort E, Monroe B and Oliviere D. (2004). Couples in palliative care. *Sexual and Relationship Therapy* **19**(3): 337–354.

34. Anath H, Jones L, King M and Tookman A (2003). The impact of cancer on sexual function: a controlled study. *Palliative Medicine* **17**: 202–205.

35. Speck P (2006). *Teamwork in Palliative Care. Fulfilling or Frustrating?* Oxford: Oxford University Press.

36. Wenger E (1998). *Communities of Practice: Learning, Meaning and Identity*. Cambridge: Cambridge University Press.

37. Payne M (2000). *Teamwork in Multiprofessional Care*. Basingstoke: Palgrave.

38. Payne M (2007). The development of health and social care. In: Adams R (ed.). *Foundations of Health and Social Care*. Basingstoke: Palgrave Macmillan, 31–37.

39. Darzi A (2007). *A Framework for Action*. London: London NHS.

40. Opie A (2003). *Thinking Teams/Thinking Clients: Knowledge-based Teamwork*. New York: Columbia University Press.

41. Payne M (2005) Adult protection cases in a hospice: an audit. *Journal of Adult Protection* **7**(2): 4–12.

42. Kristjanson LJ, Sloan JA, Dudgeon D and Adaskin E (1996). Family members perception of palliative cancer care: predictors of family functioning and family members' health. *Journal of Palliative Care* **12**(4): 10–20.

43. Waldrop DP, Milch RA and Skretny JA (2005). Understanding family responses to life-limiting illness: in-depth interviews with hospice patients and their family members. *Journal of Palliative Care* **21**(2): 88–96.

44. Zaza C and Baine N (2002). Cancer pain and psychosocial factors: a critical review of the literature. *Journal of Pain and Symptom Management* **24**(5): 526–542.

45. Randall F, and Downie R.S (2006). *The Philosophy of Palliative Care—Critique and Reconstruction*. Oxford: Oxford University Press.

46. Gomes B and Higginson IJ (2006). Factors influencing death at home in terminally ill patients with cancer: systematic review. *BMJ* **332**: 515–521.

47. Monroe B and Oliviere D (2007). *Resilience in Palliative Care—Achievement in Adversity*. Oxford: Oxford University Press.

48. Hartley N (2007). Resilience and creativity. In: Monroe B and Oliviere D (ed.). *Resilience in Palliative Care—Achievement in Adversity*.Oxford: Oxford University Press, 281–292.

49. Saunders C (1963) The treatment of intractable pain in terminal cancer. *Proceedings of the Royal Society of Medicine* **56**(3) March: 195–197.

Chapter 2

Understanding the social and cultural dimensions of family caregiving

Allan Kellehear

In the first-half of the twentieth century Western World, professional people spoke about 'families' and 'family carers' by drawing from demographic and sociological images of white nuclear families. Sometimes these family households would contain an elderly parent. Wealthier households sometimes included a live-in nanny or cook, often from a different social class or race. Since the 1960s our discussions about families have broadened to include global social and demographic changes, as well as international comparisons. Families in countries such as Britain, USA or Australia have undergone massive social, economic, political and demographic changes. Increasing numbers of people now live alone, single-parent and step-families are increasingly the norm, and workplace migration leaves many families with only distant kin support. Class, race, religion, gender or location now guide, but do not predict, attitudes, behaviour or the life course in general (1, 2).

Furthermore, during this time we have witnessed the birth and rise of global palliative care services, as well as the new forms of dying—especially AIDS and dementia dying—that have called for greater, if not equal, attention from carers, services and governments. Because specific forms of illness (cancer or dementia) or the social context of those illnesses (poverty or affluence) shape all caring conduct, it is important to acknowledge these influences on caring conduct.

This chapter will provide an overview of the key social and cultural dimensions that now influence family carers. It will summarize the background, qualifiers and mediating factors that influence caring in the modern world today. Subsequent chapters in this book should be read against this broader context to understand the most important fact about family care today—its diversity.

I will organize this chapter by reviewing the main social and cultural dimensions of family care, while also noting how less recognized influences, such as hidden relationships, might be important factors in family care behaviour.

The final section will argue for a public health response to family care that goes beyond direct service provision. I will argue that health promotion, community development and service partnerships are crucial to enhancing and supporting family carers.

Social dimensions of family care

Gender issues

Women have traditionally assumed much of the brunt of family care. Furthermore, because women tend to outlive their male partners in modern industrial contexts, two other consequences reinforce this gender inequality at the end of life. Women tend to be the main carers of their male partners because more women frequently outlive them and, secondly, more of these widows tend to be institutionalized at the end of life because there is no-one to look after them in their own homes when they begin to age and die (3).

Finally, some studies have indicated that more women than men report higher levels of perceived stress during their caring (4–6). Some of this burden of stress during care may in part be attributable to the micro-politics of gender relations during care; that is, to the possibility that men will make more demands on a female spouse than women might make on their male spouse carers. Alternatively, more women than men may feel/perceive/receive less actual support than is offered to male carers because male carers might more widely be viewed as vulnerable or unskilled in matters to do with domestic care more generally.

Financial issues

Several studies have noted the important impact that a lack of financial resources can play in the nature and level of family carer stress (7–9). Hudson (10), for example, reported that a quarter of his sample of 106 carers had stopped work or taken part-time work in order to care for dying family members at home. Although resigning from full-time work enables individuals to fully concentrate their attention on major round-the-clock care tasks, it can also have important negative consequences for a family member at home.

These problems include increasing the possibility of social isolation, reducing overall financial capacity at home, and narrowing the number of psychological and social respite breaks during the course of care. Soothill and colleagues (11) in their survey of nearly 200 carers noted that 44 per cent were retired; leaving this group, at least in principle, vulnerable to additional financial pressures and risks directly relating to caring. Furthermore, retiring or retiring early to care for dying family members can reduce capacity to deal with costs associated with long-term care. In these ways, most carers are prone to the costs of additional equipment, medications, travel costs or home care costs on their incomes, whether they are retired, working part-time or working full-time with a significant mortgage (9).

Social isolation

Social isolation is one of the most widely self-reported problems associated with family care-giving. Some of this may be attributed to the need to reduce paid employment. Other influences include the need to reduce social outings and recreational networks as the tasks of care become increasingly more complex and involving for the carer. Even a carer's own poor health has been implicated in increasing isolation, as a carer's own illness or carer-related fatigue and injury reduce social contact outside the household.

Soothill and colleagues (11) make the most pertinent observation in this literature on social isolation when they note that, although the majority of people have friends and relatives who live nearby, only a minority of these people ever offer supportive services. Clearly one of several assumptions is being made by the majority of people in communities that surround carers of dying people at home.

Perhaps people do not know what to offer other family carers or perhaps they believe that any offer would be time-consuming for them. Some may believe that offers of care would only increase a family carer's stress by having people near who are willing to help but may be less skilled. Other people might believe that family care of the dying is too private and intimate or perhaps too difficult or dreadful for distant family or friends to assist with.

Some people may also believe that formal services are adequate or indeed that some carers do not wish to accept help or support. Whatever the 'real' reason/s behind the lack of community support it is clear that an important key to relieving carer stress and burden, as well as promoting a seamless continuity of care, is the challenge of developing community capacity for this support. This challenge is, in turn, further complicated by the fact that carers' views of caring are not necessarily those of the dying person.

Dying person's views versus carer's views about care

Although it has long been recognized in Western society that most people wish to die at home surrounded by friends and family, the reality of the carer delivering this wish at home is another matter entirely. Some of the social dimensions already mentioned provide a picture of caring that is fraught with financial, interpersonal and technical problems, and one that is frequently coloured by common scenes of fatigue, loneliness and feelings of personal inadequacy. There have been conflicting complaints among research respondents that professional services and information are inadequate to many carers' needs or that broader community or family fail to support them.

Some people have traced their unmet needs to conventional care from hospitals or aged care rather than palliative care services (12). Others, however, mainly expressed satisfaction with these services compared to managing the daily personal tasks of care and life in general (11, 13). Although positive experiences are beginning to be reported in the literature (14), including the strengthening of relationships and improved levels of coping and confidence, for medical and or other social reasons dying at home may not be appropriate for both carer and dying person.

In fact, Stajduhar (9) reports that some carers feel 'pressured' to provide home care as part of a dying person's wish to die at home, as well as a growing view that dying at home 'is best'. Such views about dying at home are increasingly being enshrined in recent policy changes that encourage the dying persons to receive the majority of their care at home (4). But there are other social dimensions related to differing views between dying and their carers.

Serious illness and dying often alter one's usual roles and relationships in important and sometimes disturbing ways. Adult children who are ill or dying may experience unwelcome role reversals from parents, their children or spouses. Fluctuating states of health or illness can be ignored by an overall assumption of inadequacy in dying people by their carers. Valued roles or tasks may be prematurely given up—or taken away—from dying people (3). For fear of being viewed as ungrateful, few dying people may voice protest or criticism. From the same motives and disadvantaged position, the common overwhelming attention of friends and family who visit frequently can be a welcome source of support for carers but an added source of stress for the dying person (15). Although research comparing carers' and cancer patients' views exist in the literature (13), researches into carers' experience of the social care of dying are yet to adopt this serious comparative dimension to see which parts of these worlds overlap and which parts may collide.

Disenfranchised carers

Although much of the literature on caring attempts to scrutinize needs and satisfaction with professional support and information, or to gauge how adequate or otherwise the support is for carers, there have been few attempts to explore the problem of disenfranchised caring. The problem of disenfranchised grief has been openly acknowledged for some time now (16); including the unrecognized grief over lost animal companions, covert sexual relationships or ignored social experiences. However, the same recognition of this common problem for carers is yet to occur in the family carers' literature in any significant way. There has been some research recognition about the way in which the disenfranchised care that adults living with HIV/AIDS often receive from parents, sometimes excludes or limits the care that former or current lovers can provide. Nevertheless, this problem of unrecognized same-sex relationships also includes past or current heterosexual and bisexual relations.

Furthermore, there is little recognition that *dying people commonly also see themselves as carers* [see Vafiadis (17) for an excellent discussion of this issue]. In other words, in the matter of providing psychological and social support it is important to recognize that 'formal' professional carers, family carers and the patients are commonly engaged in what all parties view as 'caring for one another'. Therefore, hidden relationships, and the most obvious one before carers—the dying person—are frequently unrecognized relationships of care that we know little about, either because we have not adequately explored these populations in the care literature or because the dying person is always stereotypically cast as a receiver of care only and not as a population that also provides caring roles. The inadequacy of this research state of affairs notwithstanding, carers of the dying who are disenfranchised from their former and currently unrecognized relationships, and care from dying persons towards their carers, remains an important potential dimension of care to recognize in our professional practices.

Cultural and international dimensions of family care

Home versus institutional care

As mentioned earlier there is major encouragement for home care in most Western palliative care policy and ideology. The development of community-based palliative care services has made this easier to some extent, while at the same time providing consumer choice about potential locations for medically complicated or socially isolated individuals who are dying.

Nevertheless, with some historical exceptions, home care for dying people has been a long-standing desire and custom for people in the Western World for many years (18). However, both the desire and the custom of caring for dying family members at home are not cross-cultural and this is an important difference of care to consider. The Chinese and Japanese, for example, commonly view institutionalized care as a symbol of their very best care response. For some Chinese families, a death at home may bring 'bad luck' or ill fortune on a household—something both families and the dying person wish to avoid if at all possible (19). For many Japanese families, dying at home may suggest to neighbours that a family caring for their dying relative does not have the financial resources for 'better' care in a hospital—or worse—that this care is not being offered for selfish reasons.

Such values and attitudes are widespread in places such as Japan and Hong Kong but they are not universal (because in late modern circumstances, being 'Japanese' or 'Chinese' enjoys much regional, class and international variation). Japanese or Chinese diaspora in countries such as the UK, USA or Europe may display 'Western' preferences or a mixture of preferences from their national and ethnic origins. These observations highlight the need to thoroughly investigate the preferences of all carers but especially those who may not share common preferences for care in some locations or may do so but for different reasons. In this way, the reasons are as important to establish as the preferences themselves. But in this context there are even further complications worth identifying.

Care in international and mixed families

Most countries nowadays are experiencing a global form of multi-culturalism, either welcomed or forced upon them in a postcolonial, high-migrating world situation. Long-standing policies in the USA, UK, Canada and Australia have ensured that these recently settled countries have a highly diverse mixture of international peoples. The collapse of colonialism after World War Two for much of Western Europe has ensured a steady influx of citizens from their former colonies. Recent wars in Europe and Asia, and the collapse of the Soviet Union, have increased waves of refugees and human trafficking.

Global restructuring of national economies and work opportunities have increased the flow of international students, whilst at the same time offering low-paid jobs to migrants from poor economies in wealthy nations whose populations now eschew this kind of work (for example, Brazilian workers in Japan or Filipino workers in Singapore). Workplace migration is steadily increasing as globalization lowers visa requirements to support national economic agendas and needs. The consequences of these changes now see families migrating, intermarrying and adopting children from all over the globe at a historically unprecedented rate, especially in urban areas of high economic growth.

What this means for end-of-life care in general, and families in particular, is that assumptions about care are now diverse, contingent and uncertain. Definitions about what constitutes 'care' may differ even within families, as migrant spouses or parents diverge over the 'right' place to die, the 'right' people to perform intimate tasks of care or the complex problem of privacy in small ethnic communities who rely on interpreters. Families that were once large, extended and may have included servants, are now small, dislocated and may now be commonly confronted with significant communication challenges to even articulate their needs to others.

Some international communities within a country may be quite small. Longstanding social or religious divisions within these groups may be problematic. Such divisions might be ignored in the larger populations of the home country but may act as sources of embarrassment, inadequacy or resentment in dislocated contexts in a new country. Small but diverse international communities can mean that small precious items important to the comfort of the elderly, seriously ill or dying may be difficult or impossible to obtain. For example, steamed rice and some kinds of sweet jellies are important to Japanese people in illness, most especially the elderly who have very specific beliefs about the health properties of their rice. But medium-grain Japanese-style rice is absent from most supermarkets in the UK, where it is usually only obtainable from large metropolitan centres, such as London. Family care in these kinds of cultural contexts can be fraught with culture-specific complexities and difficulties, and immeasurably add to the stress of that care.

Family care in developing nations

Although tuberculosis, malaria and other infectious diseases still dog the poor nations of the world, HIV is quickly establishing itself as the most important cause of death in these global contexts. There are currently over 40 million people worldwide infected with this virus (20) with 5 million new infections annually (21). Most of these people who have reliable access to antivirals can expect some 10 years life expectancy from diagnosis but without these antivirals future prospects are considerably less (22). HIV/AIDS is now the fourth biggest killer in the world (23).

Irrespective of attempts to stop the spread of HIV, some 25 million people have already died and many millions more will suffer the same fate. For regions such as Africa, where prevalence can be 30 to 50 per cent of the population (24), end-of-life care must depend heavily on family because health services are meagre, non-existent or a causal part of the HIV epidemic itself (25). Historically, one might expect traditional customs and supports to play an important role in this care. Unfortunately, this is seldom the case because the virus itself is highly stigmatized and feared. Shame is frequently associated with the virus because various folk theories often attribute death to some moral wrong-doing or witchcraft from others (26). Furthermore, family often experience this shame, stigma and social rejection by association; leaving both dying people and their families without traditional supports (27).

In Eastern Europe, since the collapse of the former Soviet Union, villages were emptied of their working-age men and women as poverty spread and the able-bodied looked for work in foreign countries. Often this desperate search for work takes these populations to far-flung countries in Western Europe as illegal workers, refugees or unfortunate subjects of human trafficking. This leaves a major gap in the ability of families to care for their ageing and dying, as villages in Eastern Europe see a preponderance of young children and old people. The customary care provided by adult children, and especially women, is seriously compromised in these kinds of national contexts (28, 29).

Public health support for family care at the end of life

The various social and cultural dimensions of care outlined above strongly suggest the need to think outside of direct service supports for family carers. This is because professional support services, support groups, respite care and educational interventions, although important to improving the lot of family carers (12), do not address the everyday world of work, school or recreational contexts of living and dying. Professional supports occupy only a slim body of time and interaction compared to the far more numerous relationships and time that people spend with their usual social contacts and supports. This means that it is to these 'usual' and wider social supports and contexts that we must look to strengthen. This strengthening of wider supports can enhance seamless relationships with professional services before, during and after care. Furthermore, for economically poor and service-impoverished areas in developing nations, recognition of these non-professional supports may be a simultaneous recognition that these are the only supports available.

Many of the social problems of family care—isolation, lack of respite care, stigma and disenfranchisement, or cultural fragmentation—may be addressed by wider public health approaches that target misinformation, ignorance and/or community-wide fears and prejudice. For example, the importance of sex education, improved access to effective contraception and non-family supports, as well as anti-discrimination legislation and information have greatly improved the health and safety of heterosexual teenagers as well as the gay community. These health promotion improvements have complemented health service provision by ensuring that the problem of sexually transmitted diseases, unwanted pregnancies or the stigma of sexual deviance is not simply addressed by services alone. Communities are active participants in this form of healthcare and support, not only by schools, workplaces, social clubs and churches but also by mainstream media outlets such as newspapers or television, and information and education notices strategically placed in locations as different as dance venues, toilets and community noticeboards.

A public health approach not only recognizes the importance of people as users of health services but equally the importance of building health and preventing illness or disease in the social settings of the everyday life of the communities they serve.

Community development initiatives—helping communities identify and address their own health and social care needs—are valuable strategies to enhance the community capacity to support families who are supporting their dying parents, spouses, children or friends. Furthermore, in international contexts where poverty, war or meagre health services preclude a major health services response to the dying and their family carers, broader models of healthcare may need to be called forth. A public health approach to end-of-life care that incorporates health-promoting palliative care, community development and service partnerships will be crucial to the support of families in all these diverse arrangements and limitations. What are the principles of a public health approach to end-of-life care that can enhance family care of the dying?

Principle ideas driving a public health approach

Because family carers may be subject to discrimination, poor social support or personal isolation, direct support services, such as counselling, respite care or other direct professional services, can be practically helpful and of genuine value to carers. However, supports such as respite care are not designed for prevention and harm reduction efforts that would reduce the stress and lack of support at the centre of the problem itself. For example, the personal experience of bereavement may be worsened by the common belief that the bereaved should 'get over it' after a few weeks. Counselling may help the bereaved person understand misguided community attitudes and to deal with the personal pain of being a victim of such attitudes but it does not prevent the problem itself.

Identifying information that will combat ignorance about grief in the wider community—or ignorance about caring—relies heavily on community participation. In facilitating any change, identifying the barriers and incentives to that change is crucial—and few people know better what these barriers and incentives might be than the communities themselves; found in schools, workplaces, churches or families. Inside every community in schools or workplaces, for example, are people who have had direct experience of the problems of caring for the chronically ill, the aged or the dying. Encouraging communities to explore and exploit that social experience and wisdom among themselves is a crucial step in raising consciousness about a social issue that affects everyone. In these processes, the personal experiences, once identified and observed as a re-occurring experience affecting many people, soon become identified as a wider social concern to be addressed as a social task for all. Community participation then, is of paramount importance to the identification, design and, in particular, to the success of any community education and support programme.

Inside this community development approach to health promotion, education and the development of supports occur by building on existing skills and wisdom of individuals, as well as within the communities that might support those individuals. By encouraging groups and communities, such as families, schools or workplaces, to address their own perceived needs and develop strategies for dealing with them, community initiatives create 'ownership'—and therefore sustainability—of personal as well as public programmes.

Two public health examples from Australian palliative care services

Public health approaches to palliative care have been in existence for some time in Australia, where these are known as 'health-promoting palliative care' (HPPC) programmes (30, 31). Health-promoting palliative care programmes are programmes designed and developed to promote the idea that care in matters to do with death and loss is everyone's responsibility—not just from professional staff to patients and their families, but also staff to staff, staff to patients and their families, community to families and health service professionals. The goals of HPPC as defined by Kellehear (30) consist of:

* providing education and information for health, dying and death;
* providing social supports—both personal and community;
* encouraging interpersonal reorientation;
* encouraging reorientation of palliative care services;
* combating death-denying health policies and attitudes.

In this context, palliative care services think about what community partnerships, activities and roles they might play in developing their own and the wider community's capacity to cope with death, loss and care. In the city of Newcastle in the Australian state of New South Wales, the regional palliative care service covers some 350 000 residents. For some years now the palliative care service has been actively engaged in relationships with local media, schools and the community in general to promote awareness—not simply about palliative care—but how to live and live well with death, dying, loss and care.

Staff at this service have been involved with radio programmes, as well as being active contributors to the local newspapers, so they are able to promote community discussion of experiences about death, dying, loss and care by relating experiences from their workaday world of professional care. Also, inside these stories are other stories about family and community care. More directly, the Newcastle (Hunter Region) team have been involved in what is commonly termed a 'café conversation' or 'World Café'. In these social activities, a real local café is either hired or freely participates in a community invitation to discuss an important life issue, such as mortality. People dine at tables with four or five other participants and discuss several questions posed to all the people in the room. Examples include, 'Is it ever OK to die?'; 'If I had 12 months to live what would that mean to me—and my community?'. Answers or ideas are scribbled down on paper table-cloths and parties move about between different stages of the meal to read and re-examine their earlier responses in the light of other people's 'scribblings'. It is a lively, non-threatening and highly educational experience for all.

Local education authorities have been contacted and schools visited by palliative care staff to facilitate their own 'needs assessment'. Key priorities for teachers are what to say and how to be helpful to students who have parents who are living with life-threatening illness or who die. Communication issues about what to say to people affected by death or heavy care responsibilities are particularly important to teachers. Resources to help students and staff respond to these communication issues are developed.

Sometimes, the need for grief education is subsequently identified and experts are invited to conduct workshops for students or staff. Often simply reflective sessions or the combing through of institutional memory can help both staff and students identify what has helped in the past and what has not. Feedback style evaluations have affirmed that these types of efforts in community capacity building for the general public or schools have been practical and helpful in subsequent relationships encountering death-related events.

The Hume Regional Palliative Care (HRPC) team in the northern part of the Australian state of Victoria has had similar success with its health-promoting palliative care work (31). This team covers some 40 000 square kilometres and consists of five specialist palliative care units and 17 local palliative care volunteer groups.

After initial workshops on health-promoting palliative care for clinical staff, volunteers and their managers, a health-promotion resource team was brought together from both volunteers and staff who had attended the earlier in-service education workshops. This team coordinated and supported the work of other staff and volunteers in the development of community activities and partnerships across the region. The 'Big 7 Checklist' (30) was used to distinguish between possible community activities, as those that might engender a public health mission and those that might not.

A truly health-promoting initiative needed to meet one of the first three criteria documented below and then must include all of numbers 4 to 7 of this checklist:

1 Prevention of social difficulties around death, dying, loss or care.

2 Harm minimization of current difficulties around death, dying, loss or care; or

3 early intervention strategies along the journey of death, dying, loss or care experiences.

4 Changes to community settings or environments for the better in terms of our present or future responses to death, dying, loss or care.

5 Partnerships proposed, partnered and sustained by community members.

6 Sustainable impact beyond the intervention; and

7 evaluation of how successful or useful the intervention was.

Some of the practical outcomes of HRPC efforts included one larger rural town exploring how young people can communicate creatively about the reality of loss and grief in their lives. The partnerships involved developing a performance event that included local youth service workers, a school nurse, community health workers, a church minister, the local palliative care loss and grief coordinator and volunteer service, a music therapist and other community members with creative talents. The event has been linked with other youth-funding schemes, which in turn, increased its potential as a sustainable project.

Another project created an older adult day activity programme that explored how to assist their clients reflect on personal and family resources that had been used throughout their lifespan. This was done through photos, stories, memory boxes and the commencement of an illustrated journal including each participant's life-story as shared. They involved the local primary school, the adult learning centre and the community health centre as partners in the project, making it sustainable and accessible to others within their community.

Another programme involved an adult education centre in a small town that ran two courses for carers in their community. The aim was to strengthen their knowledge of available community support, to inform about loss and grief, to provide resources and skills and to provide access to a sustainable self-help network.

One palliative care volunteer service commenced discussion with their local government council to establish a reflective space at the city cemetery to shelter families and carers visiting people who have died on the palliative care programme and who are buried there. A partnership between them and the local cemetery trust, the local hospital and the palliative care service saw a rotunda and garden area built.

There were numerous World Café events across the length and breadth of the region; other projects involved church groups, palliative care service information stands at community festivals and horse racing events. Local business houses were asked to support a 'care for the carers' day, where businesses were asked to donate products or services that would help carers. Examples included food, massage, gifts or discounts to relaxing venues. Many other projects, too numerous to mention here (32), were also started and continue in this innovative health-promotion programme. The preliminary evaluation of these programmes suggest that they were enthusiastically embraced by the communities involved, were practical and helpful, did indeed build capacity to help beyond direct services and improved the relationship between palliative care services, families and the wider community (33).

Conclusion

The social history of dying indicates that human beings have always cared for their dying—and their families—as a whole community (18). Hunter-gatherer communities have shared the task of care for the seriously ill and have supported families involved more directly in that care. This is also true for peasant societies. The development of urban societies has promoted economic specialization and social diversity, and those developments have been hallmark characteristics of modernity itself.

All these developments have witnessed the rise of cross-cultural forms of reliance and dependency on professionals and their services. In the last hundred years this has made dying people more dependent on health services, at the same time as isolating families from wider community supports as folk understandings of 'care' gradually transformed itself into notions of 'expertise'. We are now seeing a major rethinking of these changes.

The recognition of the importance of family and community care is rising and this volume is testimony to this fact. The facts of family care and its common consequences—social inequalities, isolation, role ambiguities, financial strains and many other stresses—suggest the need for a wider public health approach to family care. The idea that we can prevent or reduce the harms for carers through service partnerships and community development are prompting new health service experiments in several countries, such as the ones described here for Australia. There is a greater willingness to entertain new ideas, a greater curiosity to explore the limits to public health in the context of end-of-life care. Such initiatives and desire augur well for public health developments in end-of-life care and they must surely bode well for family carers everywhere.

Key learning points

◆ The social dimensions of care that have received the most attention seem to be about the stresses of care brought about by poor social supports, social isolation and financial strain, especially for female carers. However, differing views about care between the dying person and carer can also be a source of stress and distress.

◆ Dying persons are also often overlooked as carers too.

◆ Cultural and international dimensions of care are complex factors in late modernity. People are commonly not what they seem in national, ethnic or racial terms. The desire to die at home or in hospital or hospice can arise from a diversity of social and cultural reasons related to religion, generational position or migration circumstances.

◆ Basic concepts of public health such as prevention, harm-reduction, community development, service partnerships and participatory relations are applicable to the practice of palliative care for professional and family care.

Recommended reading and resources

Beck U (1992). *The Risk Society: Towards a New Modernity.* London: Sage.

Howarth G (2007). *Death and Dying: a Sociological Introduction.* Cambridge: Polity Press.

Kellehear A (1999). *Health-promoting Palliative Care.* Melbourne: Oxford University Press.

Kellehear A (2005). *Compassionate Cities: Public Health and End-Of-Life Care.* London: Routledge.

Monroe B and Oliviere D (ed.) (2007). *Resilience in Palliative Care: Achievement in Adversity.* Oxford: Oxford University Press.

Mosley A (2004). Does HIV or poverty cause AIDS? Biomedical and epidemiological perspectives. *Theoretical Medicine* **25**: 399–421.

Payne S (2007). Public health and palliative care. *Progress in Palliative Care* **15**(3): 101–102.

Sinclair P (2007). *Rethinking Palliative Care: a Social Role Valorisation Approach.* Bristol: Policy Press.

Vafiadis P (2001). *Mutual Care in Palliative Medicine: a Story of Doctors and Patients.* Sydney: McGraw-Hill.

Wright M and Clark D (ed.) (2006). *Hospice and Palliative Care in Africa: a Review of Developments And Challenges.* Oxford: Oxford University Press.

References

1. Beck U (1992). *The Risk Society: Towards a New Modernity.* London: Sage.
2. Castells M (1996). *The Rise of the Network Society.* Oxford: Blackwell.
3. Kellehear A (1994). The social inequality of dying. In: Waddell C and Petersen AR (ed.). *Just Health: Inequality in Illness, Care and Prevention.* Melbourne: Churchill Livingstone, 181–189.

4. Payne S, Smith P and Dean S (1999). Identifying the concerns of informal carers in palliative care. *Palliative Medicine* **13**: 37–44.

5. Scott G, Whyler N and Grant G (2001). A study of family carers of people with a life-threatening illness 1: the carers' needs analysis. *International Journal of Palliative Care* **7**(6): 290–297.

6. Goldstein NE, Concato J, Fried TR *et al.* (2004). Factors associated with caregiver burden among carers with terminally ill patients with cancer. *Journal of Palliative Care* **20**(1): 38–43.

7. Neale B (1991). Informal palliative care: a review of research on needs, standards and service evaluation. *Occasional Paper* **3**. Trent Palliative Care Centre.

8. Emmanuel EJ, Fairclough DL, Slutsman J and Emanuel LL (2000). Understanding economic and other burdens of terminal illness: The experience of patients and their caregivers. *Ann Intern Med* **132**(6): 451–459.

9. Stajduhar KI (2003). Examining the perspectives of family members involved in the delivery of palliative care at home. *Journal of Palliative Care* **19**(1): 27–35.

10. Hudson P (2003). Home-based support for palliative care families: challenges and recommendations. *Medical Journal of Australia* **179**(6): S35-S37.

11. Soothill K, Morris SM, Harman JC *et al.* (2003). Informal carers of cancer patients: what are their unmet psychosocial needs? *Health and Social Care in the Community* **9**(6): 464–475.

12. Harding R and Higginson I (2003). What is the best way to help caregivers in cancer and palliative care? A systematic literature review of interventions and their effectiveness. *Palliative Medicine* **17**: 63–74.

13. Thomas C, Morris SM and Hardman JC (2002). Companions through cancer: the care given by informal carers in cancer contexts. *SocSciMed* **54**(4): 529–544.

14. Hudson P (2004). Positive aspects and challenges associated with caring for a dying relative at home. International *Journal of Palliative Care* **10**(20): 58–64.

15. Kellehear A (1990). *Dying of Cancer: the Final Year of Life*. Chur, Switzerland: Harwood Academic Publishers.

16. Doka K (ed.) (1989). *Disenfranchised Grief*. Lexington, MA: Lexington Books.

17. Vafiadis P (2001). *Mutual Care in Palliative Medicine: a Story of Doctors and Patients*. Sydney: McGraw-Hill.

18. Kellehear A (2007). *A Social History of Dying*. Cambridge: Cambridge University Press.

19. Chan CLW and Chow AYM (ed.) (2006). *Death, Dying and Bereavement: a Hong Kong Chinese Experience*. Hong Kong: Hong Kong University Press; 2006.

20. World Health Organisation (2005). *Aids Epidemic Update 2005*. Geneva: UNAIDS.

21. Economic and Social Commission for Asia and the Pacific (2003) HIV/AIDS in the Asian and Pacific Region. New York: United Nations.

22. Fleming PL (2004). The epidemiology of HIV and AIDS. In: Wormser GP (ed.) *AIDS and Other Manifestations of HIV Infection*. San Diego, Calif: Elsevier, 3–29.

23. Healey J (ed.) (2003). *HIV/AIDS*. Sydney: Spinney Press.

24. Ferrante P, Delbue S, and Mancuso R (2005). The manifestation of AIDS in Africa: an epidemiological overview. *Journal of Neurovirology* **1**: 50–57.

25. Volkow P and del Rio C (2005). Paid donation and plasma trade: unrecognized forces that drive the Aids epidemic in developing countries. *International Journal of STDs and AIDS* **6**: 5–8.

26. Liddell C, Barrett L and Bydawell M (2005). Indigenous representations of illness and AIDS in Sub-Sahara Africa. *Social Science and Medicine* **60**; 691–700.

27. Songwathana P and Manderson L (2001). Stigma and rejection: Living with AIDS in Southern Thailand. *Medical Anthropology* **20**(1): 1–23.

28. Wright M and Clark D (ed.) (2006). *Hospice and Palliative Care in Africa: a Review of Developments and Challenges*. Oxford: Oxford University Press.

29. Bingley A and McDermott E (ed.) (2007). Resilience in resource-poor settings. In: Monroe B and Oliviere D (ed.). *Resilience in Palliative Care: Achievement in Adversity*. Oxford: Oxford University Press, 261–279.

30. Kellehear A (1999). *Health-promoting Palliative Care*. Melbourne: Oxford University Press.

31. Kellehear A (2005). *Compassionate Cities: Public Health and End-Of-Life Care*. London: Routledge.

32. Kellehear A and Young B (2007). Resilient Communities. In: Monroe B and Oliviere D (ed.). *Resilience in Palliative Care: Achievements in Adversity*. Oxford: Oxford University Press, 223–238.

33. Rumbold B and Gear R (2004). *Evaluation of Health Promotion Resource Team: Hume Regional Palliative Care Caring Communities Project 'Building Rural Community Capacity Through Volunteering'*. Melbourne: La Trobe University Palliative Care Unit.

Chapter 3

Responding to family carers' spiritual needs

Rosalie Hudson

A glance at the index of many palliative care textbooks reveals an absence of attention to family carers and very few references to their spiritual needs. Are family carers' beliefs and values important and, if so, why are they so seldom explored, particularly in the context of death and dying?

This chapter explores some of the literature and raises questions about language, attitudes, standards, historical changes and contemporary perceptions regarding spiritual needs. Suggestions are offered for reflection on practice and examples provided for effective responses to family carers' spiritual needs.

The terms spiritual, religious and existential are sometimes used interchangeably in the literature; however, while they can overlap there are important differences. Speck (1) advises: 'In health care research we should differentiate between the terms spiritual and religious since, if they are used interchangeably, reports of spirituality may be describing religious practice and affiliation.' While a religious person is usually regarded as spiritual—in some religions the two are inseparable—a spiritual person may invoke no religion. For others, their search for life's meaning may be described as existential, with no spiritual or religious connotations.

Changing meanings of spirituality

It is clear from the plethora of books and articles on spirituality that there is no universally accepted understanding of the term; it is often described as a slippery concept incapable of definition. In this chapter 'spiritual' is taken to mean nothing less than the essence of life. The 'spirit' in spiritual refers to the breath that animates, the vitality that sustains life. Thus, spirituality is a term 'ancient and modern, an anachronism and a contemporary issue' (2). Spirit is not some 'thing' divorced from the body; spirit and body 'are so profoundly inter-related that every attempt to objectify either of them without the other in the end leads to absurdity (3).

Spirituality can, however, signify something so mystical that it beggars description, so ethereal as to be meaningless, so esoteric as to be superfluous or so mundane as to be unworthy of comment. Spirituality can be reduced to a generic theory or umbrella term whose meaning is presumed or it can function like 'intellectual Polyfilla, changing shape and content conveniently to fill the space its users devise for it' (4).

In its traditional meaning, spirituality included reference to the sacred and a specific alliance with organized religion; now it is regarded as an all-encompassing search for meaning described by Walter as a 'secularized version of Christianity' (5). In his earlier exposition of this trend, Walter noted 'it is also a view of spirituality which is being promoted more generally in a post-modern culture that distrusts any authority outside of the individual self' (6). This broad view of spirituality leads to the conclusion that all dying patients, and (by inference) their family carers, will have spiritual needs. Correlatively, it is widely assumed that all members of the palliative care team should be able to meet these needs.

To explore the place of spirituality in palliative care is to enter a realm where the familiar clinical language of needs, diagnosis, assessment and problem-solving does not quite fit. Although it will be argued that effective spiritual care for family carers needs to be organized if it is to be taken seriously, such organization should not replace openness to the creative initiatives of carers and their humane and imaginative responses conveyed in their own words.

Language of the spirit

As palliative care changes shape from its unapologetic Christian foundation to fit the pervasive culture of contemporary healthcare organization, it is struggling to find a place for 'the spirit'. While it is unrealistic to call for a return to the historic roots of Christian hospices, it is worth acknowledging that stereotypical views of hospices and palliative care services as religious institutions might be a barrier for some families who regard 'religious' as narrow and exclusive. In view of these cultural changes, palliative care might benefit from a more thoughtful reflection on its language. For example, the view taken in this discussion is that spirituality in family caregiving calls for an offering rather than service delivery; such a response invokes caring *about* the family carer as well as caring *for* them. While service-provision language can imply an unequal power relationship—'goods' delivered by one powerful party to another less powerful recipient—partnership language recognizes the spiritual potential of an 'exchange of power between two people' (7).

A fresh approach to the language of spiritual care also focuses on the communal rather than the exclusively private sphere, embracing the family carer's social context both within the immediate family and the wider community. This broader understanding of spirituality is an attempt to counter the widespread reductionism that sees spirituality as a soft and fluffy optional extra for those who like that sort of thing, or a catchall term for anything regarded as beyond the scientific, measurable, physical world of facts.

Taking the communal concept a step further, the health professionals' health and wholeness, as well as the family carers' well-being, can be influenced by their relationship with (and within) the palliative care team. When the team is considered a community of care, individual members might also find meaning, not merely in isolated subjective experiences but in the daily round of personal interaction. Communal language is the key to personal engagement, enabling spiritual care to take tangible form in the exchange of ordinary conversation.

Religious and transcultural issues

The contemporary proliferation of literature on spirituality in the healthcare context is largely restricted to the English-speaking world and the Judeo-Christian religion, Orchard (8) and Wright (9) being some exceptions. However, research among family carers from diverse cultural, social, and economic groups 'is sorely inadequate' (10).

It is impossible for any palliative care professional to have detailed knowledge of the wide diversity of family carers' faith perspectives or religious beliefs. Nor should it be assumed that sufficient understanding can be gained by snapshot references gleaned from a 'multi-faith folder'; as though a scant generic reference can be applied to all situations. The way each adherent to a particular religion translates their beliefs into practice will vary. One of the most important questions to be asked of the family carer is, 'Do you have any particular religious beliefs that help you in this situation?'. The conversation might also commence with, 'I am not familiar with your cultural beliefs and practices, and so, if it's all right with you, I would like to ask you a few questions to help my understanding?'.

In this way, all palliative care health professionals can make an initial assessment; the question of interventions and specific roles for particular personnel is taken up later in the chapter.

Family carer

'Family' is used here to signify the key person who is supporting the dying patient, whether in the context of home, hospice, hospital or aged care home.

It is assumed that spiritual care for every individual member of the family is generally beyond the capacity of the palliative care service. That is not to deny the importance of assessing whether the family as a whole is sustained by a particular spirituality and/or religion that supports and reinforces individual family members' beliefs. For example, one family might worship together regularly; another might welcome specific pastoral ministry to the whole family at home; others will find sustenance through music or conversation or nature. The place of spirituality and/or religion within family caregiving can also be assessed by observing non-verbal as well as verbal clues. For example, particularly in the home setting, the health professional can observe whether there are religious artefacts or other signs of beliefs and values important to the family, which might trigger discussion (11). Some family carers will regard their spirituality as inseparable from their religious beliefs and practices; others will express their spirituality in non-religious terms.

It is also important to acknowledge that specific subgroups of family carers may have widely varying spiritual attitudes and needs, which cannot be expanded here; for example, carers of dying children, people with chronic life-threatening illness such as dementia or the unique needs of young family carers.

Body/mind/spirit and impending death

Spirituality is often artificially divorced from the essential unity of the person; consequently, the whole person is divided into component parts. 'Spirituality belongs on another planet as far as I'm concerned,' claims the palliative care student. Or, from a palliative care nurse, 'I'm very comfortable with symptom management but I leave all that spiritual stuff to the chaplain.'

To suggest that spirituality belongs to some other-worldly realm is to infer it has nothing whatever to do with bodily existence, nor with the everyday realities of our lived experience. If palliative care's stated aims are to treat the patient and family holistically, then the spiritual care component cannot be disembodied or reduced to a vague and indeterminate concept, particularly in the face of impending death.

Such an approach shows little appreciation for the way in which imminent death consumes the whole person. The concept of total pain is a case in point. Twycross and Wilcock (12) list some of the non-physical factors that can contribute to pain; for example, social pain associated with feelings of abandonment and isolation; psychological pain triggered by anger, fear or helplessness; spiritual pain related to questioning the meaning of life. Similarly, Saunders (13) links spiritual pain to key issues of suffering that can consume the whole person—the family carer no less than the dying patient. This is not to suggest all family carers are totally devastated or overburdened by the experience. Many consider it a 'worthy investment or challenge' (14) where meaning is created through mutuality of relationships, goal-setting, discovering pathways to hope and optimism, and the positive lasting memories of particular words and actions. Some would interpret these responses as deeply spiritual; in whatever way they are perceived, the responses are unique to each family.

Responding to family carers' spiritual needs takes us beyond the realm of clinical certitudes and problem-solving prescriptions into a profoundly personal, and sometimes deeply disturbing, area of life. Rumbold (15) states:

> We find that spirituality is about connectedness, but also about incompleteness. It is about knowledge, but equally about what we do not know. It is about coherence and integrity, but also about vulnerability. It is about belief, but equally about doubt.

Palliative care health professionals are not beyond the vagaries of human nature in their wish to avoid their own vulnerability, thereby relegating spiritual matters to the margins. To reduce the spirit to a mere component part is, however, to objectify it. It is then a short step to adopting the problem-solving language of diagnosis, flow-charts, processes, pathways, goals, measurements, throughputs and outcomes. This step quickly leads to 'using engineering terms such as tools and instruments and other "technospeak" for the profound mystery that is the human person' (16).

To raise questions about problem-solving tools is not to decry the legitimate place for rating scales that provide a framework for understanding the concepts of spiritual care (17). However, a concentration on problems to be solved, such as interventions for alleviating spiritual distress and/or devising mechanisms for spiritual coping, can overshadow some of the very natural, joyful, creative and playful aspects of spirituality. Spirituality can be expressed through art, literature, poetry, metaphor, symbols, music and humour. A reductionist, problem-solving approach not only ignores these important factors but also leaves little room for the rich data provided through the words of family carers themselves, especially when confronting death. The paradox and ambiguity of death often comes to the fore through the words of family carers themselves. 'I want his suffering to be over but I don't want him to die.' Other issues can also come to light through careful listening when death is imminent.

Saunders recognizes the way impending death can create a sense of urgency about alleviating doubt and putting things right. 'It can also create anger, defiance, a sense of unfairness and above all a desolate feeling of meaninglessness' (13). What does it mean to 'put things right'? Rumbold cautions against an assumption that well-intended interventions will work. Rather, he argues, '... a particular question is whether end-of-life spiritual care can make up for rest-of-life neglect of spirituality' (15). The question about 'putting things right' therefore requires great sensitivity and some knowledge of the carer's attitudes and beliefs in the face of death.

Other researchers also note the paternalism that can accompany an urgency to tie up loose ends before the person dies (18). A partnership approach, rather than a unilateral focus on fixing problems, can be the means of exploring these issues with family carers.

Assessing family carers' spiritual needs

Taylor (19) identified eight categories of spiritual need for cancer patients and family carers, represented in Box 3.1 below.

While these categories provide a helpful prompt, lists of spiritual needs should not replace the valuable art of listening for the subtle nuances of other needs being expressed. Whatever form assessment takes, care should be taken not to impose a 'professional template' (18) over the family carer's own language. Even the most well-intentioned process for identifying a family carer's spiritual needs can result in satisfaction for the health professional, while leaving the family member profoundly disappointed. 'I felt they wanted me to say that,' is an all too common response. Or, worse, 'I haven't a clue what she was talking about.'

When a family carer appears reluctant to 'comply' with an assessment process relating to their spiritual needs, such silence can all too readily be misinterpreted.

Box 3.1 Eight categories of spiritual need

Relating to God or an Ultimate Other

Reviewing spiritual beliefs

Gratitude and optimism

Creating meaning and finding purpose

Loving others

Sustaining religious experiences

Receiving love from others

Preparing for death

Adapted from (19).

'I tried to raise the issue of spiritual distress with the wife, but she was resistant; I think she's in a state of denial,' reported the nurse. As Rumbold states, 'It might be better to assume that clients are unwilling to expose their concerns to practitioners who indulge in such labelling behaviours' (15).

This is not to argue against a process for identifying spiritual needs; rather, it is to focus less on codified interventions and outcomes, and more on fostering open discussion such as, 'Would you like us to talk some more about this tomorrow?'.

Conventional wisdom regarding assessment tools is that they need to be validated, and quick and easy to use; they are therefore ideally suited for assessing clinical needs such as elimination and mobility. While some spiritual assessment tools might be helpful in practice, palliative care health professionals might consider the following factors underpinning any comprehensive assessment. The need for:

- skilled communication;
- professional competence to recognize when referral is needed;
- open-mindedness;
- avoidance of hasty judgements; and
- a sensitive attitude towards different faiths and cultures.

Assessment processes might well be transformed by an attitude of discernment where the emphasis is less on prescriptive measurements and more on the language and attitudes that foster natural discussion (20).

Discernment involves dialogue and dialogue replaces the ticking of boxes. Such discernment can, for example, assist the health professional in making a decision about referral. The open question, 'I hear you expressing some concerns about your spiritual (or religious) needs; would you like me to make a referral to …?' paves the way for further dialogue, rather than hasty and potentially unwelcome directives. Discernment regarding timely referral also requires education, good communication systems and clear role descriptions for all members of the palliative care team. Health professionals need to know when, by whom and to whom referral is being advocated; not only to guard against inappropriate interventions but to avoid unnecessary duplication of resources.

Discernment also guards against reducing spiritual assessment to a once-only exercise. 'Perhaps the term "assessing" would be more appropriate in the context of spirituality, indicating a need for continual surveillance and vigilance by all health care professionals' (21). The emphasis here is on dialogue rather than documents. 'The *intent*, more than the *content*, of spiritual assessment is what matters most' (22).

An invitation to dialogue might start with, 'We believe spiritual care for family carers is important. With your permission I would like to have a brief conversation about how you understand "spiritual" and whether this issue is important to you?'. Such an open-ended question might be sufficient for one family carer to respond immediately; another person might require further prompting to elucidate the meaning of the question.

In contrast is the formulaic approach of the palliative care team member: 'I've given Mary's husband the spiritual assessment form to fill in. I don't like asking those awkward questions.' The dialogic approach allows for issues to be explored, followed up and returned to in conversation. In the formulaic approach, the issue is closed when the form is filed.

Palliative care health professionals need to be able to discern any signs of spiritual distress and to respond appropriately. Manifestations of distress might include:

- the inability to see anything good in people or surroundings;
- feelings of reduced self-worth;
- blaming others;
- fear of eternal punishment;
- feelings of abandonment by God or others; or
- lack of a reason for living.

Thorough assessment, however, involves probing more deeply. For example, a health professional might interpret a family carer's fatalistic attitude towards death as a problem, whereas fate and acceptance of fate might be central to that person's religion and a mark of virtue. Similarly, hasty judgements can easily be made either by a family carer or by a health professional, when the patient expresses a desire to die. Hudson *et al.* identified a patient's expressed desire for death as a factor that might be related to concerns in the spiritual domain, rather than a specific wish for life to end (23).

Family carers' unmet needs

Research in recent decades has demonstrated that carers' needs are largely unmet and that there is an urgent need for carer interventions, such as support and information (24). Further testimony points to the need for discerning the overlap of physical, psycho-emotional and social factors as they affect the carer's search for meaning or spiritual validation. One family carer stated, 'I was willing to do what needed to be done … but it would have been good to have felt that my role was valued … that it was seen' (25).

Questions that might help elicit family carers' less obvious spiritual needs, such as diminished self-esteem and isolation, include:

◆ What kind of information would you find most useful?

◆ What support would be most helpful to you today and in the time ahead?

◆ What makes things easier for you and what makes things more difficult?

◆ Are you experiencing any benefits, such as unexpected pleasure or satisfaction from your caring role?

◆ Is there anyone else you would like to talk to about your role as carer?

More specific prompts for the health professional in relation to spiritual needs might include:

◆ Have specific religious or cultural issues that pertain to the patient's expected death been identified?

◆ Is there a discrepancy between the family carer's understanding of spiritual needs and the patient's understanding?

◆ Is there evidence of family dynamics that interfere with the carer's role?

◆ Is the family carer aware of the scope and limitations of the health professional's role in spiritual matters?

◆ Are there any spiritual issues that might be outside the health professional's frame of reference and, if so, what support/information/referral is needed?

◆ Have the family carer's wishes for non-disclosure been respected?

Sensitive assessment, either of the family carer's broad spiritual needs or their more specific religious needs, might therefore include:

◆ Does your particular tradition offer you helpful religious or spiritual counsel in this situation?

◆ Is there a particular person you turn to for spiritual help?

◆ Do you draw strength from any particular object or symbol, e.g. art, music, poetry, religious icons?

◆ Do you have a particular place where you find solace?

◆ Are there particular people or activities that lift your spirits?

◆ Do you feel your own spiritual or religious practices are being neglected and, if so, how may we assist?

These questions help guard against potentially unacceptable bureaucratic interrogation or inappropriate interventions based on assumptions. Clear questions at the outset may also determine those situations where no interventions are being sought or required. Continuous review should uncover changing or emerging needs.

Needs and interventions

There is, at present, little evidence to guide the health professional in the realm of spiritual needs and interventions for family carers (26). A word of caution is therefore needed in relation to the hasty offering of interventions that have no proven benefit.

Health professionals need to be respectful of family carers' differences and diverse needs. For example, for some family carers the most urgent need relates to formulating advance care plans; others need relevant information before determining whether palliative care is beneficial in their circumstances; others need specific education about caregiving, including communication skills; others seek to explore options regarding meaningful activities to alleviate suffering (10). In some situations the urgent, practical needs take precedence; in others, discussion of spiritual issues might set the scene for the overall caring role. In a partnership approach the health professional's own attitudes and needs are also relevant.

Boston and Mount (27) found the 'wounded healer' concept to be fundamental to effective care. This concept encompasses self-awareness as well as staff support, and recognition that the carer (either the family caregiver or the health professional) is not expected to be perfectly 'whole' and strong at all times. Palliative care health professionals are not saviours and in this respect Nuland offers an apt reminder. ' ... [T]he central player in the drama is the dying man; the dashing leader of that bustling squad of his would-be rescuers is only a spectator, and a groundling at that' (28).

Barriers to effective spiritual care

Health professionals are generally wary of overstepping boundaries of confidentiality, causing offence or invading what is perceived as the private area of a person's life. Spiritual and religious needs can be overlooked by making hasty judgements such as, 'They've ticked "nil" in the religion box, so we can skip the spirituality question'. It has been found, however, that people are generally not offended by sensitive discussion about their spiritual and/or religious beliefs and that families appreciate this aspect of care being explored (29).

However, in spite of the best intentions, the offer of spiritual support to family carers may be rejected. Barriers from with the family might include family dysfunction/hostility, incongruence of patient and carer needs, impaired concentration and carers not wanting to bother health professionals.

Other factors focus on the helpfulness (or otherwise) of the planned interventions, so that 'families may choose to ignore supportive services if they have limited confidence that what is offered will meet their needs' (24).

Another perceived barrier may be the time factor. While the time-constraints of busy palliative care health professionals need to be acknowledged, the observant, discerning, skilled communicator will identify relevant data, not only during the admission process but throughout the course of the whole episode of care. For example, spiritual needs can arise in the course of ordinary conversation and assessment of other needs. Thus, spiritual needs may emerge over time as brief chapters in a longer narrative.

Narrative and needs

The language of 'needs' can be transformed when caregiving is regarded as entering another person's story. This is not to suggest we eradicate 'needs'; rather that we frame 'needs' in a social, reciprocal relationship, instead of in the language of an 'expert' professional carer dispensing answers to a 'care recipient'.

The language of narrative grounds the universal mode of spirituality in the individual's life story (30). Such narrative takes account of the person's family/social context, beliefs, values, rituals—either sacred or secular (2). Kellehear describes the moral and biographical, as well as the situational and the religious, as the building blocks of needs in palliative care (31). These building blocks are imbued with knowledge drawn from family carers' specific stories.

In his seminal philosophical work, Mayeroff (32) describes the knowledge needed for caring. His wisdom of nearly four decades ago has aptitude for contemporary palliative care.

> We sometimes speak as if caring did not require knowledge, as if caring for someone, for example, were simply a matter of good intentions or warm regard.... To care for someone, I must know many things. I must know, for example, who the other is, what his powers and limitations are, what his needs are, and what is conducive to his growth; I must know how to respond to his needs, and what my powers and limitations are. Such knowledge is both general and specific.

Mayeroff emphasizes qualities of humility, trust, refraining from imposing one's views and readiness to learn from the 'other' (32). Such mutual learning can be captured in the following scenario:

> Mrs M had cared for her husband, aged 82, for the 12-year course of his dementia. Due to Mr M's complex co-morbidities, and the need for expert symptom management, the time had come for referral to the local palliative care service. Without checking how Mrs M had been managing her husband's care in the past, the palliative care

nurse outlined a particular regimen for his hygiene needs. Although frail and in pain, Mr M lashed out when the nurse directed him to the shower. What had been offered as support and respite for Mrs M resulted in increased distress. 'If only she'd listened to me,' Mrs M confided to the chaplain, 'I could have explained to her in three minutes the best way of approaching him. Now he distrusts all the nurses and I'm left with the same amount of work. I had my spirits lifted when they offered all these services and now I feel more down than ever.'

Mrs M's spiritual distress is hard to miss. However, to the undiscerning, her 'problem' might have been identified merely as the need for physical assistance with her husband's hygiene. Mrs M had the power of experience and knowledge, which she was willing to share, but the sharing depended on someone hearing her story. Other carers have written about their need for a companion on their journey (33); a concept with a significant history in palliative care (34), which is often exemplified more specifically through the pastoral care role.

Role of formal clergy/pastoral carer

Traditional palliative care has always included clergy, chaplains or pastoral care workers within the team. However, along with all other care practices, spiritual and religious care requires scrutiny in order to ensure best practice. Questions that might helpfully be addressed to palliative care services regarding this role include the following:

◆ Is it important for the palliative care service to maintain a specific religious identity and discipline, while acknowledging these views and beliefs will not be shared by all who use the service?

◆ Is it preferable to adopt a more generic spirituality that attempts to cover family carers' diverse range of spiritual, cultural and religious needs?

◆ Are the patients' and family carers' needs best addressed by a 'neutral' counselor, such as a psychotherapist or a facilitator?

◆ Does the chaplain/pastoral care worker have specific responsibilities for family carers' spiritual needs and, if so, what time (and other) resources are available, particularly for home visits?

◆ Does the service distinguish between the roles of chaplain and pastoral care worker and, if so, in what way?

◆ Is it assumed that the chaplain/pastoral care worker will have a coordinating role, i.e. arranging for visits from other religious leaders or clergy of the family's choice?

◆ What evidence is available for (a) the frequency of chaplain/pastoral carer contacts with family carers and (b) their effectiveness in response to family carers' needs?

- What training and support is available for chaplains/pastoral carers, particularly regarding the needs of family carers?
- Is the pastoral care/chaplaincy service supported by relevant research?

Organization and accountability

In spite of formal standards for spiritual care, little is known about the nature and effectiveness of spiritual care offered to family carers. Palliative care services, in reviewing this area, might be prompted to reflect on the issues outlined in Table 3.1 below.

A further organizational issue relates to the timing of spiritual assessment. Is it a part of holistic assessment for every patient's family, or is it dependent on the emergence of problems? If the service regards family carers' spiritual care to be of importance, then the issue will be addressed as soon as possible after the patient is admitted to the service. Best practice suggests this should take place in a formally structured family meeting where all care planning issues are discussed.

What if harm is caused?

When spiritual care is regarded as a soft option, it often demonstrates a lack of accountability and confidence, exemplified by the awkward, embarrassed response of a chaplain when asked by the family to pray. 'Okay,' she said, 'it can't do any harm.' This prompts another question raised by Orchard as to the potential harm when there is an absence of appropriate spiritual care (35).

The issue of accountability and ethics in spiritual care is also raised by Cobb (2) who states that, while spiritual care practices are unlikely to constitute grounds for trespass or abuse, chaplains may escape such scrutiny because of their low visibility, insignificant numbers and a perception that their role is relatively benign. Increased accountability is needed to identify those (albeit rare) circumstances where harm can be caused. 'Incompetence, abuse of trust or the violation of boundaries in these circumstances can have devastating consequences and inflict life-long damage' (36). Damage can also arise when risks are not identified.

Predicting risk

Citing firsthand accounts, Hudson notes the struggle family carers experience in seeking meaning in the midst of suffering, or in expressing their fear of the future. As one 48-year-old spouse said, through her tears, 'I'm scared ... I'm tired and it's realising now the amount of care he's going to need at home. It's overwhelming to me' (37).

Table 3.1 Organization and accountability of palliative care services

Promotional material	How is spiritual care for family carers described in the palliative care service's philosophy and mission statement and/or the service's promotional literature, e.g. advertising brochure?
Assessment/Measurement/Research	How and by whom are family carers' spiritual needs assessed and documented; and is the process supported by relevant research and open to measurement and audit?
Guidelines for referral	Are there clear guidelines for referral to the chaplain/pastoral carer or other relevant counsellor; and are these processes sufficiently clear to differentiate between chaplain, social worker, family counsellor and psychotherapist?
Family carers as partners	Are family carers regarded as partners in care or merely recipients of care; e.g. is there opportunity for family carers to comment about the quality of spiritual care, including access to complaints procedures where relevant?
Equality of access	Do the care practices ensure equality of access to all family carers, regardless of specific belief, or unbelief?
Spiritual needs in relation to site of care	Is attention to family carers' spiritual needs dependent on the site of care, e.g., home, nursing home, hospice, acute hospital?
Standards, guidelines, policies, procedures	Are the organization's formal standards for spiritual care translated into realistic practice guidelines, policies and procedures which are regularly reviewed?
Education and training	What resources are available for education and training of all palliative care health professionals in the domain of spiritual care for family carers?
Family carers' needs separate from the patient's care	Are resources available for the family carers' needs to be assessed and followed up apart from the patient's care?
Role of volunteers	What role do volunteers play in this area, and what support and accountability is required?

This, and other comments from carers (38), goes to the heart of responses associated with the expectations of caring for a dying relative at home. A continuous cycle of assessment and review should, however, alert health professionals to risk factors requiring specific interventions, in order to optimize the carer's spiritual health, regardless of the site of care.

Whose task is it?

If spirituality is perceived as some generic coverall, it will be seen as requiring no particular expertise; the corollary being that anyone can provide spiritual care. In this respect, Cobb says (2):

> Not everything that takes place under the banner of palliative care needs to be carried out by professionals, but it seems reasonable to consider that the spiritual dimension of humanity is a sufficient weighty matter in the face of death to require considerable care and the utmost caution.

Walter also argues for spiritual care to be shared among the team. Such partnership, he claims, 'deepens the role of the chaplain' and 'widens the role of the nurse' (6). Walter also suggests that the matching of skills to needs might have its place, rather than assuming that every member of the team has the required competence to answer every family carer's needs.

Implications for bereavement support

'Evidence shows those who profess stronger spiritual beliefs seem to resolve their grief more rapidly and completely after the death of a close person than do people with no spiritual beliefs'(40). This finding lends further weight to the importance of addressing family carers' spiritual well-being throughout the terminal illness and after the patient's death.

Various viewpoints about the effectiveness of bereavement support in palliative care are related to, but are beyond the scope of, this discussion. There is, however, a place for caution. Best practice would urge palliative care health professionals to be guided by evidence rather than assuming bereavement counselling is always an effective response to spiritual needs.

Finally, a reflection on current practice might encourage palliative care health professionals to ensure that family carers' spiritual needs are not relegated to the periphery; rather, they are brought to the centre, the heart of holistic care.

The need for spiritual care has an impressive historical legacy, it is a recurrent theme in the contemporary explorations of many disciplines and it remains a domain that can take us closer to what it means to be human, even in the face of death (3).

Key learning points

- Interventions should match family carers' needs as articulated by the family carers, rather than being imposed by the health professional.
- To artificially separate spiritual matters from everyday bodily life is to risk objectification and fragmentation.

◆ Chaplains and pastoral care workers need to be supported by clear role descriptions and evidence-based research.

◆ Spiritual care requires skilled communication, discernment, partnership and openness towards religious, spiritual and cultural diversity.

◆ Spiritual care requires appropriate organization, resources and regular review.

◆ Spiritual care is not merely a private subjective matter, it has implications for patient, family, palliative care team and the broader community.

Recommended reading and resources

Andershed B (2006). Relatives in end-of-life care–part 1: a systematic review of the literature the five last years. *Journal of Clinical Nursing* **15**(9): 1158–1169.

Cobb M (2001). Walking on water? The moral foundations of chaplaincy. In: Orchard H (ed.). *Spirituality in Health Care Contexts.* London: Jessica Kingsley Publishers, 73–83.

Hudson R and Rumbold B (2003). Spiritual care. In: O'Connor M and Aranda S (ed.). *Palliative Care Nursing: a Guide to Practice.* Melbourne: Ausmed Publications, 69–86.

Hudson R (2006). Disembodied souls or soul-less bodies: spirituality as fragmentation. *Journal of Religion, Spirituality & Aging* **18**(2/3): 45–57.

Kellehear A (2002). Spiritual care in palliative care: whose job is it? In: Rumbold B (ed.). *Spiritual Care in Palliative Care: Spiritual and Pastoral Perspectives.* Oxford: Oxford University Press, 166–177.

MacKinlay E (ed.) (2006). *Aging, Spirituality and Palliative Care.* New York: The Haworth Pastoral Press.

Orchard H (ed.) (2001). *Spirituality in Health Care Contexts.* London: Jessica Kingsley Publishers.

Palliative Care Australia (2005). *Standards for providing quality palliative care for all Australians.* Canberra at http://pallcare.org.au

Williams M, Cobb M, Shiels C and Taylor F (2006). How well trained are clergy in care of the dying patient and bereavement support? *Journal of Pain and Symptom Management,* **32**(1): 44–51.

World Health Organization (2002). *National cancer control programmes: policies and managerial guidelines* (2nd edn) at: http://who.int/en

References

1. Speck P (2004). Spiritual needs in health care. *BMJ*, **329**: 123–124.
2. Cobb M (2002). *The Dying Soul: Spiritual Care at the End of Life.* Buckingham: Open University Press.
3. Gadamer HG (1996). *The Enigma of Health: The Art of Healing in a Scientific Age.* Cambridge: Polity Press.
4. Pattison S (2001). Dumbing down the spirit. In: Orchard H (ed.). *Spirituality in Health Care Contexts.* London and Philadelphia: Jessica Kingsley Publishers, 33–46.
5. Walter T (2002). Spirituality in palliative care: opportunity or burden? *Palliative Medicine* **16**: 133–139.

6. Walter T (1997). The ideology and organization of spiritual care: three approaches. *Palliative Medicine* **11**: 21–30.

7. Myss C (2005). *Invisible Acts of Power*. New York: Simon and Schuster.

8. Orchard H (ed.) (2001). *Spirituality in Health Care Contexts*. London: Jessica Kingsley Publishers.

9. Wright M and Clark, D (2006). *Hospice and Palliative Care in Africa: a Review of Developments and Challenges*. Oxford: Oxford University Press.

10. Allen R, Haley W, Roff L, Schmid B and Bergman E (2006). Responding to the needs of caregivers near the end of life: enhancing benefits and minimizing burdens. In: Werth JL and Blevins D (ed.). *Psychosocial Issues Near the End of Life: a Resource for Professional Care Providers*. Washington: American Psychological Association, 183–201.

11. Tanyi R (2006). Spirituality and family nursing. *Journal of Advanced Nursing* **53**(3): 287–294.

12. Twycross R and Wilcock A (2001). *Symptom Management in Advanced Cancer* (3rd edn). Abingdon: Radcliffe Medical Press.

13. Saunders C (1988). Spiritual pain. *Journal of Palliative Care* **4**: 29–32.

14. Hudson P (2003). A conceptual model and key variables for guiding supportive interventions for family caregivers of people receiving palliative care. *Palliative and Supportive Care* **1**(4): 353–365.

15. Rumbold B (2006) (ed.). *Spirituality and Palliative Care: Social and Pastoral Perspectives*. Oxford: Oxford University Press.

16. Hudson R (2006). Disembodied souls or soul-less bodies: spirituality as fragmentation. *Journal of Religion, Spirituality & Aging*, **18**(2/3): 45–57.

17. McSherry C, Draper P and Kendrick, D (2002). The construct validity of a rating scale designed to assess spirituality and spiritual care. *Journal of Advanced Nursing* **39**(4): 325–332.

18. Randall F and Downie R (2006). *The Philosophy of Palliative Care: Critique and Reconstruction*. Oxford: Oxford University Press.

19. Taylor E (2006). Spiritual assessment. In: Ferrell B and Coyle N (ed.). *Palliative Nursing*. New York: Oxford University Press, 581–594.

20. Gordon T, Mitchell A (2004). A competency model for the assessment and delivery of spiritual care. *Palliative Medicine* **18**: 646–651.

21. McSherry W (2001). Spiritual crisis? Call a nurse. In: Orchard H (ed.). *Spirituality in Health Care Contexts*. London: Jessica Kingsley Publishers, 107–117.

22. Hudson R and Rumbold B (2003). Spiritual care. In: O'Connor M and Aranda S (ed.). *Palliative Care Nursing: a Guide to Practice*. Melbourne: Ausmed Publications, 69–86.

23. Hudson P, Kristjanson L, Ashby M, Kelly B, Schofield P, Hudson R, Aranda S, O'Connor M, and Street A (2006). Desire for hastened death in patients with advanced disease and the evidence base of clinical guidelines: a systematic review. *Palliative Medicine* **20**(7): 693–701.

24. Hudson P, Aranda S and Kristjanson L (2004). Meeting the supporting needs of family caregivers in palliative care; challenges for health professionals. *Palliative Medicine* **7**(1) 19–25.

25. Kristjanson L. Hudson P and Oldham, L (2004). Working with families. In: O'Connor M and Aranda S (ed.). *Palliative Care Nursing: a Guide to Practice*. Melbourne: Ausmed Publications, 271–284.

26. Chochinov H and Cann B (2005). Interventions to enhance the spiritual aspects of dying. *Journal of Palliative Medicine* **8**(Supplement 1): S103–S115.

27. Boston P and Mount B (2006). The caregiver's perspective on existential and spiritual distress in palliative care. *Journal of Pain and Symptom Management* **32**(1): 13–26.

28. Nuland S (1994). *How We Die: Reflections on Life's Final Chapter.* New York: Alfred A Knopf.

29. Commonwealth of Australia (2006). *Guidelines for a Palliative Approach in Residential Aged Care.* Melbourne: Australian Government Department of Health and Ageing.

30. Speck P (1998). Spiritual issues in palliative care. In: Doyle D, Hanks G and MacDonald N (ed.). *Oxford Textbook of Palliative Medicine.* Oxford: Oxford University Press, 805–814.

31. Kellehear A (2002). Spiritual care in palliative care: whose job is it? In: Rumbold B (ed.) *Spiritual Care in Palliative Care: Spiritual and Pastoral Perspectives.* Oxford: Oxford University Press, 166–177.

32. Mayeroff M (1971). *On Caring.* New York: Harper Perennial.

33. Hender M (2004). *Saying Goodbye: Stories of Caring for the Dying.* Sydney: ABC Books.

34. Saunders C (1965). Watch with Me. *Nursing Times* (November 26) p. 1.

35. Orchard H (2001). Being there? Presence and absence in spiritual care delivery. In: Orchard H (ed.). *Spirituality in Health Care Contexts.* London: Jessica Kingsley Publishers, 147–159.

36. Cobb M (2001). Walking on water? The moral foundations of chaplaincy. In: Orchard H (ed.). *Spirituality in Health Care Contexts.* London: Jessica Kingsley Publishers, 73–83.

37. Hudson P (2002). Support for family caregivers of dying cancer patients; a randomized controlled trial. Unpublished PhD thesis, School of Postgraduate Nursing, Faculty of Medicine, Dentistry and Health Sciences, The University of Melbourne.

38. Payne S, Smith R and Dean, S (1999). Identifying the concerns of informal carers in palliative care. *Journal of Palliative Medicine* **13**(1): 37–44.

39. Wright M (2001). Chaplaincy in hospice and hospital: from a survey in England and Wales. *Palliative Medicine* **15**(3): 229–242.

40. Walsh K, King M, Jones L, Tookman A and Blizard R (2002). Spiritual beliefs may affect outcome of bereavement: prospective study. *BMJ* **324**(7353): 1551.

Chapter 4

Policy initiatives for family carers

Hilary Arksey and Anne Corden

Introduction

This chapter discusses policy initiatives for family carers of people with terminal illness. We focus on the situation in England with some comparisons of innovative approaches in other welfare states, including Canada, Australia and European member states.

In England and elsewhere, most people would like to die at home but for many this is not achieved (1–3). Much may depend on the availability of family carers able to work alongside health and social care professionals to help their relatives and friends achieve the best quality of life as death draws nearer. There is some evidence to suggest that having a family carer helps people achieve their wish to die at home (4).

Family carers who perceive absence of appropriate backup to deal with the issues arising may be reluctant to care for a terminally ill person at home (5). However, it is estimated that as many as 500 000 people do provide such care in the UK (6).

Carers of people who are dying have some needs in common with other groups of carers, including access to good quality, flexible, affordable and responsive service provision. Other particular issues facing end-of-life carers relate to managing complex and unpredictable conditions that may change daily; recognizing the impending onset of the terminal phase; planning for the future in the face of uncertainties; emotional demands of preparing themselves (and the ill person) for the coming death; and, sometimes, dealing with complex family relationships. There is some evidence that during the last two weeks of life, the support needs of the family may exceed those of the patient (7).

Of particular relevance for policies supporting family carers at the end of life are the impacts of different time trajectories involved. Carers thrust into a caring role where death is imminent after sudden trauma or unexpected diagnosis have little time to think about the implications or find out about, and access, services. Support needs of carers of people who have lived with chronic illness for a long time may be less intensive but more episodic. Issues of time and uncertainty have particular relevance for carers who want to continue or return to paid work.

The chapter begins by discussing the identification and position of family carers of terminally ill people within general social policy provision for carers. We then look, in turn, at employment policies and financial support for carers, including what happens after the death of the person cared for. One way of comparing policy initiatives in other countries is to create a fictional but common care scenario, and explain the different approaches. Thus, we discuss the situation of a middle-aged woman caring for her mother with terminal illness, as she might fare in England, Canada, Australia, Finland and the Netherlands. We then consider, mainly from an English perspective, the influence on policy development of 'consumer groups' representing the interests of families providing terminal care, The final part of the chapter draws together our findings, and sets out some key learning points.

Policy initiatives for carers of terminally ill people

This part of the chapter discusses policy initiatives for carers, with a particular focus on those involved in end-of-life care.

Government policy in England has traditionally taken a broad view of a 'carer' and what constitutes caregiving activities, acknowledging that carers who provide significant emotional or social support, but not instrumental care, still need support. Policies, in turn, tend to be aimed at carers in general, without identifying particular groups of carers for special provision.

Such a broad approach might be said to match the heterogeneity of circumstances in caring relationships, and the range of medical conditions of those receiving care. However, the issue that then arises is how applicable to, or relevant for, end-of-life carers are generic policy measures. While palliative care is used mainly by people with cancer, the range of other conditions of people receiving care from their family at the end of life includes motor neurone disease; cystic fibrosis; multiple sclerosis; HIV/AIDS; respiratory, cardiac, renal and liver disease, and deterioration and dementia related to ageing.

We look first at general social policy, followed by employment policy and financial support.

Social policy initiatives

England is unique in its legislative focus on carers. There are three pieces of legislation, supported by a national strategy, which is currently being revised and strengthened (see Box 4.1).

Box 4.1 Social Policy initiatives in England

Carers (Recognition and Services) Act (1995)

National Strategy for Carers (1999)

Carers and Disabled Children Act (2000)

Carers (Equal Opportunities) Act (2004)

New Deal for Carers (commitment in 2006 White Paper)

The Carers (Recognition and Services) Act (1995) provided the first legal definition of a carer, and an agreement that carers had a right to assessment of their ability to care. Subsequently, the Carers and Disabled Children Act (2000) strengthened carers' rights to assessment and amended the earlier legislation to enable carers to have services in their own right. The Carers (Equal Opportunities) Act (2004) re-focused the previous two pieces of legislation by concentrating on carers' wishes in relation to education, training, employment and leisure. This shift marks an attempt to recognize a carer holistically, as a 'total' person rather than just a carer.

The legislation is underpinned by the National Strategy for Carers, intended to improve choice and flexibility for carers (8). The Strategy was based on three elements: information, support and care for carers. Whilst the Strategy drew attention to the special needs of certain groups of carers—for example, young carers and rural carers—those caring for a terminally ill person were not singled out for any special consideration.

The National Strategy also created the Carers Special Grant through which local authorities could apply for funding to develop respite care services and short-term breaks. This kind of support can be particularly useful to end-of-life carers. Studies of carers looking after dying relatives at home emphasize their need for time for themselves and a break from the caregiving role (9–11).

Most recently, a 'New Deal for Carers', first detailed in the White Paper (12) on the future of adult social care, sets out the Government's intention to ensure short-term, home-based support for carers in emergency or crisis situations; to set up a national information service/help-line for carers; to create an Expert Carers Programme (now known as Caring with Confidence) to support and train carers, and identify lead personnel in all local authorities and primary care trusts.

On the basis of the above, it would appear that carers are well supported in England. Evaluations have shown, however, that there remain gaps in services for carers in relation to provision of information; assessments and identification of need, and provision of support (13–15). A new report by the Commission for Social Care Inspection found significant disparity between councils in the type, level and quality of services for carers (13). Financial or resource constraints were commonly cited as barriers to developing support for carers.

Other countries that have introduced legislation giving carers rights and recognition for the first time include Finland and jurisdictions in Australia (Western Australia, Northern Territory and Australian Capital Territory). Sweden is introducing legislation imminently (initially due to be enacted autumn 2007). Generally speaking, as in England, such legislation does not specifically target carers of terminally ill people, with some exceptions in terms of employment policy initiatives as discussed below.

In countries where there is no separate carer legislation, there may still be provision for addressing carers' issues. For example, in the Netherlands, home care is provided through the Exceptional Medical Expenses Act. Although Dutch carers have no entitlement to a needs assessment in their own right, the guidelines require practitioners to assess the extent and impact of caregiving on carers and to take into account their wish to work, or have some free time.

The effectiveness of many of the above policy measures depends on individuals identifying themselves as 'carers'. People who tend to view the care they give as part of normal obligations and responsibilities within relationships, and thus do not readily identify themselves as 'carers' (16), may be unaware of relevant provision. This might be a particular problem for people who suddenly find themselves in a caregiving role with a short-term time trajectory.

There are other issues to consider in relation to how far generic policy measures for carers are appropriate for carers of terminally ill people. In some situations, a caring role comes suddenly and is likely to be short-term. The kind of swift response required—for example, mandatory 'fast-track' approaches to assessment and support—might be achieved more easily by identifying specific groups of carers, rather than within generic provision.

The policy approach in England is changing rapidly, however, and recent policy documents show Government recognition that carers of terminally ill people require special recognition. The White Paper 'Our health, our care, our say', a key policy driver, highlights the importance of supporting carers of people who are dying (12). Similarly, influential guidance on supportive and palliative care for adults with cancer contains recommendations for carers (17). These include assessing and addressing the needs of family members and carers on an on-going basis, and coordination in provision of information, advice and support to match changes in clinical circumstances.

End-of-life care is now a priority, as evidenced in the new NHS End of Life Care Programme. The Programme is committed to improving the training of staff who work with patients and their carers, and is encouraging the development of ways in which primary care services can support carers (18). This is part of an overall End of Life Care Strategy, expected to be published in June 2008, to address the challenges of caring for people who are dying. Australia, in contrast to England, has had a national strategy for palliative care since 2000 (2).

Employment policies

Generally, carers find it hard to combine paid work and caregiving (19); flexibility in the workplace (as well as flexible services) is a key requirement (19–21). A literature review of carers of terminally ill people and employment issues identified a number of aspects of the palliative care setting that could affect a carer's ability to work and care (22). These included uncertainties of the caring context, especially in relation to the dying trajectory. At a time of high emotional stress, people often do not think about the long- and short-term implications of deciding to take on caring. Those who do take on this role may need to look ahead to employment opportunities following bereavement, but this may be hard to do while caring for their relative.

In England, there are no employment rights specifically for employees looking after someone who is terminally ill. However, carers' rights are protected in a number of ways (see Box 4.2).

The Employment Rights Act (1996), and later amendments in the Employment Relations Act (1999), allow people with dependents (including carers) who have a contract of employment to take a 'reasonable' number of unpaid days off to deal with certain unexpected or sudden emergencies. It also gives parent carers of disabled children under the age of 18 years the right to unpaid parental leave.

More recently, the Work and Families Act (2006) gave carers of certain adults the right to request flexible working—start and finish times, compressed working hours, part-time working and working from home. The change requested is

---

Box 4.2 Employment Policy initiatives in England

Employment Rights Act (1996)

Employment Relations Act (1999)

Work and Families Act (2006)

permanent, unless agreed otherwise with the employer. Only one request for flexible working can be made in any 12-month period. Rights to flexible working are open to all eligible carers, in line with general social policy in England. However, Government guidance for business, trade and industry suggests that, where an employee suddenly becomes the carer of someone with a terminal illness, then a temporary or time-limited period of flexible working might be more appropriate, after which they could revert back to the original pattern (23).

Australia is another country that has introduced workforce legislation covering generic carers rather than singling out any specific group. Paid and unpaid personal/carer's leave (including sick leave, carer's leave and compassionate leave) is legislated for as part of the Australian Fair Pay and Conditions Standard. Employees generally have to provide evidence, such as a medical certificate, of the illness or injury that has given rise to their application for leave.

In contrast are those countries with specific legal provision for end-of-life carers to take leave from the workplace with some income security, typically through insurance or benefits systems, rather than directly from employers. In Canada, eligible individuals caring for a family member at risk of dying within a 6-month period are entitled to 6 weeks compassionate leave during which their job and income are protected. As soon as they stop working, they need to apply for Compassionate Care Benefit (CCB) of up to 55 per cent of their average insured earnings over a 6-week period. The CCB is flexible, for instance the 6 weeks of income assistance can be taken at once or spread out over 6 months. In addition, it can be shared between family members who take turns caring for their relative.

The House of Commons Health Committee Inquiry into Palliative Care recommended the introduction of a similar initiative in England (5). This proposal was not taken up, as at the time the effectiveness of the CCB was (and still is) unproven. A small-scale pilot evaluation of the CCB found that whilst most carers viewed it positively, there were weaknesses (24). Perceived limitations included problems associated with accurate prognostication, and the requirement to have a doctor's certificate stating that the person receiving care was within 6 months of death. The definition of 'family member' eligible for CCB initially included only close relatives (since extended). The period of funding did not always match the needs of the carer.

Canada is not alone in offering financial compensation schemes and labour policies for carers of terminally ill people. Keefe and colleagues provide a useful cross-national review of labour market policies and financial compensation initiatives for carers of dependent adults in 10 countries (25). Drawing some examples from the review, the Care Leave Act (1989) in Sweden gave carers of relatives who were terminally ill the right to take up to 60 days leave from work at 80 per cent of salary. In Norway's Nursing Care Leave programme there was some relaxation of requirements for prognosis, such that employed people providing care to a family member, either permanently ill or diagnosed as terminal, were entitled to a full wage for a period of up to 20 days leave.

In her overview of these labour market policies for family carers, Keefe observes that they reduce some of the tension and stress for employees trying to balance caregiving and paid work (25). However, eligibility criteria impose some constraints; and for those who are entitled, it may take time to bring financial support on stream.

Financial support for caregiving

The financial impact for family carers may include loss of, or interruption to, their own earnings and, for some, loss of earnings of the person cared for (26). At the same time, providing home-based care may increase household bills for gas, electricity and telephone. Equipment, bedding and home alterations may be major expenses (27, 28). Paying for food may involve buying more expensive items to encourage a frail person to eat, or having to rely more on ready meals for the rest of the household. There may be travel expenses for family carers whose relative spends time in hospital or hospice. For some family carers, caring is associated with financial hardship (29, 30) and financial concerns are known to be a source of considerable stress for people with cancer and their families (31). An audit of closed patient files in a specialist hospice showed that the primary need for carers was for finance and advice about state welfare benefits (32).

Glendinning (33) provides an overview of different models of paying family carers, and explains how these are shaped by institutional and cultural traditions within different kinds of welfare states. In England, the approach is one of income maintenance—paying benefits directly to the carer to recognize and compensate for loss of other earnings. Carer's Allowance is available to people who provide regularly at least 35 hours care weekly to a disabled or older person receiving a qualifying benefit, and who have no or very low earnings. Research shows that Carer's Allowance does not act as an incentive to encourage carers to stop caring to work, to stop work to care or to combine work and care (19). The low earnings threshold can trap Carer's Allowance recipients into low-paid jobs, often below their existing skill levels and with few intrinsic rewards. Despite these shortcomings, what is important is that the benefit explicitly acknowledges the rights of carers to an independent income (33). In principle, it avoids the financial dependency of the carer on the person cared for and maintains limited protection for eventual state retirement pension entitlement for the carer. The value of the benefit is low, however, and recipients may need additional means-tested social assistance and housing benefits.

Carers in other countries can also receive benefit payments in their own right to compensate for caregiving. In Australia, for example, the Carer Payment is a means-tested income support benefit payable to people whose workforce participation is substantially constrained by caring responsibilities (34). There is also a non-means-tested Carer Allowance, a nominal fortnightly payment. Since the 2004–05 Budget, one-off lump sum bonuses have been paid annually to eligible carers in receipt of Carer Payment and/or Carer Allowance. Eligible carers in Sweden and Norway are also entitled to direct compensation through income replacement benefits, whilst carers in Canada can receive indirect compensation via various (tax) credit schemes, including the Caregiver Credit initiative (25).

Other models of financial support for carers include their direct employment by the state, as in Finland, Norway and Sweden. Glendinning (33) points out that these are all countries with high levels of both female employment and publicly funded social services. In line with movements towards self-directed care and independent living have come models in which payments to the terminally ill person are, in turn, routed to the carer. In Flanders and the Netherlands, for example, disabled and older people in need of home care have the option of receiving a 'Personal Assistance Budget' (35), which may be used to purchase care from a care agency or individual care provider. The latter includes family members and friends, who become paid informal carers. Research shows that the paid informal carer can benefit financially but there are some drawbacks. The Personal Assistance Budget is rarely used to obtain additional formal support that might reduce subjective psychological and physical burdens experienced by the paid informal carer. Models of payments to carers directly from budgets held by the person cared for depend on agreements and contracts between the parties involved. This may not be possible when people are very ill.

Some family carers in England may also receive contributions to the household budget from benefits claimed by the person receiving care. Importantly, however, the way in which these monies are made available to caring relatives remains a private matter. Disability Living Allowance and Attendance Allowance are designed to help meet the costs of care, and there are special rules to enable quick and easy access by terminally ill people. These benefits can make a valuable contribution to household budgeting for families providing palliative care. There are problems of low take-up, however (36). Research has shown considerable under-claiming of these benefits among people living with cancer, related to lack of understanding among families and professionals, practical difficulties in claiming, some reluctance to seek financial help, and wanting to maintain independence and positive outlook (26).

Financial and economic impacts for the family carer may well continue after the death. In England, bereaved people emerge as a group at particular risk of poverty and problem debt (37). Small-scale studies have shown how caring for a disabled or ill family member can adversely affect income and employment after that person dies (38–41). Little is known about whether, or when, people providing care to a terminally ill relative look ahead to their financial situation when their period of care will end. Current research on the financial implications of death of a life partner will provide some evidence here (42).

To help to ease financial transitions after the death, Carer's Allowance in England continues in payment for 8 weeks after the person cared for dies. For bereaved widows, widowers or civil partners, there are bereavement benefits. These are unaffected by earnings, other income or savings but all depend on the person who died having satisfied the National Insurance contribution conditions or having died as a result of industrial accident or disease. People who were caring for somebody other than a legal partner have no entitlement to bereavement benefits. Such people of working age who need financial support in bereavement can boost low earnings with tax credits. Those not working must make themselves available for work to claim Jobseeker's Allowance. Some may seek help for their own health condition at this stage, and may claim incapacity benefits. People who take these routes to benefits have opportunities at Jobcentre Plus (a national network of integrated offices that offer a benefits service and job search assistance to people of working age) to discuss how to get support and help in returning to, or starting, paid work.

One way of comparing across countries some of the policy initiatives discussed thus far is to create a common care scenario, and see how the carer might fare. In this section we look at the circumstances of Susan and Elizabeth.

> Susan, in her late-40s, is caring for her 80-year-old mother, Elizabeth, who lives with her. Elizabeth is disabled as a result of Parkinson's disease. Susan helps her mother with personal care and mobility. She wants to look after her mother at home for as long as possible, but is becoming increasingly tired and her health is suffering. It is hard to continue her work as a receptionist at a local hospital, but she would like to keep her job. Ten months ago, the doctor's view was that Elizabeth was close to the end of her life. The uncertainty about the likely duration of Elizabeth's terminal stage makes it difficult for Susan to plan how to best accommodate work and caregiving.

Table 4.1 sets out the policy initiatives available in selected countries to support Susan.

Table 4.1 Statutory support for Susan in different countries[a]

Is Susan's caring role recognized in law?

England	Canada	Australia	Finland	Netherlands
Yes (three pieces of legislation; see Box 4.1)	No specific legislation targeting carers	In some jurisdictions only	Yes (Family Care-giving Act, 2006)	No specific legislation targeting carers

How are Susan's needs for support assessed and met?

England	Canada	Australia	Finland	Netherlands
Legal right to assessment; entitlement to support and services as agreed in care plan. Respite may be available via local Carers Special Grant scheme.	Variable local provision of home care and nursing services, respite care, and information and support services targeted at carers.	Assessment through local coordination services such as Community Aged Care Packages. Support available through Home and Community Care Program and National Respite for Carers programme.	Legal right to assessment. Municipal authorities provide support to carers, which may include mandatory respite care.	Susan's needs should be taken into account when Elizabeth is assessed for home care, including respite care, under the Exceptional Medical Expenses Act.

Does Susan get any financial support?

England	Canada	Australia	Finland	Netherlands
Yes—Carer's Allowance.	Yes—Caregiver Credit.	Yes—Carer Payment, Carer Alowance	Yes—Home Care Allowance.	Not directly. Could be compensated from 'personal budgets' payments to Elizabeth.

What support is there for Susan's employment situation?

England	Canada	Australia	Finland	Netherlands
Right to request (unpaid) short-term emergency leave under 'Time off for dependents' initiative; right to request one change to working arrangements in a 12-month period.	Up to 6 weeks paid time off work under the Compassionate Care Benefit scheme when there is significant risk of Elizabeth's death within 26 weeks.	Paid and unpaid personal/carer's leave.	Discretionary leave, depending on employer; right to emergency short-term leave, but may not be paid leave.	Entitlement to 2 days fully paid 'calamity leave', and 6 weeks full-time or 12 weeks part-time leave without full pay.

[a] Table assumes that Susan meets relevant eligibility criteria operating in different countries.

The impact of 'consumer groups'

There is consensus that issues relevant to all groups of carers rose on the policy agenda in England through effective lobbying by carers' organizations (43, 44). It is generally recognized that focused campaigning by Carers UK (previously the Carers National Association) was instrumental in achieving the first ever legal rights for carers; increases in carers' benefits; improvements to pension provision for carers; and dedicated funding for local councils to develop services to support carers.

When we look at policy issues related specifically to carers of terminally ill people, the report of the House of Commons Health Committee Inquiry into Palliative Care (5) shows the wide range of voluntary organizations with an interest in end-of-life care who have campaigned for, and contributed to, debates about improvements in this area. These include carers' organizations, disease-specific associations, palliative care groups and organizations representing older people.

Specialist palliative care organizations in other countries have also been keen to influence Government policy. The Canadian Hospice Palliative Care Association (45) produced a discussion document designed to stimulate debate about the legal, moral and ethical issues that arise for informal carers providing hospice palliative care, and for the professionals who work with them. This Association is one of over 30 members of the Quality End-of-Life Care Coalition of Canada that in 2005 produced a framework to encourage the Federal Government to develop a strategy on palliative and end-of-life care. Likewise, the introduction of the Compassionate Care Benefit followed years of advocacy from the palliative care and caregiving communities (24).

Getting involved in strategic policy work can involve some hard choices and trade offs for voluntary organizations. For example, a choice recently facing a national palliative care organization in England was whether to campaign actively for the introduction of an equivalent of the Canadian Compassionate Care Benefit. In view of the poor evidence-base to demonstrate the effectiveness of the Benefit, the organization concerned felt it was better placed to support the flexible working initiative introduced under the Work and Families Act (2006). The importance of flexible working arrangements for carers was well documented. The organization chose to use resources to develop its own booklets on short-term, flexible working solutions for carers and employers.

Conclusion

We have seen in this chapter that English social policies for carers tend to be generic, aimed at carers in general and taking a fairly broad view of what constitutes caregiving activities, rather than targeting specific groups, such as people giving end-of-life care. There may be advantages to this approach, in that it is inclusive and does not require sensitive categorization and medical prognosis. It may be easier to provide information and advice about services generally available, and for citizens to understand their own position in relation to administrative structures and eligibility criteria. We know, however, that self-identification as a 'carer' does not come readily to many family carers providing end-of-life care, who may miss out on help available.

There might be advantages in a more targeted approach, such as fast-tracking or provision specifically designed for people providing terminal care. Looking across other countries, it is within employment policies that we find most examples of policies specifically for end-of-life carers. The need for flexible working arrangements alongside the importance of job retention and safeguarding pensions for people who face particular uncertainties about time trajectories, have led to different kinds of arrangements with employers, linked with financial compensation provision. While such arrangements can make it easier to balance care and employment, they take time to arrange and specificity of eligibility criteria means some carers are excluded.

Models of provision of financial support for carers of people who are terminally ill are diverse, and are hard to compare directly because they are individually rooted in different cultural and administrative traditions, different kinds of welfare state and varying availability of home carers. What can be said is that recent developments towards personal budget-holding by the person cared for, which originated from demands of younger, disabled people for more choice and control, may be inappropriate in some terminal care situations, where people cared for are too ill or frail to make such decisions and engage with an administrative process.

The financial and economic impact of providing end-of-life care may extend long beyond the death of the person cared for, and policy provision extends into areas such as bereavement benefits.

We conclude the chapter by looking to the future. The majority of people requiring palliative care are in the older age group (2). Population projections to 2050 suggest that in all 25 European Union member states, there will be large increases in numbers of the 'oldest' old, people aged 80 and over who have the greatest needs for care (46). Similar large growth rates for the very old are also projected for countries like Australia and Canada. Population projections of the oldest old are projections of people moving towards death. Without support from family carers it will be impossible for many dying older persons to remain at home (47).

Governments worldwide are concerned about the future supply of carers, although the debate is not usually framed from the perspective of carers of dying older people. Long-term care projections (48) show that in England care by children of the oldest old will need to increase substantially. Whether such increased demand can be met is open to question, given current decreases in family size, the reduction of co-residence of older people with their adult children and women's increasing participation in the workforce. These issues raise important questions regarding appropriate support to help carers look after terminally ill parents, relatives and friends, particularly in relation to their ability to reconcile caregiving with paid work. There is an urgent need for evaluation of the accessibility and effectiveness of services and support for carers in a palliative care setting, and research on experiences of working, or retaining jobs, whilst caring for a terminally ill person, to inform policy makers about arrangements that facilitate or constrain this harmonization.

Key learning points

- Enabling people to die at home depends largely on availability and willingness of family carers. Policies are required that provide adequate and appropriate practical, financial and emotional support for such carers.

- Policies for this group of carers must take into account the heterogeneity of terminal conditions, and uncertainties in the timing and progression of the last stages in life.

- Looking across countries, we find different models of paying family carers, and supporting those who want to combine care with paid work, or return to work afterwards. Some countries have arrangements specifically for people providing end-of-life care. The common approach in England is generic, and services are made available to carers without distinguishing particular groups.

- Carers' needs for financial information and support often extend beyond the death, when income sources and employment opportunities may change. Bereavement support services may have a role here, in provision of signposts to appropriate advisers.

Acknowledgements

The authors would like to thank Caroline Glendinning and the editors for helpful comments on an earlier version of this chapter. Marjolein Moree, and participants at the Caregivers: Essential Partners in Care conference in Toronto (June 2007) and also the Eurocarers conference in Paris (June 2007) provided valuable information about their respective countries' policies for carers.

Recommended reading and resources

http://www.ageconcern.org.uk/. Age Concern website.

http://www.direct.gov.uk/en/CaringForSomeone/index.htm. UK Government website for carers.

http://www.endoflifecare.nhs.uk/eolc. NHS End of Life Care Programme website.

http://www.helpthehospices.org.uk/. Help the Hospices website.

http://www.msvu.ca/mdcaging/policyprofiles.asp. Policy profiles for carers in ten countries. Web pages for the Maritime Data Centre for Aging Research and Policy Analysis.

http://www.ncpc.org.uk/index.html. Website for the (UK's) National Council for Palliative Care.

www.carersuk.org. Carers UK website.

Arksey H, Corden A, Glendinning C and Hirst M (2006). *Carers and the Management of Financial Assets in Later Life: Report of a Scoping Study*. York: Social Policy Research Unit, University of York.

Department of Health (1999). *Caring About Carers: a National Strategy for Carers*. London: Department of Health.

Pickard L, Wittenberg R, Comas-Herrera AKD and Malley J (2007). Care by spouses, care by children: projections of informal care for older people in England to 2031. *Social Policy and Society* 6(3): 353–366.

Acts of Parliament

Carers and Disabled Children Act (2000), (c. 16). London: The Stationery Office.

Carers (Equal Opportunities) Act (2004), (c. 15). London: The Stationery Office.

Carers (Recognition and Services) Act (1995), (c. 12). London: HMSO.

Employment Rights Act (1996), (c. 18). London: HMSO.

Employment Relations Act (1999), (c. 26). London: The Stationery Office.

Work and Families Act (2006), (c. 18). London: The Stationery Office.

References

1. Higginson IJ (2003). *Priorities and Preferences for End of Care Life in England, Wales and Scotland*. London: National Council for Palliative Care and Others.

2. Commonwealth Department of Health and Aged Care (2000). *National Palliative Care Strategy: a National Framework for Palliative Care Service Development*. Canberra: Commonwealth Department of Health and Aged Care. http://www.health.gov.au/internet/wcms/publishing.nsf/Content/palliativecare-pubs-npcstrat.htm/$FILE/Strategy.pdf. Accessed 24 June 2007.

3. Ontario Palliative Care Association (2005). It's about quality living and dying. *The Family Caregiver Newsmagazine*, summer 2007, 6. (Cited in Hospice palliative care.) http://www.thefamilycaregiver.com/pdf/TFCN_12_CCAC_TOR.pdf. Accessed 23 July 2007.

4. Klinkenberg M, Visser G, Broese van Groenou MI, van der Wal G, Deeg DJH and Willems DL (2005). The last 3 months of life: care, transitions and the place of death of older people. *Health and Social Care in the Community* **1**(5): 420–430.

5. House of Commons Health Committee (2004). *Palliative Care: Fourth Report of Session 2003–04*, Vol 1, HC 454–1. http://www.parliament.the-stationery-office.co.uk/pa/cm200304/cmselect/cmhealth/454/454.pdf. Accessed 30 June 2007.

6. Fletcher M (2006). Introduction. In: Heatley R (ed.). *Carers' Services Guide: Setting Up Support Services for Carers of the Terminally Ill*. London: Help the Hospices.

7. Higginson IJ, Wade A and McCarthy M (1990). Palliative care: views of patients and their families. *British Medical Journal* **301**: 277–281.

8. Department of Health (1999). *Caring About Carers: a National Strategy for Carers*. London: Department of Health.

9. Hudson P (2004). Positive aspects and challenges associated with caring for a dying relative at home. *International Journal of Palliative Nursing* **10**(2): 58–65.

10. Cope D (2003). Survey of carers reveals that they often need respite care. *Clinical Journal of Oncology Nursing* **7**(2): 136.

11. McGrath P, Patton MA, McGrath Z, Olgivie K, Rayner R and Holewa H (2006). 'It's very difficult to get respite out here at the moment': Australian findings on end-of-life care for Indigenous people. *Health and Social Care in the Community* **14**(2): 147–155.

12. Department of Health (2006). *Our Health, Our Care, Our Say: a New Direction for Community Services*, Cm 6737. London: Department of Health.

13. Commission for Social Care Inspection (2006). *The State of Social Care in England 2005–06*. http://www.csci.org.uk/PDF/state_of_social_care.pdf. Accessed 19 January 2007.

14. Audit Commission (2004). *Support for Carers of Older People*. London: Audit Commission.

15. Beesley L (2006). *Wanless Social Care Review. Informal Care in England*. London: King's Fund.

16. Parker G (1992). *With This Body: Caring and Disability in Marriage*. Buckingham: Open University Press.

17. National Institute for Clinical Excellence (2004). *Improving Supportive and Palliative Care for Adults with Cancer*. London: National Institute for Clinical Excellence.

18. Philp I and Richards M (2006). *NHS End Of Life Care Programme: Progress Report March 2006*. London: Department of Health.

19. Arksey H, Kemp PA, Glendinning C, Kotchetkova I and Tozer R (2005). *Carers' Aspirations and Decisions Around Work and Retirement*. Leeds: Research Report No 290, Corporate Document Services.

20. Phillips J, Bernard M and Chittenden M (2002). *Juggling Work and Care: the Experiences of Working Carers of Older Adults*. Bristol: Policy Press.

21. Yeandle S, Bennett C, Buckner L, Shipton L and Suokas A (2006). *Who Cares Wins: the Social and Business Benefits of Supporting Working Carers*. Sheffield: Centre for Social Inclusion, Sheffield Hallam University.

22. Smith P, Payne S, Ramcharan P, Chapman A and Patterson M (2006). *Carers of the Terminally Ill and Employment Issues: a Comprehensive Literature Review*. Sheffield: Palliative and End-of-Life Research Group, University of Sheffield.

23. Department for Business, Enterprise and Regulatory Reform (2007). *Flexible Working: the Right to Request and the Duty to Consider*, part 2. http://www.dti.gov.uk/employment/employment-legislation/employment-guidance/page35848.html. Accessed 23 July 2007.

24. Williams A, Crooks VA, Stajduhar KI, Allan D and Cohen SR (2006). Canada's compassionate care benefit: views of family carers in chronic illness. *International Journal of Palliative Nursing* 12(9): 438–445.

25. Keefe J, Fancey P and White S (2005). *Consultation on Financial Compensation Initiatives for Family Care-Givers of Dependent Adults: Final Report*. Halifax: Maritime Data Centre for Ageing Research and Policy Analysis, Department of Family Studies and Gerontology, Mount Saint Vincent University. http://www.msvu.ca/mdcaging/PDFs/Consultation%20Final%20Report%20English.pdf. Accessed 19 January 2007.

26. Macmillan (2004). *The Unclaimed Millions*. London: Macmillan Cancer Relief.

27. Glendinning C (1992). *The Costs of Informal Care: Looking Inside the Household*. London: HMSO.

28. Tibble M (2005). *Review of Existing Research on the Extra Costs of Disability*. Working Paper No. 21. Leeds: Corporate Document Services.

29. Holzhausen M and Pearlman V (2000). *Caring on the Breadline: the Financial Implications of Caring*. London: Carers National Association.

30. Howard M (2001). *Paying the Price: Carers, Poverty and Social Exclusion*. London: Child Poverty Action Group.

31. Quinn A (2002). *Macmillan Cancer Relief Study Into Benefits Advice for People with Cancer*. Reading: University of Reading.

32. Harding R and Leam C (2005). Clinical notes for informal carers in palliative care: recommendations from a random patient file audit. *Palliative Medicine* 19: 639–642.

33. Glendinning C (2006). In: Glendinning C and Kemp PA (ed.). *Cash and Care: Policy Challenges in the Welfare State*. Bristol: The Policy Press, 127–140.

34. Australian Institute of Health and Welfare (2003). *Australia's Welfare 2003: The Sixth Biennial Welfare Report of the Australian Institute of Health and Welfare*. Canberra: Australian Institute of Health and Welfare.

35. Breda J, Schoenmaekers D, van Landeghem C, Claessens D and Geerts J (2006). In: Glendinning C and Kemp PA (ed.). *Cash and Care: Policy Challenges in the Welfare State*. Bristol: The Policy Press, 155–170.

36. Tunnage B, Tudor Edwards R and Linck P (2004). *Uptake of Benefits in People with Cancer: a Step Forward in Understanding*. Bangor: Centre for the Economics of Health, University of Wales.

37. Kemp PA, Bradshaw J, Dornan P, Finch N and Mayhew E (2004). *Routes Out of Poverty: a Research Review*. York: Joseph Rowntree Foundation.

38. Chesson R and Todd C (1996). Bereaved carers: recognizing their needs. *Elderly Care* 8: 16–18.

39. Corden A, Sainsbury R and Sloper P (1991). *Financial Implications of the Death of a Child*. London: Family Policy Studies Centre.

40. Jenkinson A (2003). *Past Caring: the Beginning not the End*. Edinburgh: Promenade Publishing.

41. McLaughlin E and Ritchie J (1994). Legacies of caring: the experiences and circumstances of ex-carers. *Health and Social Care in the Community* 2: 241–253.

42. Corden A, Hirst M and Nice K (2006). *Financial Consequences of the Death of a Partner.* Research proposal, ESRC grant: RES-000–23–1530. York: Social Policy Research Unit, University of York.

43. Cavaye J (2006). *Hidden Carers.* Edinburgh: Dunedin Academic Press.

44. Parker G and Clark H (2003). Making the ends meet: do carers and disabled people have a common agenda? *Policy & Politics* 30(3): 347–359.

45. Canadian Hospice Palliative Care Association (2004). *The Role of Informal Care-givers in Hospice Palliative Care and End-of-life Care in Canada: a Discussion of the Legal, Ethical and Moral Challenges.* Ottawa: VOICE in Health Policy Project. http://www.projectvoice.ca/English/03%20-%20Case%20Studies/CHPCA_Case%20Study.pdf. Accessed 10 February 2007.

46. Buckner L and Yeandle S (2007). *Care and Caring in EU Member States.* Leeds: University of Leeds.

47. Ramirez A, Addington-Hall J and Richards M (1998). ABC of palliative care: the carers. *British Medical Journal* 316: 208–211.

48. Pickard L, Wittenberg R, Comas-Herrera A, King D and Malley J (2007). Care by spouses, care by children: projections of informal care for older people in England to 2031. *Social Policy and Society* 6(3): 353–66.

Chapter 5

Family carers in resource-poor countries

Jennifer Hunt

Introduction

Resource-poor countries are often characterized by widespread poverty, stagnant economies, civil unrest and political instability. In general, the label is an economic classification with accompanying social and cultural implications. Wright (1) combines the five indices of gross domestic product, the human development index (2, 3), health expenditure, overall health system achievement and morphine consumption to identify resource-poor countries in relation to healthcare. These indices describe the potential of a country to provide comprehensive health support to its citizens, the prioritization of healthcare, and the possibility of effective provision of pain control for the chronically ill and dying. Such criteria guide the identification of some countries in South America, Africa, Asia and parts of Europe as resource-poor countries. For the purpose of this chapter however, detailed scenarios from Zimbabwe will be described to provide insights into particular situations faced by family carers of chronically ill and dying relatives in the resource-poor countries of Africa. Vignettes from other African countries and Asia will complement this analysis.

A common feature of many of these countries is the role of the HIV/AIDS epidemic in shaping the development of palliative care and the impact on family care, although it is worth noting that 12.5 per cent of all deaths in resource-poor countries are caused by cancer. This is more than the total percentage of deaths caused by HIV/AIDS, tuberculosis and malaria (4). Zimbabwe and other countries in the region have some of the highest HIV/AIDS rates in the world with poor infrastructures to manage seriously ill and dying patients within mainstream health systems. UNAIDS estimates that 1.7 million people are living with HIV in 2007 in Zimbabwe and around 1.3 million children have been orphaned due to AIDS (5). The epidemic primarily affects young to middle-aged adults on whom the national economy and families depend. Women are about 1.35 times more likely to be HIV infected than men, and in the 20–24-year-old range, infection rates among young women are three times higher than men (6). These demographic details impact significantly on family carers in Africa who are generally women, young carers and older people. This chapter will examine what it means to be a family carer in such settings by starting with a review of the health environment that determines the context for care of patients, followed by a brief explanation of the role of the family carer in palliative care. In-depth portrayals of typical family carers in resource-poor settings will elucidate some of the issues facing both older and younger, commonly female, carers. These issues are then set against the holistic palliative care approach to identify obstacles to good care. An overview of interventions attempting to support families caring for the dying in resource-poor countries leads towards a conclusion offering suggestions for clinical priorities and research ideas.

Health issues affecting family carers in resource-poor countries

In much of Africa widespread problems of poverty, international debt and bad governance tend to overshadow its potential wealth. 'It is the only continent to become poorer in the last 25 years; its share of world trade has halved in one generation, and it receives less than one percent of direct foreign investment'(7). Against this backdrop, illnesses and diseases, such as malaria, TB and HIV/AIDS, thrive. As total per capita expenditure on healthcare is usually low (8), staff and bed shortages are the norm in national hospitals, and erratic supplies of medicines and diminishing numbers of health workers are recurring obstacles to provision of healthcare generally and palliative care in particular.

In resource-rich countries with established palliative care services, home is often the chosen place of death. In resource-poor countries this is sometimes the same but a home death often occurs for different reasons. Three-quarters of India's one billion people live in rural villages, often without running water or healthcare facilities. Cancer is stigmatized and many patients become social outcasts due to illiteracy, lack of awareness, fear of serious disease and subsequent treatment. Consequently, late presentation means that up to 80 per cent of people living with cancer have incurable disease at diagnosis and remain at home with the extended family, which is ill prepared to manage advanced illness (9, 10). Ugandans express a wish to die at home, close to the ancestral burial grounds with relatives to care for them (11), and this is the case in other countries sharing similar traditional values. Increasingly, palliative care services in rural areas make this possible. In Zambia, on the other hand, people expect to die in hospital because of a law requiring the family to bring the body to the hospital for death certification before burial. In Zimbabwe, where living conditions are poor and resources severely limited, a hospital death may in fact be considered preferable, even though choice of place of death in better conditions may be home (12). The wish to die in hospital can also be motivated by a fear of a death occurring at home and the risk of harassment by police if the patient has not been seen recently by a health worker. Conversely, it is expensive to transport a body from a city to the rural home for a traditional burial, leaving families to face the prospect of burying the deceased in the city without the extended family and outside of an ancestral burial ground. In general, when there are no primary healthcare teams in the community, limited local out-patient clinics and an absence of long-term care facilities nearby (13), a home death is inevitably the only option, no matter how ill-equipped the family is to manage the dying process. Table 5.1 compares the demographics of people dying at home in both resource-rich and poor settings to illustrate the divergent paths that lead to the same end.

Despite the difficulties faced by resource-poor countries, there are positive attributes of traditional community-based living and retention of family values and relationships that are often eroded in industrialized settings. In Africa, attitudes towards illness are still affected by spiritual belief systems and may involve ancestral links, which can be a great source of comfort.

Table 5.1 Demographics of home deaths in resource rich and resource poor countries

Resource-rich countries (e.g. US)	Resource-poor countries (e.g. Africa)
May choose to die at home.	Most have no option other than to die at home.
Higher social class.	Lower social class and rural dwellers.
More economic resources.	Poor economic resources.
Open disclosure of imminent death.	Secrecy, silence, minimal information.
Primary carer is healthy.	Primary carer may be ill.
Relatives manage to avoid extreme fatigue through respite.	Carers have no respite options and suffer burn-out.
Patient's self-care needs managed.	Patient's self-care needs often poorly managed.
Specialist support available at some level.	Community volunteer may be available. No specialist support.

Adapted from (14).

Consequently, both modern and traditional medicines may be used when a family member falls ill, although this is expensive (15). Prior to the introduction of Western medicine and palliative care, the seriously ill and dying were traditionally cared for by older women who attended to their hygiene, nutrition, psychosocial and spiritual needs (16). Where the social fabric has not been entirely destroyed by the impact of HIV/AIDS, the extended family and traditional support systems continue to provide an effective network of support for the sick. However, traditional family systems in Africa are changing. A rural–urban migration has resulted in overcrowding in urban areas. Accommodation is in short supply and amenities inadequate. Families are fragmented between rural areas and cities, unable to perform traditional caring roles due to geographic distance and unreliable transport facilities. Extended family mechanisms are strained and it is not uncommon for relatives to refuse to take care of sick family members, especially those showing signs of AIDS. Similarly, the extended Indian family is often mentioned as a strength in providing care for the dying, yet this again seems to be changing. More women work, families are becoming more nuclear and there are reports of some patients being abandoned by their families (17).

Palliative care, the family and the phenomenon of home-based care organizations

Perceptions of the English family system as fragmented and unsupportive of the dying led to the modern hospice movement retraining and including families in caring for their own (18); consequently shifting the focus of care to both patient and family. This element of palliative care is capitalized upon in resource-poor countries, where a burgeoning number of home-based care groups aim to bolster the efforts of family carers. Community organizations train mainly female and unemployed volunteers to offer something more than friendship. In its mission, the African Palliative Care Association (APCA) aims to promote and support affordable and culturally appropriate palliative care throughout Africa by providing training and technical assistance to non-Governmental and faith-based organizations (19). Basic training of community home-based care volunteers in Zimbabwe, Kenya, Lesotho, Swaziland and Namibia includes facts about HIV/AIDS, management of AIDS-related conditions, basic home nursing skills, environmental health, nutrition, reproductive health, psychosocial and spiritual support. Pain assessment and management, care of the dying, signs of approaching death and expanded communication skills with adults and children are added to this training by palliative care experts to enhance pain and symptom control and holistic care. A cascade model of training is used to then impart this information from health workers to family carers. There are, however, significant obstacles due to serious limitations in training capacity, support services and medical resources (20). More importantly, there is a dearth of skilled manpower to provide appropriate supervision, modelling and mentoring that could consolidate learning and practice *in situ*. This means that a much diluted version of palliative care, often no more than supportive care, is provided by family carers. Furthermore, the family support system upon which home care is based is increasingly weakened by regular illness and multiple deaths.

Carer profiles

It is well-documented that, even in well-resourced settings, family carers are at risk for physical, social and financial burdens, while caring for a dying relative at home (21). A review by Hughes *et al.* (22) of palliative care needs of rural and urban dwellers in a resource-rich country highlighted increased carer burden in rural settings as a result of lack of information, additional travel costs, family stresses and minimal palliative care support. In resource-poor countries, these problems are severely exacerbated. As in many cultures, but strongly defined in African and Indian tradition, the burden of care of the sick generally falls upon women who usually lack resources and training to provide adequate all-round care (23). In Zimbabwe and many African countries, the HIV prevalence is higher in urban than rural areas. It is common, however, for a seriously ill person to return to the rural home to die rather than remain in the city (15). There are several reasons for this beyond wanting to be with one's family. When people are suspected as being HIV positive they often lose their jobs. Poorly supplied hospitals are unable to cope with the numbers of seriously ill; they discharge patients prematurely, forcing them home to be cared for by family. Yet in the rural home, mainly female carers may also be coping with all the household chores, subsistence farming or other employment, and looking after children, older people and other dependents. A 2004 ethnographic study in Zimbabwe describes how AIDS deaths change village life. 'In Zimbabwean culture it is considered inappropriate to leave a seriously ill person unattended while continuing with the day-to-day productive activities [but] the absence of an adult labour force for productive activities [has] created a gradual depletion of the capacity to produce food resources' (15). Most carers may have HIV themselves and their own health may be deteriorating. The assumption that there is still 'an actively functioning three generation family' (24) in African rural settings is undermined by the AIDS epidemic and it is far more likely that remaining carers are few in number, overburdened, impoverished and often incapacitated by age or inappropriately young for such responsibilities.

Older carers

The demographic impact of the HIV epidemic reflects in the multitudes of grandparents looking after their sick adult children and ultimately reconstructing families for their orphaned grandchildren. Grandchildren from several deceased parents are commonly found in one home, being looked after by a grandmother. As men die earlier on average, and as there are taboos against males providing care for females, older carers are mainly women (23). Much has been written about older people caring for orphans (25) but little research seems to have been done into the effect on the older person of long-term caring for younger sick and ailing relatives. A study by HelpAge Zimbabwe (26) of older rural women looking after people living with AIDS and orphaned children, concluded that they lack the necessary resources, knowledge and support to provide effective care for the sick and are at risk of infection themselves. Instead of being taken care of, as may be traditionally expected, older people are required to rear grandchildren, look after the sick, produce food and maintain full households, often with failing health and strength themselves.

Young carers

There is ample literature about the problems of children affected by AIDS (25–28). Bourdillon categorized children who are involved in caring for sick adults as working children who are not working for an income (29). They carry out substantial caring tasks and responsibilities on a regular basis. Boys sometimes fill this role when there is no female available but girls are expected to leave school more often than boys for this purpose; taking on additional roles usually performed by adults, such as domestic cleaning, cooking, collecting water and firewood, and working in the fields. The epidemic has spawned the label 'orphans and vulnerable children' (OVC) to describe the impact of AIDS illness and deaths on children, including loss of formal and informal education, poor health, increased vulnerability to disease, exposure to opportunistic infection, fewer immunizations, increased poverty, labour demands, stigma, early sexual debut due to financial pressures and sexual abuse. Children and adolescents are heading families already strained by loss of income due to illness and the death of bread winners. They lack social support because of stigma, and are left on their own to manage this overwhelming situation.

Far less attention has been paid to investigating the needs of young carers in resource-poor countries, and this is reflected in the lack of national strategic responses in most countries. Neither the National Health Strategy for Zimbabwe 1997–2007 nor the 2004 National Plan of Action for Orphans and other Vulnerable Children make any mention of child carers (30). While there is a growing appreciation of the material needs of children and young people involved in caring for family members, there is little research to inform us of the emotional impact of this phenomenon. Where research exists, it is usually from the perspective of orphanhood (25). Many community volunteers are under-trained and seldom attend to the emotional and practical needs of young carers. Adult visitors do not routinely speak to children if there is an adult present, other than to greet them. Young people do not know how to ask for help, bound by protocol that demands respect for elders and lacking the assertiveness to approach others outside the family. Training in cooking, cleaning, bathing, lifting and understanding of the illness are needed by young carers but seldom undertaken by community organizations.

Roles of family carers

In the absence of a specialist palliative care team, it is the family carer, some-times with the help of a community volunteer, who provides care and comfort to the dying in resource poor settings. This section will review the roles of family carers in relation to the holism of palliative care (physical, emotional, social and spiritual care).

Physical care

A main challenge to provision of effective palliative care within the home in resource-poor countries is accessing appropriate analgesics for pain manage-ment. Where opioids are unavailable due to policy restrictions, and where there is lack of information about the WHO (World Health Organization) analgesic ladder, pain is usually inadequately controlled by paracetamol, the only available drug for use by home-based care providers and family carers. Unmanageable pain is debilitating for the patient and frightening for the carer. Morphine is largely unavailable in Africa and South-East Asia. Vietnam's restrictive opioid regulations permit a small number of urban-based physi-cians to prescribe limited doses for up to 7 days. For decades, the only morphine available in India was by injection and used for post-operative pain. Only in 1998 were all State Governments encouraged to apply for an improved extended licence and only 10 have done so since. It is estimated that less than 3 per cent of cancer patients in India have adequate pain relief (31).

Overly restrictive laws in Namibia and Lesotho, a weak Government administration in Zimbabwe that does not have the capacity to ensure continuity of supply, and weak health systems, infrastructure and human resource constraints in Zambia and Malawi, all create problems with accessibility and delivery of drugs. Family carers consequently have little chance of overcoming intractable pain in their loved ones. The scenario in Box 5.1 describes a home visit with a home-based care volunteer in Namibia (32) to illustrate what this means for family carers.

Recent advances in anti-retroviral treatments (ARVs), as well as improved treatment of opportunistic infections, have significantly reduced AIDS-related morbidity and mortality. These work best, however, where a comprehensive package of care is available, including nutritional guidance, emotional, social and spiritual support, physiotherapy to restore body function and occupational therapy to optimize productivity. Family carers in remote rural areas in Africa have minimal, if any, access to such services. Despite the significant advantages that ARVs can bring, there are also many difficulties that affect the patient's quality of life and consequently the role of the carer. Numerous pills need to be taken according to a strict regimen that can be disruptive to household and agricultural tasks. A special diet is recommended for people living with HIV, whether or not on ARVs, including frequent intake of green vegetables, fresh fruits, protein-rich foods and plenty of water. As with most

Field notes from Namibia: home visit to a rural-based couple

Both husband and wife are HIV positive. The wife looks in her early 30s and is the primary carer. Husband was markedly wasted and looked very ill with shortness of breath. He had not been started on ARVs but was being prepared for the treatment. He was on cotrimoxazole (a broad spectrum antibiotic) and multivitamins but no pain killers. Even in such a weak state he has to walk a distance of about 4–5 kilometers to the main road for a lift if he can get one (he has no money) to the nearby ART centre to get his supply. Wife says her husband complains of pain in legs, itching skin, swelling limbs and headaches. All she or the volunteer has is wound salve which doesn't help. The volunteer refers the client to nearest health facility where in reality, little more is done anyway. Volunteer admits to feeling badly so does what she can with 'counselling' and spiritual support, i.e. praying together.

medications, the timing of ARVs around meals optimizes the benefits and avoids unpleasant side-effects. Inadequate food supplies make such advice meaningless for many living in conditions where there is no potable water and where agriculture is limited. Family carers also have to cope with ARV side-effects, toxicities and drug interactions, all without specialist palliative care back-up. Helping children adhere to strict treatment regimens is a special challenge, as poor health or economic conditions disrupt the family unit and cause discontinuity of care. Should the primary caregiver no longer be available or be incapacitated, the HIV-positive child is at risk of defaulting on treatments for want of supervision. Where children are main carers for their ailing parents or siblings, they need information they can understand in order to properly support ARV adherence.

Physical care of the sick and dying is demanding of time and physical energy. Young carers have to forgo school to provide full-time care of the patient and the homestead. The debilitating nature of HIV/AIDS intensifies the level of work. Many children complain of aches and pains as they attempt to physically cope with parents bigger than they are. Older women too have to lift the sick and dying in their care. Someone has to be with the patient constantly, intruding on time allocated for productive work. As women provide the bulk of agricultural labour as well as caregiving, they are faced with competing demands to maintain crop production, to care for family members suffering from AIDS and other illnesses, and to protect their own health (6). This is best described in the following words of a grandmother carer (33):

> When my husband died, that is when trouble started. My husband was sick for a long time. We had no time to go to the fields. Immediately after his death, my older son fell sick too. I buried him here again and that did not give me time to engage in productive agricultural activities. For two years in a row, I could not leave the home to work in the fields. I just could not go to the field at all.

Emotional care

Emotional support is generally provided through communication between carer and patient. Personal observations of family carers and community volunteers in India, Lesotho, Swaziland and Namibia indicate that discussing life-threatening illness and imminent death is one of the hardest aspects of caregiving (33). In India, a strong extended family system continues to promote the belief that it is better for the patient not to be told of a life-limiting diagnosis (31). Consequently, open communication about the illness and death is often avoided. Although it is unlikely that anyone in African countries is unaware of HIV/AIDS, there remains a conspiracy of silence driven by stigma and discrimination. Families create narratives around AIDS that attribute the cause of death to cancer, malaria or witchcraft. Looking after family members when it is difficult to talk of the illness prohibits open communication and limits emotional support. As HIV in Africa is usually transmitted sexually, the illness raises questions of morality and infidelity. These are difficult and taboo subjects for older carers to discuss with their children and for young carers to broach with parents and adults. Older carers who are faced with the unenviable task of caring for younger people may simply withdraw, finding it too painful to emotionally engage with people who are dying too young.

An innovative study undertaken by Island Hospice Service in Zimbabwe in 2004–05 (30) involved the collection of data from group-work sessions to examine how family communication impacted on the delivery of care. It concluded that poor communication is an obstacle to effective caregiving and often leads to lasting pain and sadness in young carers. The stigma associated with HIV/AIDS, taboos surrounding discussion of sex and death generally and especially between parents and children, and the subservient role that women and young people play in this society are all major obstacles to communication. Of particular interest in this study was the significant change noted when young carers were given the opportunity to be heard and to learn about the needs of sick adults. Their improved understanding led to greater confidence in communicating meaningfully with a sick relative and there was a corresponding reciprocal response from the adults to their young.

The experiences of young carers are largely unresearched. However Foster and Jiwli (34) suggest that an increasing number of children may be frightened and traumatized by their experiences, and emotional consequences are sometimes manifested months or years later. In conditions of poverty and lack of resources, emotional care may be one of the few supports young carers can offer, yet this can be extremely difficult. Parents usually want to protect their young from distress, yet have to rely on them for physical tasks. Young carers seldom turn to relatives and neighbours for emotional support, preferring to share experiences with others in similar situations, as this reduces feelings of difference. Dramatic mood swings on the part of the patient, depression and elements of dementia associated with AIDS, may leave young and older carers unable to understand what is happening and how best to respond.

Against this backdrop, patients and family carers will inevitably suffer multiple bereavements. Adult and childhood grief is well-documented and there is a growing body of literature explaining risk indicators and helpful practice (35). However, some grief models developed in the West are challenged in situations where consecutive and concurrent deaths associated with AIDS deaths in a resource-poor country lead to overwhelming practical demands in providing for increasing dependents amongst deepening poverty. Moreover, a support network in these conditions is severely diminished by discrimination, overburdened relatives and multiple deaths.

Social care

Most people dying from AIDS in Africa and India rely on care and support from their families, friends and communities, and have limited access to other support systems. Stories abound, however, of rejection of entire families due to fear, ignorance and shame, leading to stigma and discrimination against those living with cancer or HIV/AIDS. Implicit in the transmission modes of HIV are behaviours that carry moral judgements: pre- and extra-marital sex, men having sex with men, incest, sex with children, intravenous drug use and commercial sex. Behaviours previously confined to the privacy of couples and families are publicly exposed. Family carers, moreover, face a serious financial burden in resource-poor countries. Affording food, medications and school fees is impossible for many families beset by chronic illness. Children unable to attend school for financial reasons feel socially isolated and labelled as victims of the pandemic and routinely face discrimination from their peers, relatives, teachers and the community in general. It was observed in the Island Hospice study that children who were unable to continue with education had lowered self-esteem and were markedly sadder than others (30). Teachers and other pupils may be unaware of what is happening at home and lack understanding when homework is not completed or when a child refuses to attend school in order to care for an ailing relative. There may be crises of opportunistic illnesses when a patient needs constant care, followed by periods of good health. This can be especially confusing for young carers who resent parents reclaiming their roles when healthy.

Probably one of the greatest assets of community volunteers, therefore, may be social support. Their role equips them to model caring in the community, over-riding the judgement and withdrawal that others may employ, and demonstrating that everyone in the community gains by helping people with HIV to live as fully as possible within a familiar environment. While training is important, basic support and companionship by family members and friends should not be underestimated, especially in areas where palliative care is undeveloped. By simply showing concern and spending time with the patient, morale can improve and loneliness can be reduced (36).

Spiritual care

Despite palliative care being committed to holistic care, spiritual care is generally overshadowed by the physical, emotional and social needs of patients and families, even in the resource-rich world. There may be several reasons for this, including confusion about reconciling religion and spirituality, where to place the carer's own personal beliefs, and how to explore meaning of life and death issues with patients. Murray *et al.* found in their study of rural carers in Kenya that emotional and spiritual support is usually left to the family and seldom explored in any depth by health workers (37). It concluded that the spiritual needs of patients were met by family carers rather than health workers, but the question remains whether these are explored at all or simply *avoided* and assumptions made that prayer and encouraging words of comfort are adequate.

Although the modern palliative care movement tries to maintain a secular approach, a predominantly Christian framework persists. In sub-Saharan Africa this resonates with strongly Christian communities that are characterized by religious homogeneity. Faith-based organizations have played a significant role in responding to the HIV epidemic by establishing many home-based care organizations. Lesotho is an example where church-affiliated groups play a major role in the structure and function of the public health system. Christian Mission Hospitals have been operating in Lesotho since 1863. The Christian Health Association of Lesotho (CHAL) owns 8 of the 18 hospitals and 73 of the 167 health centres in the country (38). It works closely with the Ministry of Health and leads a growing number of faith-based AIDS organizations in the country. When training of volunteers has a strong religious influence from faith-based organizations, volunteers and family carers may run the risk of making assumptions about beliefs rather than enquiring about the impact of the illness on spirituality. In Box 5.2, field notes on a home visit in Namibia illustrate this tendency (33).

Impact of roles

Much of the stress experienced by carers of the terminally ill is in the nature of the work itself. This is compounded by the regularity and complexity of AIDS-related deaths in ill-equipped environments, often leading to burn-out. Family carers in resource-poor countries walk a lonely and frightening road with little or no specialist palliative care support when dealing with a stigmatizing illness that predominantly kills young people. It is vital that these carers take time to care for their own needs but this is difficult because of the workload brought on by HIV.

A multitude of implications for family carers arise from caring for the dying at home in these situations. A survey in Zimbabwe found that agricultural output declined by nearly 50 per cent among households affected by HIV/AIDS (6). In both urban and rural areas women and girls sacrifice the

Home visit to a 44-year-old HIV-positive woman who is on anti-retrovirals

She looks after several nephews and nieces whose parents have died or who are working in distant towns. She has not told the children she is ill, and neither has the carer helped her to do this. When I discussed later with the carer the need for the children to be informed what is happening and involved with the patients care, the carer admitted that dealing with emotional issues is too hard to do.

I asked the volunteer to explore whether this illness has changed the client's beliefs. The client responded that she was accepting and repentant. This response was not followed up in any way by the carer. The silence seemed to reinforce the moral judgement that the client has absorbed from church/community/family. I witnessed no exploration whatsoever of a spiritual nature. Emotional support and spiritual care were dealt with by means of talking, preaching and advising rather than asking and listening. Spiritual support especially seems to be based on assumptions especially if the client is of the same faith, rather than asking questions about the meaning of life and death.

opportunity to generate income or improve education by being unpaid carers. Many adolescents are faced with ill or dying parents, bereavement, difficulty in continuing their education, change of financial and social status, poverty and all the complexities of becoming sexually active and making and maintaining peer relationships (23). Rural grandmother households rely heavily on younger family labour to produce food, and when this is diminished by illness and death, food supplies are affected and impoverishment sets in, exacerbated by expensive medications and funeral costs. Lack of transport between rural and urban homes means respite to primary carers cannot be offered. All these factors contribute to a change in the traditional way of caring for the sick. Roles and responsibilities become confused, blurring gender relations and age-appropriate behaviours. A synthesis of obstacles to provision of good palliative care in these settings is provided in Table 5.2.

Efficacy of interventions to support family-based palliative care

The move towards greater provision of ARVs as a treatment for HIV/AIDS has unfortunately resulted in the lower prioritization of care, including

Table 5.2 Barriers to good palliative family care in resource poor countries

Care	Roles of family carer	Barriers to implementation
Physical	Lifting	Age-related weakness (young and old)
	Feeding	Restricted food options
	Bathing and hygiene	Mobility/water availability
	Management of pain, illness and infections	No opioids/lack of medications and supplies
Emotional	Discussion of illness with patient	Secrecy due to fear of stigma
	Disclosure of illness to all family members	Fear of stigma
	Share worries and concerns	Poverty/practical needs take precedence over emotional needs
	Griefwork with all family members	Unsure how to talk of the deceased
Social	Help maintain: normal relationships	Rejection and social isolation
	Ensure children attend school	Poverty
	Engage network of helpers	Association with HIV leads to stigma
Spiritual	Explore impact of illness on faith/meaning of life and death	Assume religious homogeneity. Own beliefs take precedence
	Examine fears of dying	Own fears unexamined: too threatening

palliative care. The most recent WHO guidelines on palliative care, symptom management and end-of-life care that has implications for resource-poor countries is included in the Integrated Management of Adult Infections (IMAI) training package, which was developed in 2001–02 (39). Central to this is a public health approach that places home-based care at the cornerstone of essential HIV/AIDS integrated services (40). This is viewed as a cost-effective response to the crisis (41). It places family carers firmly at the centre of care, yet adequate training, support and supplies, including ARVs are woefully neglected.

The Global Fund also strengthens community-based support for the chronically ill. Latest figures indicate 1.2 million orphans receive home-based care and 23 million receive community outreach services as a result of Global Fund activities (42), although no data specifically relate to palliative care. Various other donors provide funding for home-based care organizations that claim to deliver palliative care services but which fall short of the WHO definition (39).

The USAID managed Presidents Emergency Plan for AIDS Relief (PEPFAR) uses a broadened definition of palliative care. Prevention and treatment of TB, gender issues, human capacity development, policy development and supply chain management are also funded as essential components of palliative care (43). In 2006, the number of people who received palliative care/basic healthcare support under this definition totalled 2.4 million, the majority being cared for in their homes by family carers.

Communities with networks of health and church volunteers have the capacity to care for patients at home but lack resources and expertise. Home healthcare is one model that can be implemented in resource-poor settings, as described in this chapter, but interventions beyond home-based care are needed. Some components of caring skills are woven into projects aimed at enhancing life skills for young carers but more needs to be done. The 'Young People We Care' programme (44) is designed to encourage groups of young people to support peers, younger children and adults living in households affected by HIV/AIDS. Tips for caring in the home and some helpful guidelines for preparing for death are included. Work is also currently in progress in Zimbabwe on a child-friendly ARV literacy tool kit to help children understand issues surrounding ARVs in the home.

Clinical priorities and future research

The urgency to manage large numbers of dying people in resource-poor countries has understandably driven the response towards empowering families to care for their own with the help of trained community volunteers. The cascade training approach needs to be evaluated for dilution of information and skills along its journey to educating family carers in palliative care skills.

The voices of older people and young carers need to be heard to establish what caring for the dying in resource-poor countries is really like, to guide donors and policy makers in implementing effective palliative care in home settings. Great strides have been made in materially supporting orphans and grandmother-headed households, but a fresh emphasis on the emotional and spiritual impact of family caring is required.

Most palliative care research has focused on deaths at home for cancer patients. The unpredictable nature of HIV/AIDS and the social implications of this illness may create different issues. The effects on the older person of caring for their dying young and the emotional impact on young carers of caring for parents and other relatives are currently unknown. This information could guide interventions that are culturally and psychosocially appropriate.

In resource-poor countries with high death rates it is tempting to focus on the practical and quantifiable needs of affected families. Multiple deaths within families mean that, even during the illness trajectory, a patient is likely to be bereaved several times and may have suffered previous losses of loved ones. If care is to be truly holistic, priority needs to be paid to ensuring a supportive environment for grieving patients and family carers. Innovative programmes for community volunteers and families to raise awareness of bereavement issues are urgently needed to ensure this aspect of family caring is not ignored.

Children continue to be invisible and under-acknowledged despite their increased roles and responsibilities in caring for ill relatives. A focus on children's needs as carers and not only as AIDS orphans is required. Children in the Island Hospice study reported more criticism than help was received from neighbours and relatives. Child carers, simply because they are children, are generally not consulted in decisions concerning treatment or care plans. A child's understanding of and involvement in the illness and dying process affects grief outcomes, yet seldom do family or community volunteers talk to children about death and sadness. These topics are harder to raise than practical issues but research confirms that young carers want and need to talk about these issues, even though they are painful (30).

In a rare study that asks patients and carers about the problems of home care, patients in Kenya (37) were concerned they were becoming a physical and financial burden to their family. Clinical priorities can be drawn from the concerns of the carers who identified their greatest difficulties as lack of drugs in the home, inadequate medical knowledge and fear of not knowing what to do if the patient deteriorated. Resource-poor countries have a variety of barriers to accessing opioids that continue to prevent effective home-based palliative care. A positive exception is Uganda, where the Ministry of Health signed a ground-breaking statutory instrument in 2004 authorizing palliative care nurses and clinical officers to prescribe morphine. This significantly increases accessibility to rural patients.

Life-saving medication for people living with HIV is meaningless when food, needed to be taken in conjunction with it, is unavailable. Similarly, when there is no transport to facilitate ARV re-supplies or visits by health workers to assess and manage care, the system of palliative home-based care collapses. These systems need to be integrated into home-based care programmes, drawing also on the resilience of rural communities that often develop their own ways of managing these situations.

Knowledge of illness and symptom management can be increased by integrating home-based care training into mainstream health systems.

Uganda and South Africa have successfully achieved this. Effective communication with Government, established national palliative care associations, access to pain-relieving medications, curricula for training health professionals and a growing body of trained home-based care volunteers, are some of the elements that contribute towards increased palliative care delivery in these countries. Despite attempts to replicate this model elsewhere, serious problems remain in cascading the skills and resources to remote villages. Quality of care is likely to improve significantly with good training in counselling and nursing. This is especially true for men who do not traditionally perform caring roles. Although family carers are predominantly female, there is a growing advocacy for male involvement, which could expand the numbers of carers and spread responsibility.

Conclusion

The experiences of family carers in resource-poor countries—often puzzling, heart-rending and confusing—need to be woven into a coherent story that can help construct positive accounts of how families cope with illness and dying in harsh conditions. There are many positive aspects to family care in resource-poor settings that can be strengthened, if knowledge and support are available. Increasing the skills of other carers in the community in a meaningful and sustainable manner is one approach. Exploring alternative channels to provide good palliative care in the home, no matter how resource poor, is mandatory.

Key learning points

- HIV/AIDS drives palliative care development in resource-poor countries.
- Home-based care is the main setting for delivery of palliative care with support provided by community volunteers.
- Erratic drug supplies, low income, food insecurity, transport shortages and diminished human resources increase the burden of care on families.
- Adequate training and sustained practical and emotional support for family carers is mandatory for effective palliative care in the home.
- Research should focus on efficacy of training models to ensure that family carers have all they need to provide home-based palliative care.

Recommended reading and resources

Brakarsh J, Le Breton J, O'Gorman M and Stally A (ed.) (2004). *The Journey of Life*. Bulawayo: Regional Psychosocial Support Initiative (REPSSI).

Clark D and Wright M (2006). *Hospice and Palliative Care in Africa*. Oxford: Oxford University Press.

Jackson H. (2002). *AIDS Africa*. Harare: SAfAIDS.

Mallman S-A (2003). *Building Resilience in Children Affected by HIV/AIDS*. Windhoek: Catholic AIDS Action/Maskew Miller LongmanReferences.

Matshalaga N (2004). *Grandmothers and Orphan Care in Zimbabwe*. Harare: SAfAIDS.

Sherman J and Davies M (2005). *Young People We Care!* (2nd edn). Harare: JSI UK.

Smith T (Salvation Army Masiye Camp) (2004). *A Child Headed Household Guide*. Bulaway: Regional Psychosocial Support Initiative (REPSSI).

Winiarski M (2004) *Community-Based Counselling for People Affected by HIV and AIDS*. Windhoek: Catholic AIDS Action/Longman.

References

1. Wright M (2003). *Models of Hospice and Palliative Care in Resource-Poor Countries: Issues and Opportunities*. London: Hospice Information.

2. http://en.wikipedia.org/wiki/Resource poor countries (accessed April 2007).

3. The HDI is a summary composite index that measures a country's average achievements in three basic aspects of human development: longevity, knowledge and a decent standard of living. Longevity is measured by life-expectancy at birth: knowledge is measured by a combination of the adult literacy rate and the combined primary, secondary, and tertiary gross enrolment ratio: and standard of living by GDP per capita.

4. Global Health Council Newsletter (2007), Email newsletter, conference@globalhealth.org. (accessed 14 May 2007).

5. http://www.unaids.org/en/Regions_Countries/Countries/zimbabwe (accessed April 2007)

6. Ministry of Health and Child Welfare, National AIDS Council (2004). The HIV and AIDS Epidemic in Zimbabwe (booklet): 14.

7. Clark D and Wright M (2006). *Hospice and Palliative Care in Africa*. Oxford: Oxford University Press, 5.

8. Total health expenditure per capita is the per capita amount of the sum of Public Health Expenditure (PHE) and Private Expenditure on Health (PvtHE). The international dollar is a common currency unit that takes into account differences in the relative purchasing power of various currencies. Figures expressed in international dollars are calculated using purchasing power parities (PPP), which are rates of currency conversion constructed to account for differences in price level between countries.

9. Chaturvedi P (2003). Letter. *British Medical Journal* **326**: 1146.

10. Burn G (1997) From paper to practice: quality of life in a developing country. In: Surbane A and Zwitter M (ed.). *Communication with the Cancer Patient. Information and Truth*. New York: The New York Academy of Sciences.

11. Gwyther L, Merriman A, Mpanga Sebuyira L and Schietinger H (2006). *A Clinical Guide to Supportive and Palliative Care for HIV/AIDS in Sub-Saharan Africa*. African Palliative Care Association. Kampala: CD version produced in collaboration with National Hospice and Palliative Care Association (USA) and Foundation for Hospices in Sun-Saharan Africa (USA).

12. Hunt J (2003). From Micro to Macro. A comparative analysis of views on how India and Zimbabwe Use the British Hospice Model. Unpublished MA dissertation. University of Reading.

13. Shvartzman P and Singer Y (1998). Community education in palliative medicine. *Journal of Palliative Care* **14** (3): 75–78.

14. Adapted from Vachon M (1998). Psychosocial needs of patients and families. *Journal of Palliative Care* **14 (3)**: 49–56.

15. Matshalaga N (2004). *Grandmothers and Orphan Care in Zimbabwe*. Harare: SAfAIDS.

16. Munodawafa A (2001) Zimbabwe. In: Ferrell B and Coyle N (ed.). *Textbook of Palliative Nursing*. New York: Oxford University Press, Inc., 718–726.

17. Burn G (1997) Palliative care in India. In: Clark D, Hockley J and Ahmedzai S (ed.). *New Themes in Palliative Care*. Buckingham: Open University Press.

18. Clark D and Seymour J (1999). *Reflections on Palliative Care*. Buckingham: Open University Press.

19. Powell R and Downing J (ed.) (2007). *Mentoring for Success*. Kampala: African Palliative Care Association, 6

20. Hunt J (2004). Questions for hospice in resource poor settings. *Progressin Palliative Care* **12**(4): 4.

21. Stajduhar K and Davies B (1998). Death at home: challenges for families and directions for the future. *Journal of Palliative Care* **14** (3): 8-14

22. Hughes P, Ingleton C, Noble B and Clark D (2004) Providing cancer and palliative carein rural areas: a review of patient and carer needs. *Journal of Palliative Care* **20**: 44–49.

23. Farrell C (2005) Bearing witness to stories of substitute mothers to girls orphaned by AIDS in Zimbabwe. Unpublished PhD. University of East London in conjunction with the Tavistock Clinic.

24. Stjernsward J and Pampallona S (1999). Palliative medicine—a global perspective.In: Doyle D, Hanks G and MacDonald N (ed.). *Oxford Textbook of Palliative Medicine* (2nd edn). Oxford: Oxford University Press, 1232.

25. Grainger C, Webb D and Elliott L (2001). *Children affected by HIV/AIDS: Rights and Responses in the Resource-poor World*. Working paper 23. London: Save the Children.

26. Farrell C (2005). Bearing witness to stories of substitute mothers to girls orphaned by AIDS in Zimbabwe. Thesis submitted as fulfillment of Doctorate of systematic therapy, the University of East London in conjunction with the Tavistock Clinic (unpublished).

27. SAfAIDS News (2004). Addressing the needs of OVCs. SAfAIDS News **10**(3): 15–16.

28. Southern Africa HIV/AIDS Action (2004). Malawi: Orphan Crisis a Challenge to Communities **62**: 8. Newsletter

29. Bourdillon M (2000). *Earning a Life: Working Children in Zimbabwe*. Harare: Weaver Press.

30. Martin R (2006). Children's perspectives: roles, responsibilities and burdens in home based care in Zimbabwe. *Journal of Social Development in Africa* **21**(1): 106–129.

31. http://www.eolc-observatory.net/global_analysis/india_current_services (accessed on April 2007).

32. Hunt J (2007). Field notes for African Palliative Care Association assessment in Lesotho. Unpublished.

33. Hunt J (2006/7) Field notes for African Palliative Care Association assessment in Namibia. Unpublished.

34. Foster DG and Jiwli L (2001). Psycho-social Support of Children Affected by AIDS: an evaluation and review of Masiye Camp, Bulawayo, Zimbabwe (unpublished). Report.

35. Dryregrov A (1991) *Grief in Children*. London: Jessica Kingsley Publishers Ltd.

36. Jackson H (2002). *AIDS Africa*. Harare: SAfAIDS.

37. Murray S, Grant E, Grant A and Kendall M (2003) Dying from cancer in resource rich and resource poor countries: lessons from two qualitative interview studies of patients and their carers. *British Medical Journal*: **326**: 368–371.

38. Capacity Project (2006). Scope of Work for Inter-church Medical Assistance (IMA) project consultancy.

39. Collins K., Dickinson C., Goh C., Harding R. Hunt J., Krakauer E., Morris C., Pahl N. (2007). *Review of Global Policy Architecture and Country Level Practice on HIV/AIDS and Palliative Care*. London: DFID Health Resource Centre.

40. Collins K., Dickinson C., Goh C., Harding R. Hunt J., Krakauer E., Morris C., Pahl N. (2007). *Review of Global Policy Architecture and Country Level Practice on HIV/AIDS and Palliative Care*. London: DFID Health Resource Centre.

41. Collins K., Dickinson C., Goh C., Harding R. Hunt J., Krakauer E., Morris C., Pahl N. (2007). *Review of Global Policy Architecture and Country Level Practice on HIV/AIDS and Palliative Care*. London: DFID Health Resource Centre.

42. Collins K., Dickinson C., Goh C., Harding R. Hunt J., Krakauer E., Morris C., Pahl N. (2007). *Review of Global Policy Architecture and Country Level Practice on HIV/AIDS and Palliative Care*. London: DFID Health Resource Centre.

43. Office of the United States Global AIDS Coordinator (2006). HIV/AIDS Palliative Care Guidance for the US Government in Country Staff and Implementing Partners.

44. Sherman J and Davies M (2005). *Young People We Care!* (2nd edn). Harare: JSI UK.

Chapter 6

Family carers: ethical and legal issues

Michael Ashby and Danuta Mendelson

Introduction

Given the fundamental emotional, social, spiritual and religious dimensions to the biological process of death and dying, it is perhaps not surprising that end-of-life issues are often the subject of ethical deliberation, and that the law will become involved at times. Disagreements may arise concerning sensitive personal issues such as beliefs and values, or what constitutes a person's best interests, and who should determine and communicate these if a person is unable to do so themselves. These differences may arise within families themselves, between families and health service personnel, and between members of the healthcare services involved.

The emphasis in ethics, law and professional conduct is on respect for the autonomy of the patient, and this has primacy in all aspects of clinical and theoretical work, and there would be little dissention on this point. However, a rigid interpretation of what ethics and law have to say about autonomy would leave little or no place for the family. As the growing field of palliative care has always recognized, few people live or die in a social vacuum, and the family and social context must be recognized and worked with (1, 2). The extent to which this is done, and the balance between the needs and wishes of patients, and those of their families and communities, is often a delicate one, where sensitive case work and pragmatism will be argued to be more useful than rigid ethical or legalistic interpretation. The family may be considered as having a number of roles worthy of ethical consideration in palliative care: they may be seen as primary or principal carers, as subjects of care themselves, as decision-makers and, hopefully rarely, as litigants.

Ethics and law tend to be invoked in clinical work when something has been thought to have gone wrong, or where there is difference in approach or perception, as reflected in the expression ethical 'dilemma'. The challenge is to so integrate ethical awareness into practice that ethical and/or legal scrutiny is rarely, if ever, needed. It will, therefore, hopefully become clear that ethics in practice is a process, consisting most importantly of clear, honest, compassionate and realistic communication from (and amongst) the health team, rather than knowledge of the subject of ethics *per se*.

It is a major challenge to see family work as being more than just dealing with negative situations and discord, particularly where ethics is invoked. One way to do this at a practical social policy level is to adopt the principles articulated by Allan Kellehear in his concept of health-promoting palliative care (3, 4). Central to this approach, is to encourage interpersonal reorientation towards a 'natural' death and combating death-denying health policy and attitudes. A wider application of these principles, which aim to open up death and dying within the broader community, would do a lot to prepare families to deal with death in their midst, and allow them to take back responsibility, and some control, from the professional arena.

There has been an important theoretical and empirical move, within nursing, to better understand the role of family caregiving and how to support it. Nolan's typology of care in 1995 set an agenda for this area of research, and suggested that older conceptual approaches were limited, and some nursing interventions may even have been obstructive (5). There is now high-level evidence of the value, for instance, of caregiver education that targets a wide range of empirically derived carer needs, with a strong focus on psychological and emotional need, coupled with clear practical assistance, such as adequate provision for respite care (6).

There has also been some limited work in bioethics to move away from the sole focus on the individual and encompass the family as well, and to view the family as more than just a potential problem. Kuczewski has challenged the bioethical tendency to view families as conflicting interests, which result, in his view, from an impoverished understanding of informed consent (7).

In order to discuss the key issues encountered in practice, it will be necessary first to discuss ethics in relation to family caregiving in palliative care in general, to look at the various ethical approaches on offer and to describe ways to proceed— the ethical 'process'. The most common issues for family carers in palliative care practice that may be framed as 'ethical' will be considered under the headings of 'death talk' and truth-telling, capacity and competence, causing death, litigation, cardio-pulmonary resuscitation and requests for assistance to die.

Ethics and family caregiving in palliative care

Palliative care services everywhere tend to pride themselves on a three-part all-embracing ideological approach: caring *for* the whole person, *and* their family, *with* a multidisciplinary team. Indeed so prominent is the focus on the family care-giving component that it is often stated that 'the family is the unit of care'. With such a broad claim, there is potential for a significant rhetoric-reality gap, between the so-called 'philosophy' or ethos of care, and putting it into operation.

Some caution is required with the stance of the family as the 'unit' of care, as pointed out by Randall and Downie (8). Firstly, the primary ethical and legal duty is owed to the patient, and it is the patient, if competent, who determines whether anyone else, and if so, who, is involved and consulted about what happens. Secondly, with such an all-embracing multidisciplinary model of care, it may be found that the patient wishes to 'cherry-pick' components of a given service, and some carers, family, and close friends may not wish to be included as recipients of care themselves at all. If family and friends are reluctant to receive care or counselling from the palliative care team, then it is important that these secondary duties are offered with care, and initiated with explicit consent. This is particularly relevant to grief and bereavement work. It is important to recognize the enormous public mental health impact of grief, and the healing possibilities of working these through with models such as David Kissane's family-focused therapeutic approach (9). Community capacity-building is also important here too, as grief should not be over-professionalized, and there are logistical limits to such professional inputs anyway.

It is clear that there is an inherent tension between an inclusive and an holistic view of any form of healthcare and the intense contemporary preoccupation with the wants, needs, privacy and entitlements of the individual. If this is coupled with the social and demographic trends underway in most Western societies, then a much more complex and challenging picture emerges.

It is important to firmly emphasize the centrality of the patient, whilst acknowledging that death and the process of dying are socially constructed events, and that the person's memory lives on in the community and in the lives of the bereaved (10). Any social and family work will inevitably be based on a balance between individual patient and family, and consent of all parties: patient and family is required to engage in this manner. It should be clear that the patient's interests have primacy in ethics and law, but no more in one's dying than at any other time of life does one get all one's needs and wishes met. Indeed it is incumbent on the team to be mindful of the needs of carers too. The main work centres on negotiation; the aim is to reach the best compromise plan that accommodates all parties to some extent. There is no place here for ideological purity, where theoretical principles trump compassionate pragmatism.

Health workers often seem to resort to ethics in much the same way as they do to any other subject or area of expertise, namely as a body of knowledge or set of techniques that can be mobilized to 'solve' what are seen to be difficult or complex situations. Ethical analysis of a situation or case is a dynamic process, and must be distinguished from reference to set rules for conduct, such as might be found in professional codes of conduct. The academic subjects of medical ethics or bioethics are, of course, full of robust disagreement, and offer diverse techniques of determining what is right and wrong, and differing views about the course of action to be followed in any given situation.

The main division in ethics is between the deontological approach, where it is adherence to rules and duties (often, but not exclusively, derived from religious traditions) that determines the rightness or wrongness of a course of action, and the consequentialist approach, where the outcome determines this. Virtue ethics places the emphasis on the good character of the practitioner, and sees good ethical conduct arising from, and being intrinsic to, virtuous professional practice. The principles-approach of Beauchamp and Childress (11), where actions are matched against, and balanced between, the principles of autonomy, beneficence, non-maleficence and justice has found wide popularity. While all having their relative merits, and some awareness of these major ethical techniques is important, it is not necessary for practitioners to engage with the dialogue between these different approaches unless they wish to, as this is more properly the province of academic ethics and bioethics.

Clinical work is self-evidently case-based. This is not to say that the rightness or wrongness of a course of action is always determined by the case (a 'casuistic' approach), but rather that casework is what happens, regardless of the favoured ethical theory in question. The ethical process in clinical practice starts with the basics of communication (12, 13). Healthcare workers, especially doctors and nurses, have the pivotal role of explaining the medical facts to the patient and, where appropriate, to those whom the patient identifies in their immediate social context as carers and supports, and to other members of the health team. No ethical deliberation of any quality or meaning can take place without a clear exposition of the facts of the patient's case.

It is always important to identify the true nature of the difficulty or complexity, as this may be obscured by strong feelings associated with entrenched views and positions. Ethical deliberation can clarify language and arguments. It is very helpful to distinguish between the facts of a situation and any values or beliefs at play. It is then possible to obtain agreement as to the facts, and then separately address conflicts between values and beliefs, and hopefully work these through. Often, fairly straightforward ethical analysis can demonstrate flaws in arguments, such as contradictions and false inferences.

It will often also emerge that there is no demonstrable ethical 'dilemma' as such, and that the concerns resulted from the framing of the problem, and false perceptions about what law and ethics have to say, rather than any true conflict of ethical principle or legal requirement. Actions based on professional judgment relating to invasive treatment (including intake of medication) that provides overall clinical benefit, tend to be legal, if they respect the wishes of a competent patient. However, there will be situations where the patient either refuses all proposed treatments or insists on a treatment that the medical team considers inappropriate. If it is clear that the patient's refusal of treatment is a result of family pressure, it may be prudent to ask, where the jurisdiction permits it, a guardianship tribunal or court to determine the issue in the patient's best interests. Medical teams need to take into account, but are not under a duty to comply with, patient or family requests for treatments that are not clinically indicated.

Where, despite the best efforts of the team, conflict with the patient or family cannot be resolved by negotiation, and the issues at stake are of real importance to the patient's comfort and welfare, legal advice may need to be obtained before any action is taken. Medico-legal officers or corporate legal advisers are now available in most major healthcare organizations. Social workers are also an important resource in these matters.

In relation to incompetent patients, unless there are compelling medical or ethical considerations to the contrary (for example, a request for treatment that, in the clinical team's judgment, is inappropriate), where known and documented, the wishes of such persons should be followed. In situations where the patient's wishes are not known and documented, treatment decisions should be guided by the patient's best interests.

Health workers involved in palliative care are primarily subject to the law and their codes of professional conduct. In most respects, palliative care is subject to the same generic ethical standards that apply to care at any other point of the life cycle; for example: confidentiality; honest and clear communication; accurate record-keeping; statutory (legally required) duties (including those that relate to prescription of opioid medications in a given jurisdiction); standards of competence; integrity and professional etiquette. Palliative care practice itself is not usually generically subject to any special or separate ethical or legal standards, although there may be local laws or guidelines of relevance, such as those that provide for advance care-planning, living wills and appointment of agents (see below).

In pluralist liberal democratic societies, reference to a single rigid core set of beliefs and ethical principles is not possible. While religious and cultural diversity makes such a monochrome approach unwise and inappropriate, two important unifying forces are also at work. Firstly, despite fundamental differences in belief, it is usually possible to agree on many core common values and attributes of good and compassionate care at the end of life. Very few people disagree, for instance, with relief of suffering and maintenance of dignity. Secondly, in clinical work, as in law, clear decisions are required that, in a given situation, will result in only one course of action being pursued. A generic approach to the promotion of values that results in a clear course of action for patients and their families, using family meetings and based on conflict-resolution principles, is set out below.

Family meetings and dealing with difference: conflict-resolution approaches

It is often helpful to use generic modern conflict-resolution approaches when dealing with differences of opinion, particularly between patients and families, and families and palliative care practitioners. This consists of a series of steps as set out by Wertheim *et al.* in a 1992 book, that follow the principles of conflict resolution as an approach to dealing with difference and disagreement in a wide range of contexts (14). The core process is to identify and abandon positions, focusing instead on common interests. It should usually be possible to place the interests of the patient at the centre of these deliberations but in the brain-storming of solutions, the needs and wishes of the family may need to be accommodated as well.

A common way of communicating in palliative care practice, especially where there are contentious issues, is to call a family meeting. These can be effective, healing and a source of clarification and decision-making, and where there is difference, the conflict-resolution approach is to be commended. An approach to running family meetings is set out in Box 6.1.

Box 6.1 Conduct of family meetings

Preparation

- Choose a quiet venue free from interruptions.
- Nominate a chairperson prior to the meeting.
- Agree to a time limit.
- Brief staff participants and interpreter (if needed) prior to the family arriving.
- Arrange where the interpreter sits in relation to the patient and family.

Box 6.1 Conduct of family meetings *(continued)*

Greeting and introductions

- ◆ Introduce staff members.
- ◆ Ask family members to introduce themselves.
- ◆ Set out the agenda and a rough time limit.

Content

- ◆ Provide an update on the patient's current medical condition.
- ◆ Explore the prognosis.
- ◆ Allow each family member dedicated time to express his or her concerns.
- ◆ Brainstorm future care options.
- ◆ Deal with any specific issues. Meeting may have one specific purpose, which must not get lost in the proceedings, e.g. death at home, children, open discussion of dying.

Closure

- ◆ Thank carers for their attendance.
- ◆ Advise them that they can raise other concerns, which they have forgotten, with team members at a later date.
- ◆ Debrief and reflect, with other team members and the interpreter, on how the meeting went.
- ◆ Confirm the tasks of each team member.
- ◆ Nominate a case manager if the case is complex.
- ◆ Ensure that the patient and family have space and privacy, and access to immediate staff support if they want it.

Reproduced with permission from: Palliative Care Expert Group (2005). Components that may be included in a family meeting. In: *Therapeutic Guidelines: Palliative Care*, Version 2. Melbourne: Therapeutic Guidelines Limited, 48

Until recently, family meetings have received little research attention, and have not enjoyed a high priority within hospitals. They may, therefore, be initiated and run by relatively junior staff, with scant support and a lack of clarity of purpose and procedure. It is important for practitioners who convene and run them to be clear about why the meeting is proposed, what its goals are and who should be there. Inadequate planning and key absences, or wrong inclusions, can spell disaster. The conduct of the meeting requires skill and experience.

If a patient is competent, then their permission for a meeting to take place is required. They should also be asked for permission, specifically, for their health and, just as importantly, personal information to be discussed. Patients need to have a choice about whether or not they attend themselves, but many patients will be too sick or tired to participate, and very commonly they will be also be incompetent to do so. The role of the family may vary in different cultural settings. It is especially important to find out who the patient wishes to be their spokesperson, and to ensure that senior family members are shown appropriate respect in the communication process.

Where patients are not competent and cannot provide permission for the disclosure of their clinical records, the professional who is convening the family conference will need to be clear about relevant privacy principles and rules that govern the handling of health records in such circumstances. A clinical case conference may be needed prior to meeting the family to clarify the clinical situation and to resolve any differences of opinion between teams or practitioners. This should not be done in front of the family; a united front and clear message is essential, even if that means acknowledging that a difference of opinion exists among the health service personnel.

'Death talk' and truth telling

It is now well-established in ethics and law that truth telling is the accepted standard in communication between health workers and both patients and families, although there are cultural variations in this. Guidelines that incorporate good evidence of what works in this sensitive area of professional practice are now available (12, 13). The balance between veracity and maintenance of hope is a delicate one, which must ultimately rest with each practitioner and be modified for each particular situation (15). In the spirit of health-promoting palliative care, this is termed 'death talk', as a frank reminder of the matter in hand. Palliative care workers have experience and skills to help families who may be dealing with their first death in a generation. Rather than being prescriptive, they can try to empathize and tell family members how, more often than not, dealing frankly with reality and impending mortality can bring peace and clarity. At the very least, palliative care workers can be the repository of stories that back up veracity and reality against false hope that obstructs care and adaptation of patient and family to the process of dying.

It is, however, not uncommon for a family meeting to have to address situations in which family members express the wish that the patient not be told their diagnosis and/or prognosis. In common law countries, while in the exercise of their professional skill and judgment doctors are under a comprehensive duty to inform patients about their condition and appropriate treatment choices (including attendant risks), this duty is subject to the therapeutic privilege. Under the therapeutic privilege, doctors do not need to disclose all relevant information, if in their professional judgment there is a danger that such disclosure would prove damaging to a 'nervous, disturbed or volatile' patient (*Sidaway v Governors of Bethlem Royal Hospital*; *Rogers v Whittaker*).

Thus, whilst there are ethical and legal requirements for patients to be told the truth, some sensitive negotiation may be necessary if the family objects. The matter is straightforward where patients express a clear wish to be appraised of their situation, but this may not occur, and there may also be a language barrier. Some tips to assist in these discussions are set out in Box 6.2.

Statements to families about the patient's right to know, whilst in principle justified, will often only increase family suspicion and antagonism. A gradual process of negotiation will usually unlock the situation, and sometimes agreement to disagree is the best avenue. This is particularly advisable where the patient does not show any sign of wishing to know more and may be complicit with the family's view. Challenging of this dynamic by the palliative care team may be counter-productive. The degree to which this is challenged will also depend on the issues at stake: if it is mere knowledge of one's specific medical condition and fate that is being resisted, this is understandable and should be respected. However, it is harder to back away from confronting realities when consent is required for medical or surgical treatment from a competent patient who is not 'nervous, disturbed or 'volatile', and who indicates a wish to know; for the legal duty to inform may prevail over the exception provided by the therapeutic privilege. The acknowledgment that the patient is dying is also vital in cases where the failure to do so will leave major problems for the individual or the family; for example, executing a will or the appointing of an agent with medical powers of attorney or a guardian, while the patient is still competent.

Capacity and competence

Cognitive impairment of varying degrees of severity is very common in dying patients, and is often resistant to therapeutic endeavours. Patients' capacity to express their wishes may vary depending on the issue at hand, but will diminish

Box 6.2 Some tips to assist in working with family members who do not wish to see frank discussion about poor prognosis with a patient

◆ Enquire about the basis for the wish for non-disclosure.

◆ Acknowledge concerns.

◆ Demonstrate the benefits of honest and open communication by illustrations from previous experience, e.g. how common it is for people to know that they are dying; peacefulness that can ensue from open acknowledgment of impending death.

◆ Identify social, cultural and ethnic differences in approach to these issues.

◆ Offer to ask open questions in the presence of family members (and interpreter when appropriate), and be prepared to back off if the patient does not wish to know any more.

◆ Advise the family that direct questions from the patient should be answered truthfully if and when they arise, but that these issues will not be raised if there is no request from the patient.

Reproduced with permission from: Palliative Care Expert Group (2005). Ethics of disclosure. n: *Therapeutic Guidelines: Palliative Care*, Version 2. Melbourne: Therapeutic Guidelines Limited, 24–25

and may disappear as death approaches. Capacity refers to the medically assessable ability to receive and process information, and make decisions. Competence is a legal determination of whether a person can manage their own affairs, including appointing agents or guardians and making a will, or signing any legal documents (16). The law assumes competence, and requires rigorous assessment before a person may be deemed incompetent. Recent work suggests that a person may have capacity for some things and not others; in other words that it is variable with the task required, and over time (17).

There is increasing international interest in advance care-planning due to the challenges of decision-making at the end of life for incompetent persons (18). The utility of advance care-planning has, however, often been doubted, in that, despite widespread public and policy support for the concept, the uptake of these instruments has been low, their actual practical role in decision-making has been minimal, they may be ignored and they may not adequately cover the situation that actually arises. Some have also questioned whether advance directives will deprive certain people of treatment that might be beneficial to them, particularly some groups within society that are seen as disadvantaged, such as the aged, disabled and mentally ill. It is arguable that the interests and welfare of incompetent patients may be better served by 'focusing directly on their current interests rather than by diverting attention to questions, such as what the patient had or would have chosen when competent, which address a situation very different than that faced by the incompetent patient'(19).

Peter Singer of the University of Toronto Joint Centre for Bioethics has addressed some of the concerns relating to advance directives in the following way. Firstly, he and his group have developed disease-specific advance directive documents (20). Secondly, they have pointed out that if you look at the issue from the point of view of the patient, the family and social aspects of making an advance directive are very important. Whilst the emphasis has often seemed to be on the directive being a way to talk to healthcare professionals, patients emphasize that these instruments are a way of talking to their families and friends about their values and beliefs, as well as their views about future treatment options (21). Given the fact that many patients referred to palliative care services may be some time away from death, and will continue to access the rest of the health system, the routine use of jurisdiction-appropriate advance care-planning at, or soon after, referral to the service may be useful, especially if this facilitates communication within the family of the realities of the situation and patient wishes, where known (22).

Where an incompetent patient has not executed a binding advance directive, and no agent or guardian has been appointed, attending physicians, in consultation with the family, may decide to withdraw or not initiate medical treatment on the basis that continuation of treatment is inappropriate and not in the best interests of the patient. It should be remembered that most 'next of kin' roles assumed in hospitals probably have little force *per se* in most jurisdictions, although common sense usually prevails if there are no grounds to question good faith, and the closest blood relative is usually consulted if the patients are incompetent to make decisions themselves. However, in some jurisdictions there is now recognition of a 'person responsible' who will be approached to give consent to medical treatment, or treatment abatement (23),[1] if the patient

---

[1] Robert Weir, a bioethicist from the Medical College of Iowa, adopts the term 'abatement'. This term, which is used throughout this chapter, encompasses both non-initiation and cessation of medical treatment. This appears to be an important distinction in clinical decision-making behaviour, but not in terms of outcome, where death can clearly result from both non-initiation and cessation of medical treatment.

is deemed to be incompetent. In many jurisdictions, the hierarchy of substitute decision-makers is set out and the first person on the list who is reasonably available, willing and able, will be approached by the hospital to assume the role of 'person responsible'. This list will vary according to the jurisdiction concerned, depending on the legal provisions in place, but it usually gives priority to legally appointed agents or guardians (when appointed) over blood relatives, starting with spouses and then nearest relatives. Carers, although not paid professional ones, are usually included in this hierarchy.

Causing death

It is particularly important to be clear that death is not of itself an ethical issue. It seems self-evident to point out that death is an inevitable consequence of having life; that, in that sense, it is a natural event (24). Whilst healthcarers have a duty to attempt to save and sustain life, acknowledgement of dying and relief of suffering are required when this is no longer possible. Death is the inevitable outcome of an inexorable underlying process, it just *is*, it is nobody's responsibility. False perceptions of what the law and ethics require have been found to be significant barriers to care and decision-making at the end of life, and this has been found in both professional and, particularly for the family carer perspective, amongst the public submissions (24).

Health professionals and members of the public usually have a narrow empirical view of causation, and they should be made aware that the law takes a common sense and multi-factorial view, and indeed will often not even apply a causal analysis, focusing more on legality of actions and presence or absence of duties instead (25.) Clarification of what law and ethics really say about death causation, in the setting of the care of dying people, will show that causal anxiety is largely misplaced, inflated and inappropriate. Providing the prevailing standards of palliative care are adhered to, there is no basis for health professionals to be in fear of legal sanction when dealing with dying persons. Similarly, there is no reason for family members to feel that they are under any legal or ethical obligation to endorse continuing curative treatment where this is no longer clinically appropriate; nor that they should be concerned about appropriate palliative interventions, for which they may also have or perceive that they have some responsibility, causing death.

Litigation

Occasionally, there is such a fundamental stand-off between a family and the healthcare system, or lack of clarity about the lawfulness of treatment abatement, that a legal action is initiated. It is noticeable that recent litigation by families in several countries has resulted in a number of court decisions in favour of treatment abatement and the deployment of appropriate palliative care rather than futile and burdensome medical care that has no prospect of success. These cases usually concern treatment or life-support cessation in a patient believed to be hopelessly ill with no prospect of recovery, or in a post-coma unresponsive state.

Since in almost all cases, the result of termination of artificial nutrition and hydration or mechanical ventilation is death, in some cases, the hospitals have asked courts to declare the abatement of these treatments lawful, such as in the cases of *Airedale NHS Trust v Bland, Cruzan v Director, Auckland Area Health Board v Attorney-General.* Other legal cases were a result of a conflict between the relatives or guardians of the patient and the medical personnel in relation to the abatement of life-sustaining treatment (26–30). In some cases, the family wished for the treatment to be continued (*Northridge v Central Sydney Area Health Service, Glass v United Kingdom*), while in others, the request was to withdraw or withhold further treatment (*Gardner; Re BWV*) (31–33). There are also situations where the conflict within the family—between relatives and guardians regarding abatement of treatment—may end up in litigation, such as the internationally reported case of *Schindler v Schiavo* (34). In situations of conflict, it is helpful for practitioners to be able to differentiate their clinical judgment on the one hand from attitudes on news relating to the patient and the family, and one's own beliefs, likes and dislikes on the other.

Medical provision of hydration and alimentation

Provision of artificial hydration and alimentation is widely held in ethics, law and public policy, to be medical treatment like any other, and there is no medical, ethical or legal requirement for these to be administered to dying persons, unless indicated for comfort. For this reason, Beauchamp and Childress (11) favour the unambiguous term 'medically-administered nutrition and hydration' (MN&H). They conclude that there is:

> ... no reason to believe that medically administered nutrition and hydration is always an essential part of palliative care or that it necessarily constitutes, on balance, a beneficial medical treatment.

It is a normal part of the dying process for there to be a gradual reduction, and eventual cessation of oral intake. In palliative care units, food and drink, and assistance with eating and drinking, are always available to satisfy a patient's thirst and hunger, but MN&H is not routinely used when oral intake ceases (35). All treatments that are not required for comfort are stopped when a person is dying. MN&H, for example, subcutaneous fluid infusion, is only used for symptomatic thirst or hunger that cannot be adequately treated by other means. Clinical experience shows no basis for believing that patients receiving palliative care are experiencing symptoms of starvation and dehydration, which would be lessened or abolished by the routine provision of MN&H. Such symptoms, especially poor appetite and lack of energy, are intrinsic effects of the underlying condition, and are usually resistant to any treatment.

Health workers, particularly those in acute hospitals and aged care facilities need not feel that they are legally or ethically required to provide medically-administered nutrition and hydration, regardless of the clinical situation. Benefits and risks must be carefully evaluated in each case, and these intervention(s) are only usually indicated if the patient has a reasonable chance of recovery, with eventual restoration of normal oral intake. Where this is not the case, then quality and comfort issues must be addressed. There is now a growing realization that insertion of percutaneous gastrostomies for patients with advanced dementia and impaired swallowing after severe stroke give poor clinical outcomes, and are usually contraindicated (36, 37).

Nonetheless, it would be wrong to underestimate the amount of concern that family members may have about the failure to feed and hydrate people who are dying. There are profound social, cultural and emotional dimensions to the provision of food and drink, even to very sick people. It is a necessary part of palliative care practice to work closely with families who may feel that they are inflicting a cruel dying, or that they are neglecting their social or religious duties by non-provision of nutrition and hydration.

Cardio-pulmonary resuscitation

Cardio-pulmonary resuscitation (CPR) is a medical treatment that is indicated to re-start normal respiration and circulation when these have stopped due to a potentially reversible cause. On common sense grounds, the issue of resuscitation of individuals who have a terminal illness should not give rise to controversy, but sometimes it does, particularly for medical and nursing staff (38). Many patients are well aware of their conditions and that their quality of life, should resuscitation be successful, will be very limited. The success rate of resuscitation in previously healthy individuals who arrest is low. In the presence of advanced incurable disease, outcomes of resuscitation are likely to be significantly worse. Unless patients are cared for in situations where resuscitation equipment exists, the decision to resuscitate or not is irrelevant, although ambulance services often have policies that resuscitation is required when attending or transporting patients, even for palliative care purposes. The wider use of advance directives and dialogue with these services is necessary to prevent such problems.

Discussion of CPR with patients is required if a 'not for resuscitation' (NFR) order is being considered in an acute care facility. Rightly or wrongly, this is often the moment when referral to a palliative care service is first considered. The presence or absence of such orders is often a source of anxiety for junior members of medical and nursing staff. For dying persons, resuscitation is inappropriate and irrelevant, and should not be the focus of care and decision-making. CPR is a medical treatment like any other and subject to the same criteria for implementation as any other. It is neither a patient right nor a last rite. In many palliative care units it is not specifically discussed as it is usually not available, and will only be addressed if explicitly requested by patient or family. However, owing to the referral of patients at earlier stages of their disease process, this is being questioned by some units, and such discussions may result in patients not being transferred or the offer of limited resuscitative measures to certain patients. For instance, it may be appropriate to treat respiratory obstruction or insufficiency in some circumstances; for example, in narcosis after pain-interventions.

Local health guidelines and laws may dictate that resuscitation status be directly and specifically addressed with patients, their agents of families. Ideally, it should be part of the palliative care admission process, and can often be merged into general discussion of the patient's needs and wishes. Unfortunately, it will often fall to families to agree to an NFR order, even in situations where the patient's condition renders it a non-decision. This will need sensitivity and an understanding of the great weight this may place on the shoulders of those who are asked.

Requests for assistance to die

The incidence of requests for assistance to end life is not precisely known, but the limited data available suggest that sustained requests are uncommon in palliative care practice (39, 40). However, intermittent requests occur and practitioners should not be alarmed but should explore the thinking behind the request, especially with regard to whether there is an underlying depression or inadequate pain management.

Most patients understand the ethical and legal limitations incumbent upon health professionals with regard to causing death. They will usually accept the offer of optimal palliative care and assurances that no futile and unwanted attempts will be made to prolong their dying, that their pain and suffering will not be abandoned and that there will be no compromise on symptom control, including the offer of heavy sedation during the final dying process, if they wish.

Some patients will seek the confidential assistance of those who offer more proactive assistance to die (41) and it is best for palliative care practitioners to offer continued support and care, but also to refrain from involvement in this process. The vast majority of patients will respect this stance. Family requests to 'speed things up', with accompanying remarks about the way animal suffering is dealt with, can only be met with reassurance that symptom control will be worked at attentively until death, and that there will be no attempts to prolong the dying process by medical means.

Conclusion

Death is not *per se* an ethical issue, and false perceptions of what the law and ethics require have the capacity to obstruct good care and decision-making at the end of life. The law and parliaments have been very supportive of palliative care, and their deliberations have hitherto opposed the prolongation of the dying process and supported good pain and symptom management.

Ethics in palliative care is mainly about good process rather than theory. Effective, appropriate and sensitive work with families is necessary for good palliative care to be delivered. It is self-evident that this can only occur where communication is given the time and attention it deserves. Well-conducted family meetings (with clear purpose) can be valuable, and conflict-resolution principles help where there is difference. There are jurisdiction-specific procedures and bodies that are charged with the responsibility of assisting or intervening where there is disagreement or uncertainty, and practitioners should be aware of these. Health-promoting palliative care and death education within the community can assist families and carers to prepare for dealing with death and dying.

Key learning points

- Death is not an ethical 'dilemma' in its own right.
- Death is the whole community's business. Broadly-based health-promoting palliative care work has the capacity to help families to avoid death-denying attitudes that obstruct necessary decision-making and care at the end of life.
- Ethics is a process more than a knowledge base.
- Good communication is at the heart of good ethics.

- Clarity about clinical facts and realities of the situation are important.
- Law does not require the dying process to be prolonged needlessly.
- The patient must come first; the family cannot be ignored. It is a balance.

Acknowledgement

Parts of this paper can be found, with some small differences in *Palliative Care Expert Group. Therapeutic Guidelines: Palliative Care*, Version 2 (2005). Melbourne: Therapeutic Guidelines Limited, 19–28.

Recommended reading and resources

Beauchamp T and Childress J (2001). *Principles of Biomedical Ethics*. New York: Oxford University Press.

Ethox Centre, Department of Public Health and Primary Health Care, the University of Oxford, Badenoch Building, Old Road Campus, Headington, Oxford, OX3 7LF at http://www.ethox.org.uk/

General Medical Council (2002). *Withholding and Withdrawing Life-Prolonging Treatments: Good Practice in Decision-Making*. www.gmc-uk.org

The Hastings Centre (an independent and non profit Bioethics research institute), 21 Malcolm Gordon Road, Garrison NY 10524–4125 at http://www.thehastingscenter.org/

Journal of Medical Ethics. http://jme.bmj.com/

Randall F and Downie RS (2006). *The Philosophy of Palliative Care: Critique and Reconstruction*. Oxford & New York: Oxford University Press.

Singer P (ed.) (1991). *A Companion to Ethics*. Oxford: Blackwell.

Therapeutic Guidelines. Palliative Care, Version 2 (2005). Melbourne: Therapeutic Guidelines. Limited at http://www.tg.con.au/index.php?sectionid=47.

Legal citations

Sidaway v Governors of Bethlem Royal Hospital (1985) AC 871

Rogers v Whitatier (1992) 175 CLR479.

Cruzan v Director, Missouri Dept of Health (1990) 497 U.S. 261.

Auckland Area Health Board v Attorney-General (1993) 1 New Zealand LR at 235.

Airedale NHS Trust v Bland (1993) AC 789.

Northridge v Central Sydney Area Health Service (2000) NSWSC 1241, #674

Glass v United Kingdom (2004) 39 EHRR 341; [2004]1 FLR 1019

Gardner; Re BWV (2003) VSC 173

Schindler v Schiavo (Re Schiavo) 780 So 2d 176 at 176; 26 Fla L Weekly D305 (2001)

References

1. World Health Organization (2004). *The Solid Facts. Palliative Care*. Copenhagen: WHO.
2. National Institute for Clinical Excellence (2004). *Guidance on Cancer Services: Improving Supportive and Palliative Care for Adults with Cancer. The Manual*. London: NICE. http://guidance.nice.org.uk/csgsp

3. Kellehear A (1999). *Health-promoting Palliative Care*. Melbourne: Oxford University Press.

4. Kellehear A (2005). *Compassionate Cities: Public health and End-of-life Care*. London: Routledge.

5. Nolan M, Keady J and Grant G (1995). Developing a typology of family care: implications for nurses and other service providers. *Journal of Advanced Nursing* 21(2): 256–265.

6. Hudson P, Aranda S ans Hayman-White K (2005). A psycho-educational intervention for family caregivers of patients receiving palliative care: a randomized controlled trial. *Journal of Pain and Symptom Management* 30(4): 329–341.

7. Kuczewski MG (1996). Reconceiving the family: the process of consent in medical decision-making. *Hastings Center Report* 26(2): 30–37.

8. Randall F and Downie RS (2006). *The Philosophy of Palliative Care: Critique and Reconstruction*. Oxford & New York: Oxford University Press.

9. Kissane DW and Bloch S (2002). *Family Focused Grief Therapy*. Buckingham: Open University Press.

10. Walter T (1999). *On Bereavement*. Buckingham: Open University Press.

11. Beauchamp T and Childress J (1994). *Principles of Biomedical Ethics*. New York: Oxford University Press.

12. Fallowfield L and Jenkins V (2004). Communicating sad, bad, and difficult news. *Lancet* 363: 312–319.

13. Clayton JM, Hancock KM, Butow PN, Tattersall MN and Currow DC (2007). Clinical practice guidelines for communicating prognosis and end-of-life issues with adults in the advanced stages of a life-limiting illness, and their care-givers. *Medical Journal of Australia* 186(12): S77–S108.

14. Wertheim E, Love A, Littlefield L and Peck C (1992). *I Win You Win*. Melbourne: Penguin.

15. Kirk P, Kirk I and Kristjanson LJ (2004). What do patients receiving palliative care for cancer and their families want to be told? A Canadian and Australian qualitative study. *British Medical Journal* 328: 1343–1349.

16. Mendelson D (2006). Assessment of competency: a primer. *Journal of Law and Medicine* 14: 156–166.

17. Darzins P, Molloy DW and Strang D (ed.) (2000). *Who Can Decide? The Six Step Capacity Assessment Process*. Adelaide, Australia: Memory Australia Press.

18. Cartwright C (2007). Advance care-planning in Australia: challenges of a federal legislative system. *Progress in Palliative Care* 15(3): 113–117.

19. Robertson JA (1991). Assessing quality of life: a response to Professor Kamisar. *Georgia Law Review* 25: 1243–1253 at 1248.

20. *University of Toronto JCfB. Living Wills* (2006). [cited 2007 6/08/07]; Available from: http://www.utoronto.ca/jcb/outreach/documents/JCB_Living_Will.pdf

21. Martin DK, Emanuel LL and Singer PA (2000). Planning for the end of life. *Lancet* 356: 1672–1676.

22. Brown M, Fisher JW, Brumley DJ, Ashby MA and Milliken J (2005). Advance directives in action in a regional palliative care service: 'Road testing' the provisions of the Medical Treatment Act 1988 (Vic). *Journal of Law and Medicine* 13(2): 186–190.

23. Weir R (1989). *Abating Treatment with Critically Ill Patients*. New York: Oxford University Press.

24. Ashby M (2001). Natural causes? Palliative care and death causation in public policy and the law. Unpublished MD thesis. University of Adelaide.

25. Somerville MA (1997). Euthanasia by confusion. *University of New South Wales Law Journal* **20**(3): 551–575.

26. Dyer O (2005). Judges support doctors' decision to stop treating dying man. *British Medical Journal* **331**: 536.

27. Dyer C (1995). Girl with leukaemia will be treated privately. *British Medical Journal* **310**: 687.

28. Dyer C (2004). Doctors need not ventilate baby to prolong life. *British Medical Journal* **329**: 995.

29. Dyer C (2004). Baby should be allowed to die, UK court rules. *British Medical Journal* **329**: 875.

30. Dyer C (2007). Judge will not intervene as dying woman denied life support. *British Medical Journal* **335**: 119.

31. Ashby MA and Mendelson D (2004). Gardner; re BWV: Victorian Supreme Court makes landmark Australian ruling on tube feeding. *Medical Journal of Australia* **181**(8): 442–445.

32. Faunce TA and Stewart C (2005). The Messiha and Schiavo cases: third party ethical interventions in futile care disputes. *Medical Journal of Australia* **183**(5): 261–263.

33. Thiagarajan M, Savulescu J and Skene L (2007). Deciding about life support: a perspective on the ethical and legal framework in the United Kingdom and Australia. *Journal of Law and Medicine* **14**: 583–596.

34. Gostin LO (2005). Ethics, the constitution, and the dying process: the case of Theresa Marie Schiavo. *The Journal of the American Medical Association* **293**(19): 2403–2407.

35. Van der Riet P and Brooks D (2006). Nutrition and hydration at the end of life. *Journal of Law and Medicine* **14**: 182–198.

36. Gillick MR (2000). Rethinking the role of tube feeding in patients with advanced dementia. *The New England Journal of Medicine* **342**(3): 206–209.

37. Finucane TE and Bynum JP (1996). Use of tube feeding to prevent aspirational pneumonia. *Lancet* **348**: 1421–1424.

38. Willard C (2000). Cardiopulmonary resuscitation for palliative care patients: a discussion of ethical cases. *Palliative Medicine* **14**: 308–312.

39. Hudson PL, Schofield P, Kelly B, Hudson R, O'Connor M, Kristjanson LJ, Ashby M, and Aranda S (2006). Responding to desire to die statements from patients with advanced disease: recommendations for health professionals. *Palliative Medicine* **20**(7): 703–710.

40. Hudson PL, Kristjanson LJ, Ashby M, Kelly B, Schofield P, Hudson R, Aranda S, O'Connor M, and Street A (2006). Desire for hastened death in patients with advanced disease and the evidence base of clinical guidelines: a systematic review. *Palliative Medicine* **20**(7): 693–701.

41. Magnusson RS (2002). *Angels of Death: Exploring the Euthanasia Underground*. Melbourne: Melbourne University Press.

Chapter 7

Assessing family carer satisfaction with healthcare delivery

Kevin Brazil

Since the early 1980s, healthcare organizations have become increasingly focused on the quality of services provided. Much of the interest around quality of care has developed in response to dramatic advances in medical sciences in recent years. Despite the rapid transformation in medical care, the healthcare delivery system struggles in its ability to provide consistent quality care.

A recent report released by the Institute of Medicine (IOM) (1) reported that there is a 'quality chasm' between average care (the care we have) and the best quality care (the care we could have). The authors of this report identified a combination of overuse, underuse and misuse of the healthcare system as contributing factors in the uneven provision of quality healthcare. Overuse involves the unnecessary use of particular interventions or treatments. Underuse is characterized by insufficient use of particular interventions or preventive measures, while misuse describes the poor implementation of clinical care. The IOM report acknowledged that the challenges of achieving quality care in the healthcare system are not because of a lack of effort but due to the fundamental shortcomings in the way care is organized. Research on the quality of care reveals that the healthcare system frequently falls short in its ability to translate knowledge into practice and to apply technology safely and appropriately (1, 2).

To most readers, quality healthcare is about delivering the best possible care and achieving the best possible outcomes for people every time they encounter the healthcare system or use its services. Efforts to define standards of quality care in palliative care have been undertaken by several organizations (3). Within these standards it is recognized that the notion of quality requires multiple considerations such as access, equity, efficiency, appropriateness, effectiveness, acceptability, and relevance (4, 5).

Defining quality care also depends on the viewpoint from which it is examined. For patients and their family carers, high-quality healthcare means their needs and expectations are being met. For healthcare providers, quality healthcare means their diagnoses are accurate, they are part of a well-functioning system and the care they provide is appropriate and effective. This chapter will examine the considerations that must be made when assessing family carer perceptions on the quality of healthcare delivery at the end of life.

A conceptual framework to assess quality palliative care

It has been suggested that to effectively assess the quality of healthcare it is useful to have a conceptual framework that assists in specifying and defining relevant domains appropriate for evaluation (3). While several conceptual approaches are available, the most popular model is that developed by Avis Donabedian (5). Donabedian assumed quality as a multidimensional concept that could be evaluated on service structure, process and outcomes. This threefold framework, long considered the backbone of a sound quality assessment and service improvement, promotes the evaluation of the structures, the processes and the outcomes of healthcare delivery.

Stewart *et al.* adapted the Donabedian framework for application to assess quality of life and care for the dying person (3). The Stewart framework provides a dynamic and integrated model to assess quality palliative care that consists of four broad themes: personal and social environment; structure; process; and outcomes of care.

Personal and social environment considerations address the context within which the patient and family seek palliative care. These considerations include the patient's and family's ethnic/cultural background, financial resources, concurrent life issues, and social support. All of these contextual factors can affect the structure, process, and outcomes of care. Structure of care describes the characteristics of a programme or service the patient and family receive. Features may include the organization of care, the comprehensiveness of care, the distribution and qualifications of the personnel involved in delivering palliative care, and the physical environment of care. For example, site of care and site of death have both been associated with quality of care and satisfaction with care (6). Satisfaction with in-patient hospice care, home hospice care and specialist community outreach teams is generally high; while hospital, nursing home and community care receive a greater number of criticisms by family carers (7).

Process of care describes how care is delivered in the last phase of life. Stewart *et al.* (3) described process of care to include:

- technical aspects, such as the timing and appropriateness of care;
- decision-making processes for both the patient and family, such as the information provided about care options;
- the provision of psychosocial counselling to the patient and their family carers; and
- the interpersonal and communication style of providers, which includes respectfulness and compassion.

Given that patients may be cared for across multiple sites, by many providers and through a variety of services, continuity and coordination of care is an important process issue to consider when evaluating the quality of palliative care.

Outcomes in palliative care (the final theme) can include a variety of factors related both to the patient (e.g. physical comfort, spiritual well-being) and family (e.g. burden, well-being and grief resolution). Satisfaction with health-care is viewed by many as an essential outcome of clinical care. Based on the premise that palliative care is both patient-focused and family-centred, this framework considers family carers as an important source to assess the quality of palliative care.

At least two considerations have fuelled the interest in assessing family carer satisfaction with palliative care. First, researchers, policy-makers and direct care providers are widely aware of the pivotal role that the family plays in caring for the dying patient. Simply put, formal healthcare relies on family carers. Second, family caregiving is now widely understood to be potentially stressful; several studies have documented the burden family members experience when they are often ill-prepared to provide the level of care required by a terminally ill person. The resultant burden can have significant psychological, physical and financial consequences for family carers (8–11). Recognizing the high burden involved in caregiving, the importance of assessing family needs and satisfaction with service delivery has grown in importance.

Need identification and satisfaction assessment

Seen from the family carer's perspective, quality palliative care is viewed as the extent to which needs are addressed and met. Identification of needs, therefore, has a direct effect on satisfaction with care (12). The IOM report on EOL (13) identified several key patient needs including: support for fears of abandonment and protracted death; the need for reliable, respectful care; and the need for advance care planning that promotes 'norms of decency'. Assessment of palliative care needs has been identified as problematic (14). In part, this may be due to the ambiguity in the notion of 'need', which includes a broad spectrum of considerations within the patient–family experience (14, 15). It may also rest in the difficulty healthcare providers and patients/families have in communicating with one another (16, 17). When there is no systematic assessment of the needs of patients and families, planning and setting priorities is difficult, if not impossible, to achieve. The findings that some patients and families are dissatisfied with the care they receive, feeling they are not getting what they need, is most likely associated with inadequate needs assessments by healthcare providers (14). Wen and Gustafson (12) developed a model that explores the relationship between health needs and satisfaction with care in cancer patients. Their work stresses the importance of a comprehensive, systematic approach to needs assessments that gives patients and families the opportunity to identify the issues they want recognized and addressed by healthcare providers. Understanding patient and family expectations can help service providers to identify the value they place on options that are available in care.

The recognized importance of understanding patient and family needs, including their experiences in palliative care, has increased the value of measuring satisfaction with healthcare. Assessing satisfaction with healthcare has its roots in the consumer movement of the 1960s, where provider omnipotence and beneficence gave way to principles of patient autonomy and shared decision-making (18, 19). The shift towards the importance of a user's perspective on healthcare delivery influenced the definition of 'quality healthcare', where satisfaction has become a key attribute of quality healthcare. Consequently, satisfaction has become a key outcome in palliative care (20).

The importance of assessing satisfaction with care is valued from several perspectives. From a clinician's point of view, satisfaction is known to have a significant impact on compliance—whether or not the user will carry out a treatment plan (21). Satisfied healthcare users are more likely to carry out the treatment plan—to continue using medical care services, to comply with medical regimens and to maintain a relationship with a specific provider (18).

For researchers and policy makers, assessing satisfaction with care may be used as an evaluative outcome. High levels of dissatisfaction with a programme may be an early indicator of problems with programme design or implementation. Assessing satisfaction has become increasingly important from an administrative point of view in this era of Continuous Quality Improvement (CQI) and Total Quality Management (TQM). In this framework, quality is often defined as meeting the needs and expectations of the customers. Regular measurement of satisfaction also assists organizations in meeting regulatory requirements. Thus, the ability to measure satisfaction precisely in a valid and reliable manner is important. Many healthcare institutions are beginning to use satisfaction information as a basis from which to compare all future improvements and services. For some healthcare organizations, satisfaction data are used for the purposes of customer relations and marketing. In this context of heightened importance in the use of satisfaction assessment, close scrutiny of its role is required.

What is satisfaction with healthcare?

While many view satisfaction as an important criterion to assess the quality of palliative care, a significant critique in the research literature has been the lack of consensus regarding the meaning associated with the word (20, 22). The most commonly used conceptual model to describe satisfaction works on the discrepancy perspective. Pascoe (23) viewed satisfaction as an individual's reaction to salient aspects of the context, process and the result of their service experience. According to this definition, patients and families evaluate a directly received service by comparing their personal experience to a subjective standard, which is related closely to their expectations regarding their healthcare.

While patients' and families' expectations and values are involved in the evaluation of care, it is not a straightforward relationship. Strasser (24) suggests that an individual's values and expectations, which are influenced by life experiences, are modified by the experience of the care they receive. Williams (19) argues that to understand satisfaction we must understand the role that families and patients perceive themselves to have within the healthcare system. Both these positions stress that to assess and interpret satisfaction we must first understand patients' and families' perceived needs and roles within the healthcare system.

The lack of a widely accepted conceptual framework for satisfaction complicates attempts to examine satisfaction with care. Dimensions included in the measurement of satisfaction can vary from study to study, as different satisfaction measures are developed to deal with different aspects of healthcare. There have been several attempts to define quality care at the end of life. While a number of professionally derived taxonomies of the domains and outcomes variables that comprise quality palliative care have been developed, recent efforts have focused on identifying the patient and family perspective on quality palliative care (25, 26). These research studies have identified many similar attributes of quality palliative care, yet variation is noted across them, creating confusion as to what are the right domains.

In a recent study by Howell and Brazil (27) a meta-synthesis was conducted to derive a comprehensive and integrated understanding of the attributes of quality palliative care from the patient and family perspective. The results of this study identified common domains that appeared important to patients and families across age groups, gender and disease populations. Patients and families expect that a dying experience will ensure that pain and symptoms are controlled, that they will be assisted to prepare for death emotionally and spiritually, that the patient will die in the place of their choice with loved ones present, that they will have the opportunity for sustained relationships with family and friends, that their treatment preferences and decisions will be assessed and respected, and that the moment of death will be consistent with their choices.

Factors related to family carer satisfaction

Given the variety of approaches to measuring satisfaction, it is difficult to draw firm conclusions on factors that are associated with satisfaction with palliative care. With the exception of age, few consistent demographic variables have been associated with satisfaction in palliative care. It has been found that older respondents are less likely to express dissatisfaction with care (28). The reasons for this are unclear, although they may relate to different expectations or experiences with the healthcare system (28). With regard to disease, a recent systematic review by Lorenz and Lynn (29) reported little evidence that satisfaction differed by disease.

Research conducted by Fakhoury (30) found that family carers who perceived care as rewarding, had no unmet needs while caring for patients at home, expressed a positive health status post-bereavement and were more likely than others to be satisfied with care. These findings highlight the importance of patient and family carer characteristics in the interpretation of results from satisfaction surveys.

Several studies have investigated the relationship between satisfaction and interventions designed to improve the delivery of palliative care. Grande *et al.* (31) evaluated a hospital at home service that involved specialist palliative nursing care during the final weeks of life. Informal carers who received the intervention reported better satisfaction with care than those who received usual care. Kane *et al.* (32) reported similar results from informal carers who received enhanced home hospice care compared to those who received usual care. Ringdal *et al.* (33) evaluated an intervention that included community education and the integration of a hospital-based palliative care programme with local provider activities. Carer satisfaction scores favoured the intervention with regard to improved pain management and communication with the family. Riegel (34) reported higher levels of satisfaction for treatment among those who participated in a case management programme for congestive heart failure compared to those who received usual care. In other studies, the relationship between satisfaction and service delivery is more ambiguous. Molloy *et al.* (35) conducted a study on advance care-planning in nursing homes and reported that family satisfaction did not differ between those families who participated in the advanced care-planning intervention and those who received usual care.

A systematic review conducted by Wilkinson (7) identified that in the UK, patients and families were more satisfied with palliative care that was provided in specialist in-patient palliative care units or in the community, than palliative care provided in general hospitals. Criticisms directed to general hospital care included the psychosocial aspects of care, communication and coordination with other community services. While the research has shown satisfaction to be high with home-care services, informal carers have expressed concerns that included inadequate sleep while caring for the patient, as well as the need for more overnight help and access to respite services. Lorenz and Lynn (29) reported an association between satisfaction and interventions that improved communication or addressed other aspects of care. Important attributes of care associated with satisfaction included effective pain management, practical support, enhanced caregiving and provider accessibility. Harding and Higginson (36), who undertook a systematic review around the effectiveness of interventions for informal carers, determined that existing studies suffer from small sample sizes and untested measures, making the determination of effectiveness problematic.

Several studies have compared satisfaction across different settings of care (29). Teno (6) evaluated the US dying experience based on location of death, through interviews with family members. Sixty-seven per cent of care recipients died in an institutional setting, while 33 per cent died at home. The results of this study suggests that those dying in institutions have unmet needs for symptom management, physician communication, emotional support and being treated with respect. Family members of those who died with home hospice services were more likely to report a favourable dying experience.

Methodological issues in assessing satisfaction

The accuracy of measuring family carer service satisfaction can be affected by a number of methodological factors. A key factor is the quality of the instrument in terms of reliability and validity (37). Reliability concerns variability in measurement—the extent to which measurements in satisfaction obtained under different circumstances provide similar results. There are a variety of ways of assessing the reproducibility of a satisfaction measure; for example, having the family carer complete the instrument on two occasions separated by an interval of time (test–retest reliability). Inter-observer reliability describes the degree of consistency of assessment between different interviewers. This calculation of reliability is relevant for those instruments that are interviewer administered (28, 37).

When internal consistency has been estimated for a satisfaction instrument, traditional psychometric standards have been applied to that instrument. Internal consistency calculates reliability on the basis of the average correlation among items in the assessment instrument. Measurement using Cronbach's coefficient alpha is a popular approach. Unfortunately, most instruments developed to assess satisfaction do not report on the reliability of their measures. In a review of satisfaction measures, Sitza (38) reported that only 46 per cent of the studies reported some reliability and validity data.

Determining if the instrument is measuring what it intended to measure crosses into validity issues. Face validity indicates that the instrument appears to be assessing satisfaction and its associated dimensions. Content validity is a closely related concept, representing the judgement that the instrument includes questions that represent the relevant or important domains of family carer satisfaction. Both forms of validity can be assessed on the basis of expert judgement to determine whether the instrument appears appropriate for the purpose of measuring family carer satisfaction.

Most satisfaction instruments have not been validated beyond content or face validity (28, 38). Criterion validity describes the correlation of a newly developed scale with a pre-existing measure or an existing 'gold standard'. In the absence of criterion validity, construct validity may be conducted to demonstrate that the measures are indeed measuring what is intended. One approach to assessing construct validity is to compare family carers' assessment of satisfaction with other variables that are theoretically related to satisfaction. Unfortunately, very few satisfaction measures have been validated. Smith (28) suggests that this may be due to the absence of well-developed conceptual models of satisfaction.

The response format for individual questions in a family carer satisfaction instrument can have a substantial impact on the reliability and validity of the results (37). Satisfaction questions typically use a statement of opinion and a five-point Likert 'agree/disagree' response scale. These types of instruments are easy to design and are easily understood by survey respondents. However, scales that are scored on a continuum like the Likert scale, are prone to several types of biases, which include: central tendency bias that refers to people's difficulty in making absolute judgement, placing their responses to questions toward the centre of the scale; and positive skew, which describes the phenomena where responses to questions of satisfaction with care skew toward the favourable end of the scale producing a ceiling effect. To manage these biases, it is important to follow general guidelines to ensure clarity in how questions are asked, as well as the format used for responses when developing a family carer satisfaction instrument or choosing among alternative instruments (37).

It is assumed that when a family carer completes a satisfaction questionnaire they will answer honestly. However, there are numerous factors that may influence a family carer's response. Family carers may wish to be seen in a good light, they may wish to get the help they need or they may simply want to complete the questionnaire as quickly as possible so they can move on with their life. There are a number of biases that can influence the response a family carer will provide on a satisfaction instrument.

Social desirability is a bias where the family carer has the tendency to answer questions they believe are consistent with the expectations of the interviewer (37). Social desirability depends on a number of factors including the respondent's sex, cultural background, the specific question and the manner in which the question was asked (face-to-face interviews versus anonymous questionnaire). If responses on a satisfaction questionnaire are affected by social desirability, the validity of the instrument may be jeopardized.

Related to social desirability are family carers' potential fears of retribution or being stigmatized as a 'complainer' if they express dissatisfaction with care (39). These potential biases may be responsible for the typically high approval ratings found in many satisfaction surveys. Criticisms of hospice and specialist palliative care services are particularly rare, owing to their high standing in public opinion (7). Respondents may feel pressured to provide socially desirable answers to sensitive questions, especially those that deal with the care provided to a family member. Recognizing the high ratings in satisfaction surveys, it has been recommended that the focus be directed to those respondents who do report dissatisfaction. By exploring the minority expression of dissatisfaction, more substantive efforts toward improving service quality may be accomplished (39–41).

Acquiescent bias describes the tendency of a family carer to agree with a statement in a satisfaction questionnaire, regardless of the content. It has been suggested that this bias operates most strongly for older respondents or those who are seriously ill (28). Acquiescence poses a real threat to validity and must be considered when developing a survey instrument. For example, positively worded items may result in higher ratings of satisfaction. To correct for this potential bias, instrument developers may have an equal number of items phased in positive and negative directions. Non-response bias is a significant problem in family carer satisfaction surveys as response rates are typically low. Given evidence that non-respondents may evaluate care differently than those who complete satisfaction surveys, survey results must be interpreted cautiously when the response rate is low.

The timing of administrating a family carer satisfaction survey can also influence the results. Consideration needs to be paid to the possible ways in which retrospective accounts on quality care are subject to change due to the emotional impact of bereavement or simply by virtue of memory. There is some evidence that the views of family carer assessment of care may change over time (42). On this issue, further research is required.

The most common method of measuring satisfaction is with a closed-question format questionnaire administered through either face-to-face interview, over the telephone or through the mail. The relationship between mode of administration and response patterns has not been well studied. There is no one method of administration that is ideal in all circumstances. Factors such as cost, completion rate and the type of questions asked, must be taken into account (43).

It is recognized by a number of authors that a quantitative survey approach to satisfaction with care may overlook the complexity of the family carer experience (44). Rather, it has been argued that a qualitative approach allows for more of an in-depth exploration on matters of quality in service delivery. The goal of qualitative methods is to help understand family carer satisfaction with care by giving due emphasis to the meaning, experiences and views of the family carer. For example, a qualitative approach would be well-suited to explore the reasons why family carers do not use formal services when available.

Most qualitative studies that have explored satisfaction with palliative care have employed either focus groups or unstructured interviews. Qualitative research has provided important insights on family carers' perception of care at the end of life. Qualitative studies have identified the desired attributes of quality palliative care (e.g. effective pain and symptom management, continuity of care, adequate information, respectful empathetic support and practical support). They have supported the idea that the relationship between service delivery and satisfaction are mediated by contextual characteristics that include the healthcare setting and patient family carer characteristics (29). It has also been noted that where qualitative approaches have been used, family carers show greater inclination to express dissatisfaction with care (44). The open-ended approach that is offered in qualitative methods allows family carers to express themselves in their own words. Alternatively, researchers can consider the benefit of integrating both qualitative and quantitative strategies (45).

There is evidence that family carers' reports of patients' experiences may differ from patients' reports of their own experience, particularly in relation to emotional and physical state (46). For example, it has been reported that relatives tend to rate symptoms more severely than patients (46). Family carers are often viewed as a proxy respondent on the behalf of patients. This is unfortunate as family carers can offer important insights on service-delivery issues. Given their unique position, criteria for selecting the appropriate family carer respondent must be considered. Family carer satisfaction should be investigated for its own sake and not considered as secondary to assessing patient satisfaction.

Instruments measuring family carer satisfaction

There has been progress in the development of satisfaction instruments to measure patient and family carer perceptions on the quality of palliative care. Teno (47) conducted a systematic review of measures relevant to EOL care that included a review of satisfaction instruments. The Toolkit of Instruments to Measure End of Life Care (TIME), current to 2000, is a web-based resource of instruments for evaluating EOL care. Teno reviewed measures of satisfaction with ambulatory care and hospitalization to determine if existing instruments would be applicable to palliative care. On the basis of this review, several instruments were identified as worthy of further consideration to assess satisfaction with palliative care. Teno (47) identified the satisfaction surveys developed by Ware and colleagues as having application to assess quality palliative care. These instruments have measured patient satisfaction in terms of the physical environment, access to care, technical aspects of care and interpersonal support. The Toolkit After-Death Bereaved Family Interview, developed by Teno (48), is a telephone survey for family members that has versions for various settings of care. A third instrument identified by Teno that assesses family carer perceptions of care is the FAMCARE (49), a 20-item questionnaire that is interviewer-administered and asks family carers to assess various dimensions of care that include availability of care, physical patient care, psychosocial and information giving.

Subsequent to Teno's review, additional family carer satisfaction instruments that report psychometric data have been developed. The Quality of Dying and Death (QODD) instrument is a 31-item family after-death interview that addresses six domains (50). Mystakidou developed a 21-item questionnaire to assess families' attitudes, perceptions and patterns of choice in the management of terminally cancer patients (51).

Volicer *et al.* reported on the psychometrics of an instrument completed by family carers on the quality of care provided to dementia patients receiving palliative care (52). A postal questionnaire to examine carer satisfaction with palliative care was described by Jacoby *et al.* (53). Vohra *et al.* (54) reports on the development of the Family Perception of Care Scale (FPCS), which was intended to assess family perceptions of care for a dying family member in a long-term care facility.

While progress has been made in developing family carer satisfaction instruments specific to assessing the quality of palliative care, further psychometric development is required for many commonly used instruments that assess satisfaction.

Ethical considerations in assessing family carer satisfaction

While satisfaction surveys are being used increasingly, administrators are guided by different rationales for their use. It is important to distinguish between two general purposes of satisfaction surveys: marketing versus assessing the quality of care provided to the patient and family (55). The use of satisfaction surveys as a marketing tool is linked to the growth of a consumer-centred approach in the healthcare system. As a marketing tool, satisfaction surveys may have little application to improving quality of care. Using satisfaction surveys exclusively as a marketing tool may result in serious ethical violations, such as deception or denial, where isolated remarks may be used to market a service that has numerous problems with its delivery of care.

To maximize the benefit of satisfaction assessment, attention must be given to producing sound methodology that includes the quality of the instrument and its implementation (19). Poor data collection practices are not only a waste of time and money but are also unethical, as they do not contribute to the well-being of the intended population. Too often, an organization that conducts satisfaction assessments will cite budgetary concerns and settle for low response rates. However, low response rates do not reflect the opinions of the majority of service users. In this context, satisfaction surveys are little more than marketing a positive image that the organization 'is doing the right thing'. To circumvent this ethical dilemma experienced by well-intentioned service providers, it must be recognized that assessing family carer satisfaction is simply one quality indicator among a host of many. The onus on service providers is to identify multiple indicators that allow triangulation in the determination of quality palliative care. Further, alternate strategies to the traditional quantitative survey approach should be considered (39).

This may include qualitative strategies, such as in-depth interviews or focus groups (56).

One of the underlying principles of satisfaction surveys is to increase the involvement of family carers in the delivery of healthcare and to make health services more democratic and accountable (56). One of the main ethical dilemmas for service providers and researchers is whether this principle is feasible for family carers in palliative care. Typically, family carers are in a situation in which they have, if any, limited options and are unable or unwilling to express expectations or preferences for care. Related to this point is the paternalistic view that some service providers adopt based on the justification that families cannot make their own decisions involving care of their family member. The concern is that satisfaction assessment and the values that drive their use promote an illusory image of how formal care actually operates and what families really experience.

A primary ethical concern in assessing family carer service satisfaction is confidentiality. Confidentiality requires that the information pertaining to an individual will not be revealed publicly. Failing to secure family carers' trust regarding confidentiality may result in biased answers. An ethical issue can arise as a consequence of the conflict between assuring confidentiality and addressing revealed risk or wrongdoing. What happens when patterns of negligence or wrongdoing are revealed? Family carers may be distressed if the information they provide in confidence is made known.

Ethical guidelines should be an integral part of the planning and implementation of satisfaction assessment. While traditional academic researchers are expected to be well versed in principals of ethics, many organizations who pursue family carer satisfaction surveys as part of their quality improvement strategy may lack guidance in planning ethically responsible data collection practices.

Conclusion

Family carer satisfaction with care has emerged as a key outcome variable for evaluating the quality of palliative care. However, satisfaction has limitations as a measure of quality of care. While promising developments have occurred in the development of satisfaction instruments, a number of methodological challenges need continued attention. Given the limitations of conventional quantitative strategies, novel approaches to assessing quality and evaluating family carer perceptions of care are needed. Underlying these points is the emphasis that the study of family carer satisfaction with healthcare is guided by ethics based practice.

Key learning points

♦ The shift towards the importance of a user's perspective on healthcare delivery in North America, Northern Europe and Australia has influenced the definition of 'quality healthcare' in these regions, where satisfaction has become a key attribute of quality healthcare.

♦ Seen from the family carer's perspective, quality palliative care is viewed as the extent to which needs are addressed and met. Identification of needs, therefore, has a direct effect on satisfaction with care.

♦ While progress has been made in developing family carer satisfaction instruments, further methodological issues need to be addressed.

♦ A quantitative approach to assessing satisfaction with care may overlook the complexity of the family carer experience. A qualitative approach allows for more in-depth exploration on matters of quality in service delivery.

♦ Ethical guidelines must be an integral part of the planning and implementation of satisfaction assessment.

Recommended reading and resources

Aday LA, Begley CE, Lairson DR and Balkrishnan R (2004). *Evaluating the Healthcare System: Effectiveness, Efficiency, and Equity* (3rd edn). Chicago (IL): Health Administration Press.

Donabedian A (2004). *The Definition of Quality and Approaches to its Assessment.* Ann Arbor (MI): Heath Administration Press.

Howell D and Brazil K (2005). Reaching common ground: a patient-family-based conceptual framework of quality EOL care. *J Palliat Care* **21**(1): 19–26.

Lorenz K and Lynn J (2004). *Evidence Report/Technology Assessment*, No. 110. Prepared for the Agency for Healthcare Research Quality (AHRQ). End-of-life care and outcomes. [Online]. 2004 Dec [cited 2007 Apr 10];[651 screens]. Available from: URL: http://www.ahrq.gov/downloads/pub/evidence/pdf/eolcare/eolcare.pdf

Sinding C (2003). Disarmed complaints: unpacking satisfaction with end-of-life care. *Soc Sci Med* **57**(8): 1375–1385.

Smith MA (2000). Satisfaction. In: Kane RL and Kane RA (ed.). *Assessing Older Persons: Measures, Meaning, and Practical Applications.* Oxford (UK): Oxford University Press, 261–299.

Stewart AL, Teno JM, Patrick DL and Lynn J (1999). The concept of quality of life of dying persons in the context of healthcare. *J Pain Symptom Manage* **17**(2): 93–108.

Streiner DL and Norman GR (2003). *Health Measurement Scales: a Practical Guide to their Development and Use* (3rd edn). Oxford (UK): University Press.

Teno JM (2004). *TIME: Toolkit of Instruments to Measure End-of-Life Care.* [Online]. [Cited 2007 Apr 10]; available from: URL: http://www.chcr.brown.edu/pcoc/toolkit.htm

Williams B (1994). Patient satisfaction: a valid concept? *Soc Sci Med* **38**(4): 509–16.

References

1. Institute of Medicine (US) (2001). *Crossing the Quality Chasm: a New Health System for the 21st Century.* Washington (DC): National Academy Press.

2. Romanow RJ (2002). *Commission on the Future of Healthcare in Canada. Building on Values: the Future of Healthcare in Canada.* [Online]. 2002 Nov [cited 2007 Apr 10]; [392 screens]. Available from: URL: http://www.cbc.ca/healthcare/final_report.pdf

3. Stewart AL, Teno JM, Patrick DL and Lynn J (1999). The concept of quality of life of dying persons in the context of healthcare. *Journal of Pain and Symptom Management* **17**(2): 93–108.

4. Aday LA, Begley CE, Lairson DR and Balkrishnan R (2004). *Evaluating the Healthcare System: Effectiveness, Efficiency, and Equity* (3rd edn). Chicago (IL): Health Administration Press.

5. Donabedian A (2004). *The Definition of Quality and Approaches to its Assessment.* Ann Arbor (MI): Heath Administration Press.

6. Teno JM, Clarridge BR, Casey V, Welch LC, Wetle T, Shield R and Mor V (2004). Family perspectives on end-of-life care at the last place of care. *Journal of the American Medical Association* **291**(1): 88–93.

7. Wilkinson EK, Salisbury C, Bosanquet N Franks PJ, Kite S, Lorentzon M and Naysmith A (1999). Patient and carer preference for, and satisfaction with, specialist models of palliative care: a systematic literature review. *Palliative Medicine* **13**(3): 197–216.

8. Covinsky KE, Goldman L, Cook EF, Oye R, Desbiens N, Reding D, Fulkerson W, Connors AF Jr, Lynn J and Phillips RS (1994). The impact of serious illness on patients' families. SUPPORT Investigators. Study to Understand Prognoses and Preferences for Outcomes and Risks of Treatment. *Journal of the American Medical Association* **272**(23): 1839–1844.

9. Emanuel EJ, Fairclough DL, Slutsman J, Alpert H, Baldwin D and Emanuel LL (1999). Assistance from family members, friends, paid care givers, and volunteers in the care of the terminally ill. *The New England Journal of Medicine* **341**(13): 956–963.

10. Brazil K, Bedard M, Willison K and Hode M (2003). Caregiving and its impact on families of the terminally ill. *Aging Mental Health* **7**(5): 376–382.

11. Hauser JM and Kramer BJ (2004). Family caregivers in palliative care. *Clinics in Geriatric Medicine* **20**(4): 671–688.

12. Wen K and Gustafson DH (2004). Needs assessment for cancer patients and their families. *Health and Quality of Life Outcomes* **2**: 11.

13. Institute of Medicine (US) Field MJ and Cassel CK (ed.) (1997). *Approaching Death. Improving Care at the End of Life.* Washington (DC): National Academy Press.

14. Osse BH, Vernooij-Dassen MJ, de Vree BP, Schade E and Grol RP. Assessment of the need for palliative care as perceived by individual cancer patients and their families: a review of instruments for improving patient participation in palliative care. *Cancer* **88**(4): 900–911.

15. Asadi-Lari M, Tamburini M and Gray D (2004). Patients' needs, satisfaction, and health related quality of life: towards a comprehensive model. *Health and Quality of Life Outcomes* **2**: 32.

16. Maguire P (1985). Barriers to psychological care of the dying. *British Medical Journal* **291**(6510): 1711–1713.

17. Holland JC and Almanza J (1999). Giving bad news. Is there a kinder, gentler way? *Cancer* **86**(5): 738–740.

18. Carr-Hill RA (1992). The measurement of patient satisfaction. *Cancer* **14**(3): 236–249.

19. Williams B (1994). Patient satisfaction: a valid concept? *Social Science and Medicine* **38**(4): 509–516.

20. Aspinal F, Addington-Hall J, Hughes R and Higginson IJ (2003). Using satisfaction to measure the quality of palliative care: a review of the literature. *Journal of Advanced Nursing* **42**(4): 324–339.

21. Kincey J, Bradshaw P and Ley P (1975). Patients' satisfaction and reported acceptance of advice in general practice. *Journal of the College of General Practioners* **25**(157): 558–566.

22. Sitzia J and Wood N (1997). Patient satisfaction: a review of issues and concepts. *Social Science and Medicine* **45**(12): 1829–1843.

23. Pascoe GC (1983). Patient satisfaction in primary healthcare: a literature review and analysis. *Evaluation and Program Planning* **6**(3–4): 185–210.

24. Strasser S, Aharony L and Greenberger D (1993). The patient satisfaction process: moving toward a comprehensive model. *Medical Care Review* **50**(2): 219–248.

25. Singer PA, Martin DK and Kelner M (1999). Quality end-of-life care: patients' perspectives. *The Journal of the American Medical Association* **281**(2): 163–168.

26. Steinhauser KE, Christakis NA, Clipp EC, McNeilly M, McIntyre L and Tulsky JA (2000). Factors considered important at the end of life by patients, family, physicians, and other care providers. *The Journal of the American Medical Association* **284**(19): 2476–2482.

27. Howell D and Brazil K. Reaching common ground: a patient-family-based conceptual framework of quality EOL care. *Journal of Palliative Care* **21**(1): 19–26.

28. Smith MA (2000). Satisfaction. In: Kane RL and Kane RA (ed.). *Assessing Older Persons: Measures, Meaning, and Practical Applications*. Oxford (UK): Oxford University Press, 261–299.

29. Lorenz K and Lynn J (2004). *Evidence Report/Technology Assessment*, No. 110. Prepared for the Agency for Healthcare Research Quality (AHRQ). End-of-life care and outcomes. [Online]. 2004 Dec [cited 2007 April 10];[651 screens]. Available from: URL: http://www.ahrq.gov/downloads/pub/evidence/pdf/eolcare/eolcare.pdf

30. Fakhoury W, McCarthy M and Addington-Hall J (1996). Determinants of informal caregivers' satisfaction with services for dying cancer patients. *Social Science and Medicine* **42**(5): 721–731.

31. Grande GE, Todd CJ, Barclay SI and Farquhar MC (2000). A randomized controlled trial of a hospital at home service for the terminally ill. *Palliative Medicine* **14**(5): 375–385.

32. Kane RL, Wales J, Bernstein L, Leibowitz A and Kaplan S. A randomized controlled trial of hospice care. *Lancet* **1**(8382): 890–894.

33. Ringdal GL, Jordhoy MS and Kaasa S (2002). Family satisfaction with end-of-life care for cancer patients in a cluster randomized trial. *Journal of Pain and Symptom Management* **24**(1): 53–63.

34. Riegal B, Carlson B, Kopp Z, Le Petri B, Glaser D and Unger A (2002). Effect of a standardized nurse case-management telephone intervention on resources use in patients with chronic heart failure. *Archives of Internal Medicine* **162**(6): 702–712.

35. Molloy DW, Guyatt GH, Russo R, Goerce R, O'Brien BJ, Bedard M, Willan A, Watson J, Patterson C, Harrison C, Standish T, Strang D, Darzins PJ, Smith S and Dubois S (2000).

Systematic implementation of an advance directive programme in nursing homes: a randomized controlled trial. *The Journal of the American Medical Association* **283**(11): 1437–1444.

36. Harding R and Higginson IJ (2003). What is the best way to help caregivers in *Cancer* and palliative care? A systematic literature review of interventions and their effectiveness. *Palliative Medicine* **17**(1): 63–74.

37. Streiner DL and Norman GR (2003). *Health Measurement Scales: a Practical Guide to their Development and Use* (3rd edn). Oxford (UK): University Press.

38. Sitzia J (1999). How valid and reliable are patient satisfaction data? An analysis of 195 studies. *International Journal for Quality in Health Care: Journal of the International Society for Quality in Health Care/ISQua* **11**(4): 319–328.

39. Coyle J (1999). Understanding dissatisfied users: developing a framework for comprehending criticisms of healthcare work. *Journal of Advanced Nursing* **30**(3): 723–731.

40. Rogers A, Karlson S and Addington-Hall J (2000). 'All the services were excellent. It is when the human element comes in that things go wrong': dissatisfaction with hospital care in the last year of life. *Journal of Advanced Nursing* **31**(4): 768–774.

41. Sinding C (2003). Disarmed complaints: unpacking satisfaction with end-of-life care. *Social Science and Medicine* **57**(8): 1375–1385.

42. McPherson CJ and Addington-Hall JM (2004). How do proxies' perceptions of patients' pain, anxiety, and depression change during the bereavement period? *Journal of Palliative Care* **20**(1): 12–19.

43. Addington-Hall JM, Walker L, Jones C, Karlsen S and McCarthy M (1998). A randomized controlled trial of postal versus interviewer administration of a questionnaire measuring satisfaction with, and use of, services received in the year before death. *Journal of Epidemiology and Community Health* **52**(12): 802–807.

44. Vohra JU, Brazil K and Szala-Meneok K (2006). The last word: family members' descriptions of end-of-life care in long-term care facilities. *Journal of Palliative Care* **22**(1): 33–39.

45. Tashakkori A and Teddlie C (ed.) (2003). *Handbook of Mixed Methods in Social and Behavioral Research*. Thousand Oaks (CA): Sage Publications.

46. McPherson CJ and Addington-Hall JM (2003). Judging the quality of care at the end of life: can proxies provide reliable information? *Social Science and Medicine* **56**(1): 95–109.

47. Teno JM (2004). *TIME: Toolkit of Instruments to Measure End-of-Life Care*. [Online]. [Cited 2007 Apr 10]; available from: URL: http://www.chcr.brown.edu/pcoc/toolkit.htm

48. Teno JM, Clarridge B, Casey V, Edgman-Levitan S and Fowler J (2001). Validation of toolkit after-death bereaved family member interview. *Journal of Pain and Symptom Management* **22**(3): 752–758.

49. Kristjanson LJ (1993). Validity and reliability testing of the FAMCARE scale: measuring family satisfaction with advanced cancer care. *Social Science and Medicine* **36**(5): 693–701.

50. Patrick DL, Engelberg RA and Curtis JR (2001). Evaluating the quality of dying and death. *Journal of Pain and Symptom Management* **22**(3): 717–726.

51. Mystakidou K, Parpa E, Tsilika E, Kalaidopoulou O and Vlahos L. The families evaluation on management, care and disclosure for terminal stage cancer patients. *BMC Palliative Care* **1**(1): 3.

52. Volicer L, Hurley AC and Blasi ZV (2001). Scales for evaluation of end-of-life care in dementia. *Alzheimer Disease and Associated Disorders* 15(4): 194–200.

53. Jacoby A, Lecouturier J, Bradshaw C, Lovel T and Eccles M (1999). Feasibility of using postal questionnaires to examine carer satisfaction with palliative care: a methodological assessment. *Palliative Medicine* 13: 285–298.

54. Vohra JU, Brazil K, Hanna S and Abelson J. Family perceptions of end-of-life care in long term care facilities. *Journal of Palliative Care* 20(4): 297–302.

55. Cleary PD and McNeil BJ (1988). Patient satisfaction as an indicator of quality care. *Inquiry* 25(1): 25–36.

56. Avis M, Bond M and Arthur A. Questioning patient satisfaction: an empirical investigation in two outpatient clinics. *Social Science and Medicine* 44(1): 85–92.

Chapter 8

Family caregiving in hospitals and palliative care units

Betty Ferrell, Tami Borneman and Chan Thai

Introduction

This text on family caregiving addresses the many dimensions of providing physical and emotional support for a family member. The increased emphasis on family caregiving over the past decade has been prompted in large part by the shift in healthcare to the home-care setting. The focus in research and literature on home care is justified given the enormous responsibility that family members assume in managing the complex demands of chronic and terminal illness at home.

The in-patient setting and acute hospitalization, while less frequently addressed from a caregiving perspective, also offers unique demands. This chapter provides an overview of the significant challenges imposed by admission of a patient to an in-patient setting and strategies for supporting family carers in these settings.

In-patient settings of care

To illustrate the family issues related to in-patient settings, we offer three case illustrations representing the settings of medical surgical/oncology units, intensive care units and in-patient palliative care units. Viewing the experience of caregivers in these settings illuminates their needs for support.

Medical surgical or oncology units

Case 1: Mr Wertz

Mr Wertz is 78-year-old retired music teacher who has been treated for colon cancer at the University Hospital Cancer Center in Los Angeles, California (US) for the last 3 years. He has undergone surgery, chemotherapy and radiation therapy for metastatic disease but has previously been hospitalized only once for his initial surgery. Mrs Wertz (age 77), his wife of 58 years, has been his constant caregiver at home and has meticulously performed his ostomy care, met his special dietary needs and organized his extensive out-patient care. She has also worked intently to manage his multiple symptoms, including pain, constipation, frequent nausea and ongoing anxiety and depression. Mr and Mrs Wertz are of German descent and their only child, a son, was killed in combat during the war. They are intensely private and stoic, never complaining about Mr Wertz's cancer treatment.

Mr Wertz is now admitted to the in-patient oncology unit with an admission diagnosis of bowel obstruction. Further diagnostic evaluation reveals that his colon cancer has metastacized to the liver and lungs and that his bowel obstruction is almost complete. He is nauseated, in pain and febrile, and Mr Wertz's oncologist is shocked to see how much he has declined since he was last seen in the clinic 8 weeks ago. Mrs Wertz, very uncharacteristically, begins to cry and apologizes for 'failing' to care for her husband. She is exhausted and overwhelmed with the new information about his progressive disease.

Mr Wertz's oncologist does not believe that he is a candidate for surgery and implements a conservative attempt to relieve the bowel obstruction through the use of steroids, hydration and nasogastric decompression. Mr Wertz shows slight improvement over the following days, but Mrs Wertz is described by the staff as 'out of control'. She refuses to leave her husband's bedside, constantly criticizes the nursing care, persists in giving him sips of soup 'to help him get stronger', even though he is not allowed any liquids, and she often refuses care, insisting 'he just needs his rest to get well'.

Intensive care units

Case 2: Mrs Thomas

A retired school teacher, beloved wife, mother of four children and a grandmother, Mrs Thomas is a 68-year-old African American woman living in St Louis, Missouri in the US. She is an active woman whose days are filled with cooking, babysitting, extensive volunteer work and being the primary caregiver of her 90-year-old mother-in-law who has Alzheimer's and has resided with her for the past 8 years. Mrs Thomas has had mild hypertension and well-controlled diabetes, but is otherwise healthy. One morning while Mrs Thomas is gardening, she experiences severe chest pain and collapses. A neighbour finds Mrs Thomas, who is then transported to the hospital cardiac care unit, where it is determined that she has had an extensive myocardial infarction and brain anoxia resulting in neurological damage. She is on a ventilator and has remained non-responsive.

Mrs Thomas and her family are deeply religious and they hold a constant vigil in the Intensive Care Unit (ICU) waiting room, praying for a miracle. Her husband, a very quiet man, remains isolated and simply weeps at her bedside, but her three sons seem to compete for control of her care. Their anxiety and demands to 'save our mother' have resulted in numerous medical specialists called in for consultation including cardiology, pulmonology, neurology, endocrinology and nephrology.

On the eighth day of hospitalization, Mrs Thomas' daughter arrives from across the country where she has lived for the past several years. The daughter, Denise, is a nurse; she was told by her brothers over the past few days that their mother was getting better. She is shocked to find her mother in a critical condition, unresponsive and clearly with poor prognosis. Denise speaks to the cardiologist and ICU nurses, who confirm her sense that her mother will not survive. The situation was made more complex by the nephrologist who had spoken with the family earlier in the day and reported that 'things are much better', referring to Mrs Thomas' renal status, while ignoring her overall status.

A major confrontation occurs in the ICU in which Denise accuses her brothers of torturing their mother, while the sons angrily accuse Denise of 'giving up' and having no faith. Mr Thomas, embarrassed by the behaviour of his family, leaves the unit. The sons become angry at the ICU staff, believing they are siding with their sister because she is a nurse.

In-patient palliative care

Case 3: Ms O'Malley

Helene O'Malley is a 60-year-old Irish spinster living in the US who has had chronic renal failure and diabetes over the past 10 years. Four years ago she began dialysis and she has been supported by a strong network of friends and neighbours in New York City, New York. She is a lively character who has enjoyed dancing, travel and bridge; she describes herself as a 'fun-loving broad'. Over the past year, her health has declined significantly and progressive renal failure has resulted in a life limited to dialysis, frequent hospitalizations and total dependence on friends and a hired caregiver. She has been hospitalized again for dialysis complications and after extensive discussion with her physician, social worker, and a psychologist, she decides to stop dialysis. She says that she has lived a wonderful life and would like to spend her final days on the palliative care unit where she can be visited by her friends. She also insists that these years of 'clean living' have been boring and she also hopes to have time in these last days for beer and pretzels, forbidden in her strict dialysis diet in recent years.

Helene is admitted to the palliative care unit (PCU) and her care is focused on management of mild nausea, itching and progressive weakness. She is visited by her family and friends, all of whom are greatly saddened by the impending death, but are comforted to see her free of what they all have come to know of as her 'damn dialysis'. Her home caregiver/nursing assistant arranged to bring in Matilda, Helene's 12-year-old cat and the PCU staff have also arranged for telephone calls with Helene's siblings in Ireland to say goodbye.

Case commentary

As evidenced in the above studies, family carers are involved in the patient's care in many ways, and the demands and expectations of caregivers fluctuate from case to case. In the case of Mr Wertz, hospitalization results in extreme anxiety for his wife who feels helpless and out of control. The sudden transition from their life at home to the foreign hospital environment evokes intense loss for Mrs Wertz of her role as sole support for her husband and she panics at the possibility that he will not recover. How can the hospital staff benefit from the knowledge that Mrs Wertz holds regarding the intricacies of the care she has provided to Mr Wertz? On the other hand, how can the healthcare team better support the needs of Mrs Wertz as her role as a carer shifts and changes?

The case of Mrs Thomas serves as an example of the many factors that influence family dynamics in illness. Her children and spouse share their common bond of concern for her, yet each person holds a unique relationship to her. There seems to be disagreement between Mrs Thomas' family members concerning her care plan. How can the hospital staff and care team better assist this family in arriving at an agreement regarding their family member's care?

In the case of Ms O'Malley, her family carers are not blood relatives but rather a social network of friends. Yet their presence and support are vital to Ms O'Malley's final days, which will be spent in the in-patient setting. How can Ms O'Malley's family carers be incorporated into her care plan and become a part of the healthcare team that will ensure a comfortable end of life?

Each family situation presents a unique set of circumstances and different challenges to healthcare professionals. Transition into the in-patient setting is sometimes perceived as the end of the family member's role as a carer. Yet the argument has been made that admission into the in-patient setting still requires the family carer to be highly involved but in a different environment (1). Admission into the hospital is not a relinquishment of the duties of caregiving; rather it marks the renegotiation of the carer's role (2).

A fundamental issue that deserves some discussion is understanding how the family carer fits into the care setting: is the carer a resource or is the carer a recipient of care? Perhaps the family carer fits into both roles. Family carers often contribute to the provision of care to the patient, through providing direct care or by acting as a liaison between the patient and the healthcare team. Yet as the family carer becomes an integral part of the care team and the care plan, he or she also inevitably becomes a care recipient, as the burdens of caring for a family member begin to take their toll on the caregiver. Understanding this dual role the family carer can play will allow the healthcare team to better situate the family carer in the in-patient or hospital setting.

Benefits of family caregiving in in-patient settings

Family carers play an important role in supporting the hospitalized patient as exemplified in the above cases. The presence of family carers in the in-patient setting can provide many benefits for the patient and hospital staff. It is often a challenge for hospital staff and family carers to determine how the carers can best be included in the patient's care. Speice and colleagues (3) conducted a multi-institutional study in eight US cancer centres, whereby 19 focus groups (11 patient and 8 provider) were held with the purpose of examining doctor–patient communication with regard to the inclusion of family members in the patient's care. The patients ($n = 96$) were either currently receiving treatment or considered survivors. The focus groups were approximately 90 minutes in length, the questions for patients and providers at each focus-group session were similar in structure, and the sessions were audiotaped and transcribed verbatim. Results indicated three categories concerning the inclusion of family members in patient care: creating a welcoming environment; integrating family needs; and family as resources. It is this third category that is of particular relevance to the benefits that family carers can bring to the in-patient setting and from which three sub-themes emerged.

The first sub-theme was the carers' functioning as an 'extra set of ears.' Family members were helpful in clarifying information for the patient, asking questions, assisting the patient with reporting symptoms or other issues the patient may have forgotten. In the second sub-theme, family carers were a source of comfort and support to the patient. This was especially helpful when bad news was received. Third, family carers were used as a resource by patients for treatment-related decisions. They helped the patient by providing a sense of objectivity when the patient was too overwhelmed to make a decision. This study indicated that family carers can contribute positively to the hospitalization experience by acting as liaison between the patient and hospital staff by providing direct patient care and assisting in patient decision-making.

Family carer involvement in direct patient care and comfort

Family carers can provide a great deal of direct care, which can benefit the hospital staff as well as the patient. When nursing staff is limited, the family member may be willing and/or prefer to bathe the patient or provide other personal care (4). Caregiver involvement is often essential in communicating vital information, as family carers often provide clarification for information exchanged between the healthcare team and the patient. Family carers also play a vital role in making the transition from home to hospital, and back to the home, as smooth as possible, as they are able to communicate the patient's needs and facilitate the process.

As patients encounter the often sterile and highly technical hospital setting, having a family member present is very comforting. They share the journey, however long or short, bear witness to the experience, respond to the patient's needs and many times view their presence with the patient as a sign of fidelity (4). In providing comfort to the patient, the carer may in turn be comforted by the assurance that their family member is receiving the best of care, such as in a dedicated palliative care unit, where therapies are given under supervision of the palliative care team (5).

There are many intricacies of symptom management and family carers are often key experts in the control of symptoms. Family members provide rich historical data as they have been involved in the patient's comfort and titration of medications to achieve optimum relief. Carers have biographical expertise, with a detailed understanding of the likes and dislikes of the patient, their hopes and aspirations, and other knowledge that can be highly beneficial to care staff (1).

Decision-making

Family carers frequently assist the patient in making decisions and/or act as a surrogate decision-maker, supporting and upholding the patient's wishes (3, 4). Evans and colleagues (6) conducted a study evaluating reasons caregivers transferred their family member to either a hospital, in-patient hospice or a nursing home, while enrolled in hospice. Patients were transferred due to one of several reasons: acute event requiring hospitalization, uncontrolled symptoms, imminent death or issues related to safety. Although the caregivers preferred to have the patient at home, they wanted the patient to have the best care to address the issues at hand. In many respects, family carers provide much needed information and assistance in the provision of care to the patient. However, as the family carer's role increases, many obstacles arise as a result of this responsibility.

Challenges of family caregiving in in-patient settings

Caregiving in the in-patient setting presents several challenges. The most prominent among those challenges is the failure of the healthcare team and hospital staff to understand and address the needs of family carers. Within this realm are the sub-themes of lack of privacy and intimacy in the in-patient setting, and its impact on bereavement; conflicts between family carers and staff members; and the burdens of caregiving on the family carer, including physical exhaustion and economic strain.

Unmet needs of family carers

Life-threatening and chronic diseases often affect the entire family and not just the patient (7). Family members experience both physical and psychological changes in their well-being when a family member is ill. As the patient declines, his or her distress and uncontrolled symptoms can have a negative impact on the well-being and quality of life on his or her family members (8). When this occurs, family carers need the support of the healthcare team and hospital staff; often, however, this support is non-existent or found to be deficient.

In a cross-sectional, descriptive and comparative study conducted in Iceland (9), the investigators sought to understand the perceived care needs of family members of patients receiving palliative care, to what extent these needs were met, and whether needs differed based on background characteristics and site of care. They surveyed 67 family members of patients from four different acute and palliative care settings. The investigators extracted 20 key needs that were considered as important or very important by the participants, and found that, although the needs did not differ based on where the patient received palliative care services, the extent to which needs were met differed between settings. The needs of family members were more likely to be met in specialized palliative care settings (67 per cent) than on acute units, where only half (52 per cent) of perceived needs were met.

One explanation the Icelandic researchers offered for this discrepancy is that, while the acute units receive consultations from a specialized palliative care team, the day-to-day care is mostly provided by the unit staff. Healthcare workers in acute settings are ill-equipped to provide quality palliative care, as they work in settings where this is not the focus or priority of care (9). Additionally, they suggest that by the time a patient is admitted to a specialized palliative care unit, decisions about shifting from curative to palliative treatment have already been made, whereas it is usually in the acute setting that these difficult decisions are made.

Lack of privacy and intimacy, and impact on bereavement

Lack of privacy and intimacy is one of the biggest challenges to caregiving in the hospital setting. Dunne and Sullivan (10) interviewed eight family caregivers in a general hospital without the services of a palliative care team. Four themes emerged from the data: the hospital environment as a place to deliver care; needs and feelings expressed by family members; the family's experience of the patient in pain; and communication as experienced by family members. All eight family carers stated that the hospital was a poor place for their loved one to die because the environment was so rushed. They were rushed to leave soon after the death to make room for another patient. There was little to no privacy and families feared intrusion. The focus on cure in the acute care setting created a culture with no attention to palliative care, as though death never occurred.

A loss of intimacy was also found to be problematic in a study of 233 caregivers at a Southern US site and an inner-city Northeastern US site (11) that identified predictors of multiple dimensions of caregivers' subjective stress. Hawker *et al.* (12) found noise in community hospitals to be problematic for the patient and caregiver, and to be highly intrusive. While some might assume that sexuality concerns would be less important to patients with advanced disease, the recognition of life coming to an end may in fact evoke a heightened need for intimacy.

Family/staff conflict

Family/staff conflicts can occur when the patients and family members are not clearly communicating for any number of reasons. Family members may seek information from the healthcare provider to avoid talking with the patient, and dysfunctional family dynamics often divide family members and interfere with the patient's care (3). Conflicts can also occur when families fail to conform to the expected behaviour of the medical system and are therefore labelled as dysfunctional (4). Lack of communication regarding the patient's health situation is another source of conflict, possibly preventing caregivers and patients from seizing the final days or weeks of life as valuable time; it often impedes the opportunity to use time for resolving conflicts or expressing love and the opportunity to say goodbye (10, 13–14)

Burdens of caregiving

Family carers' exhaustion and burnout is well documented in the literature (11, 15–16). An interesting study by Weitzner and colleagues (16) included 267 family carers of cancer patients receiving curative treatment and 134 family carers of cancer patients receiving palliative treatment. Findings show that family carers of patients receiving palliative care have lower quality of life than family carers of cancer patients receiving curative treatment. Additionally, the carer's quality of life directly correlates with the patient's physical status.

Other caregiving factors that cause fatigue are worry, situations requiring around-the-clock care, hypervigilance, fears and lack of sleep (13, 15, 17). Professionals should address exhaustion with family members and encourage them to care for themselves during hospitalization.

According to the Family Caregiver Alliance (18), caregivers suffer many work-related problems. Two-thirds have had to rearrange their work schedule, decrease their work hours or take unpaid leave to meet their caregiver responsibilities. In a 1994 survey, 62 per cent of 1247 caregivers in the US reported having to make accommodations in their work as a direct result of caring for a family member (19)

Meehan and colleagues (20) studied 40 caregivers of autologous stem cell transplant recipients during hospitalization. Each caregiver completed a one-page survey inquiring about their time commitment and out-of-pocket expenses. Results show that caregivers travelled a median of 829 miles over 17.8 hours. Expenses for those who stayed in local accommodations ($n = 11$) were US \$849.35 (housing, gas, and food). For caregivers who stayed in the patient's room, their expenses totalled US \$181.15 (gas, food). Each caregiver who stayed in local accommodations lost a median of 43.5 hours of work and those who stayed in the patient's room lost 8 hours.

Another study by Yun *et al.* (21) analysed responses of 704 family caregivers who completed questionnaires. The carers were from six university hospitals and the National Cancer Center in Korea. As a result of the money spent on healthcare, most of the families had to move to less expensive homes, change educational plans for a member of the family or delay medical care for another family member. They found that most of the burdens of caregiving were associated with loss of family income.

Suggestions for improving family caregiving in in-patient settings

Family caregiving is undoubtedly a challenging task and is further complicated in an in-patient setting. Patients and their family carers, no longer in the comfort of their own homes, often find themselves in an unfamiliar environment that operates under a different set of rules. It is extremely important that those who understand the rules—the hospital staff and members of the palliative care team—do what they can to provide support and guidance for the family caregivers, as they redefine their roles in a hospital setting. As family carers are utilized as a resource in the care plan of the patient, they concurrently become recipients of care, as the burdens of watching their families decline may take an emotional and economic toll on them.

Family/staff communication

In order to improve the experience of the family carer, open and honest communication is essential and is frequently cited as the most important need of families. In the foreign environment of the in-patient setting, patients and their caregivers need to be constantly informed about what is going on and about the status of the patient. Patients and their family carers generally want more information, but sometimes feel too overwhelmed to ask. They need to be offered opportunities to ask questions and to have their questions answered in a language and in terms that they can comprehend and understand (22). It is therefore imperative that hospital staff be proactive about providing information and support about where to find out more information and answer questions.

The needs of patients and their carers change over time as the condition of the patient changes. Carers want information on the trajectory of the disease as this allows them to know what to expect. Dealing with the unknown or with the uncertainties of illness is often described as the most difficult aspect of the caregiving experience. In a study to assess the informational needs of patients living with advanced cancer and their family carers, Wong *et al.* (23) surveyed 144 respondents and found that, although both patients and carers cited the desire for information about the pain management, symptom management and home care services, the carers additionally cited that they wanted more information about the aetiology of the cancer and the disease trajectory.

A study conducted by Dellesega and Nolan (1) further corroborates this finding. In a study conducted on family carers involved in their family member's placement process in nursing homes in both the US and the UK, the investigators explored the issue of what would have been helpful to the carers during the admission process. Two main themes emerged: the carers cited that some form of emotional support would have been helpful and that more information regarding the institution and finances would have been beneficial.

It is the responsibility of the hospital staff and members of the care team to determine the informational needs of family carers and to provide accurate and understandable information to meet these needs. Providing written information is vital since verbal communication may be difficult to recall as family carers attempt to share the information with other family members or recall details for their own information or decision-making.

Open communication between team members is also of great importance, as this ensures that there is the same understanding of the patient's condition between all staff members and that patients and their family carers receive consistent information. The complexities of a given case can be further exacerbated if patients and their caregivers are receiving conflicting information. Hospital staff and care team members need to dedicate the time and effort to ensure that open communication is flowing between all parties involved, while keeping in mind the privacy of the patients and their families.

Family conferences

Understanding and improving communication about end-of-life care between care hospital staff and family carers is an important component to improving quality of care. Families communicate with each other differently, and research has shown that most patients and families facing end-of-life decisions want help in opening up the lines of communication about these topics (24). Holding family conferences offers an opportunity for family members to discuss their concerns with clinicians and for clinicians to better understand the concerns and needs of the family.

Each family is dealing with a unique set of circumstances and family members have vastly different communication abilities. Holding a family conference will allow for clinicians and care team members to assess the specific circumstances and communication style of each family. Although formal, planned conferences provide for the most thorough discussion and assessment, conferences will sometimes occur informally at the bedside or in the hallway. Care team members must be prepared at all times to facilitate these discussions about end-of-life issues with patients, their families and other care team members.

In a comprehensive review on the utilization of family conferences to address end-of-life issues in the ICU setting, Curtis and colleagues discuss the pivotal roles nurses, doctors and social workers play in helping families understand end-of-life issues. Care team members must be adept at communicating openly and explaining new ideas and concepts to patients and their families. They must carefully prepare ahead of time by reviewing the patient's diagnosis and medical history (25). As families respond to the rapid changes occurring around them, they need help with role transitions and decision-making. Family conferences provide a venue for these concerns to be addressed (26). Doctors, nurses, social workers and other members of the care team need to develop the listening and communication skills necessary to facilitate these meetings.

Family conferences, while recommended as a fundamental intervention in palliative care, are complex and challenging. Common mistakes include failure of all healthcare professionals to be informed about the patient's status and failure to have clear objectives for the conferences. Other problems include failing to allow adequate time for questions and discussion or planning for follow up communication. Nurses can play a vital role in helping families to understand the information provided, share the information with other family members and to be accessible to families as they make decisions following the conferences. It is also important for all professionals involved in the patient's care to know when a family conference is scheduled and for a summary of the conference to be documented on the medical record (27–29).

Family support and education

Hospitalization of a family member often leaves family carers in a state of helplessness and feeling a loss of control. Education and support programmes are effective ways to help family carers learn about the disease process, symptoms and treatment options, as well as how to care for their family member and cope with the disease process. Carers have been shown to benefit from education about disease trajectory and aetiology, as well as information about strategies to reduce pain. Furthermore, education and support programmes can serve to promote caregiver confidence and reduce helplessness (30).

Wong *et al.* surveyed advanced cancer patients and their carers ($n = 144$) about whether or not patients and their carers would attend an educational workshop (23). They found that 31 per cent of respondents replied positively, and an additional 40 per cent said they would consider attending. For those who responded tentatively, access barriers were often cited as the reasons for their uncertainty. In the overwhelming environment of the in-patient setting, caregivers may not know where or how to find information, and providing them with materials or resources can help to improve their experiences. A list of several key resources that offer information relevant to family carers can be found at the end of the chapter.

Educational interventions can also include teaching family carers self-care strategies. Carers should be encouraged to rest when needed, to share their concerns with others and to seek help when they need it. Carers have been shown to respond favourably to learning distraction and relaxation techniques, which reduce anxiety and help to promote their confidence and to reduce helplessness (30). Members of the care team should be proactive in encouraging these activities among carers and remind the carers that maintaining their own health will allow them to continue providing care for the patient.

In 2006, the Oncology Nursing Society (ONS) conducted a review of evidence on the topic of caregiver strain and burden. Their evidence review concluded that psycho-education interventions are likely to be effective, as were psychotherapy and supportive interventions. Full details on this evidence review are available on the ONS website (www.ons.org) and are summarized on the Putting Evidence into Practice (PEP) card on this topic (31). Two meta-analyses, one by Martire and colleagues (32) and one by Sorensen and colleagues (33) are cited on the PEP card. The ONS review of evidence acknowledged that most of this literature is in non-cancer populations, such as dementia, with only 10 per cent of the studies in cancer populations.

In addition to education programmes, counselling or support interventions may also help caregivers in their coping and adjustment to the in-patient setting. Counselling or group support interventions can help enhance morale, self-esteem, coping and sense of control, while reducing levels of anxiety and depression among family carers (30). By discussing their problems and fears with healthcare professionals and others facing the same issues, carers may be better able to cope with the challenges they face. There may also be carers who respond better to individual counselling, for whom staff should be prepared to offer support. Whether at the group or individual level, providing emotional support to family carers is an invaluable tool in improving the carer's experience.

In assessing the effectiveness of a support programme in New York City at Mount Sinai Medical Center's Department of Social Work Services, Dubrof and colleagues reported that when carers are engaged in psychosocial services, and when social workers make special efforts to follow up with the carers, they are better able to cope with their responsibilities and have a better understanding of how to acquire necessary resources (34).

Role of palliative care teams

Palliative care teams are the foundation of quality care in the in-patient setting. They serve as the resources for the family carer, who may be feeling overwhelmed and helpless. To provide the optimum level of support and care to patients and their families, members of the palliative care team must recognize the importance of their role as part of the care team, rather than as individual healthcare professionals. The physical, social, psychological and spiritual needs of the family carer should be assessed and supported by all members of the team.

Each team member brings a different perspective to the table, and each member has a role to play in meeting the needs of carers. Physicians offer information about the disease and its symptoms. Nurses, who have the most direct contact with the patients and their family carers, can integrate carers into the care plan and serve to reinforce education efforts. Social workers can provide information relating to financial difficulties, counselling services and other resources carers may need. Chaplains can meet with the family and determine the role of spirituality and religion within the family and provide the counselling or guidance necessary to address spiritual concerns (30).

Palliative care teams should meet frequently to discuss and exchange new information regarding each family. In the hospital setting, developments unfold at a rapid rate, and optimum support can only be provided when all team members have an accurate understanding of the patient and family carer's situation. Teams should set up a system to ensure that all team members receive up-to-date information about each patient as new developments occur. Additionally, teams should reach a consensus about prognosis and a care plan before sharing it with families to ensure consistency.

Summary

This chapter has reviewed some of the unique challenges imposed by the in-patient setting for family carers of the chronically or seriously ill. While most family caregiving literature and research has focused on the home environment, and justifiably so given the burden of care assumed by families, there are also challenges in the hospital setting.

Care delivered in the in-patient setting that includes clear communication between staff and family can offer relief and bereavement support. The in-patient setting is often a place of serious decision-making, as the goals of care shift and families consider decisions about disease-focused care versus palliative care. There are opportunities to help families in navigating these pivotal decisions. Referring back to the case study of Mr Wertz, the care team and hospital staff members can provide a tremendous amount of support to Mrs Wertz by educating her and guiding her through the disease process. As she has been the sole carer for her husband, she has come to understand his illness and her role as his carer in a certain way. Yet Mr Wertz's disease has clearly progressed, and Mrs Wertz needs the correct information and support to understand and cope with this change.

A key intervention in the in-patient setting is a well-orchestrated family conference. Coordination of the interdisciplinary team and family perspectives is vital to preserving patient goals of care and supporting the family. In the case of Mrs Thomas, there is a discrepancy between her family members in the understanding of her disease trajectory. In this case, it would be extremely beneficial to hold a family conference, where all of the family members and all the members of the care team can sit together to clarify the status of the patient and the disease so that the family members can ask questions to acquire the appropriate knowledge to make the most informed decision with regard to the next step.

In the case of Ms O'Malley, where the decision has been made to focus on palliative treatment rather than curative treatment, the emphasis should be placed on how best to provide the support needed for a comfortable and dignified death. It is often in the setting of a palliative care unit where the fundamental principles of palliative care can be best applied and adhered to and where patient and carer needs are most frequently met.

Key learning points

◆ Family carers face unique challenges imposed by admission of a patient to an in-patient setting.

◆ The Intensive Care Unit is an especially stressful environment for family carers.

◆ Family carers often experience a sense of helplessness and a loss of control during hospitalization.

◆ Strategies that enhance professional-caregiver communication are essential during hospitalization.

Recommended reading and resources

Caregiver Resource Directory. http://www.netofcare.org/crd/resource_form.asp

Carers Alliance. http://www.carers.org.au/index.html

Confederation of Family Organizations in the European Union (COFACE): Charter for Family Carers. http://www.coface-eu.org/en/basic435.html

Curtis JR and Rubenfeld GD (2001). *Managing Death in the Intensive Care Unit. The Transition from Cure to Comfort.* New York City: Oxford University Press.

Education in Palliative and End-of-Life Care Project (EPEC). http://www.epec.net/EPEC/webpages/index.cfm

End-of-Life Nursing Education Consortium (ELNEC). http://www.aacn.nche.edu/elnec/

Medical Ethics Committee of the British Medical Association (1998). *Withholding and Withdrawing Life-Prolonging Medical Treatment. Guidance for Decision Making.* London: BMJ Books, BMA House, 84.

National Family Caregivers Association (NFCA). http://www.nfcacares.org/

National Family Carer Network. http://www.familycarers.org.uk/

Nolan M, Lundh U, Grant G and Keady J (2003). *Partnerships in Family Care: Understanding the Caregving Career.* Berkshire, England: Open University Press.

References

1. Dellasega C and Nolan M (1997). Admission to care: facilitating role transition amongst family carers. *Journal of Clinical Nursing* 6: 443–451.
2. Anehensel CS, Pearly LI, Mullan JT, Zarit SU and Whitlach CJ (1995). *Profiles in CARE-GIVING: the unexpected career.* Academic Press, San Diego.

3. Speice J, Harkness J, Laneri H, Frankel R, Roter D, Kornblith AB, Ahles T, Winer E, Fleishman S, Luber P, Zevon M, McQuellon R, Trief P, Finkel J, Spira J, Greenberg D, Rowland J and Holland JC (2000). Involving family members in cancer care: focus group considerations of patients and oncological providers. *Psychooncology* **9**(2): 101–112.

4. Levine C and Zuckerman C (2004). The trouble with families: toward an ethic of accommodation. In: Levine C (ed.). *Always on Call: When Illness Turns Families into Caregivers*. Nashville (TN): Vanderbilt University Press. 147–148.

5. Fischberg D and Meier D (2003). Hospital-based palliative care. In: Morrison S, Meier D and Capello C (ed.). *Geriatric Palliative Care*. New York: Oxford University Press. 402–412.

6. Evans WG, Cutson TM, Steinhauser, KE and Tulsky JA. Is there no place like home? Caregivers recall reasons for and experience upon transfer from home hospice to in-patient facilities. *Journal of Palliative Medicine* **9**(1): 100–110.

7. Kristjanson LJ and Ashcroft T (1994). The family's cancer journey: a literature review. *Cancer Nursing* **17**: 1–17.

8. Borneman T, Chu DZ, Wagman L, Ferrell B, Juarez G, McCahill LE and Uman G (2003). Concerns of family caregivers of patients with cancer facing palliative surgery for advanced malignancies. *Oncology Nursing Forum* **30**: 997–1005.

9. Fridriksdottir N, Sigurdardottir V and Gunnarsdottir S. Important needs of families in acute and palliative care settings assessed with the Family Inventory of Needs. *Palliative Medicine* **20**: 425–432.

10. Dunne K and Sullivan K (2000). Family experiences of palliative care in the acute hospital setting. *International Journal of Palliative Nursing* **6**(4): 170–178.

11. Gaugler JE, Hanna N, Linder J, Given CW, Tolbert V, Kataria R and Regine WF(2005). Cancer caregiving and subjective stress: a multi-site, multi-dimensional analysis. *Psychooncology* **14**(9): 771–785.

12. Hawker S, Kerr C, Payne S, Seamark D, Davis C, Roberts H, Jarrett N, Roderick P and Smith H (2006). End-of-life care in community hospitals: the perceptions of bereaved family members. *Journal of Palliative Medicine* **20**(5): 541–547.

13. Ferrall S (2006). Caring for the family caregiver. In: Carroll-Johnson RM, Gorman L and Bush NJ (ed.). *Psychosocial Nursing Care Along the Cancer Continuum* (2nd edn). Pittsburgh: Oncology Nursing Society. 603–610.

14. Prendergast T (2007). Palliative care in the intensive care unit setting. In: Berger A, Shuster J and Von Roenn J (ed.). *Principles and Practice of Palliative Care and Supportive Oncology* (3rd edn). Philadelphia: Lippincott Williams & Wilkins. 849–868.

15. Gaston-Johansson F, Lachica EM, Fall-Dickson JM and Kennedy MJ (2004). Psychological distress, fatigue, burden of care, and quality of life in primary caregivers of patients with breast cancer undergoing autologous bone marrow transplantation. *Oncology Nursing Forum* **31**(6): 1161–1169.

16. Weitzner MA, McMillan SC and Jacobsen PB (1999). Family caregiver quality of life: differences between curative and palliative cancer treatment settings. *Journal of Pain and Symptom Management* **17**(6): 418–428.

17. Schumacher KL (1996). Reconceptualizing family caregiving: family-based illness care during chemotherapy. *Research Nursing and Health* **19**(4): 261–271.

18. Family Caregiver Alliance (homepage on the internet) (2007). *Fact Sheet: Selected Caregiver Statistics*. Retrieved April 3, 2007.

19. Hunt G (2004). Caregiving and the workplace. In: Levine C (ed.). *Always on Call: When Illness Turns Families into Caregivers*. Nashville (TN): Vanderbilt University Press. 101–112.

20. Meehan KR, Fitzmaurice T, Root L, Kimtis E, Patchett L and Hill J. The financial requirements and time commitments of caregivers for autologous stem cell transplant recipients. *Journal of Supportive Oncology* **4**(4): 187–190.

21. Yun YH, Rhee YS, Kang IO, Lee JS, Bang SM, Lee WS, Kim JS, Kim SY, Shin SW and Hong YS (2005). Economic burdens and quality of life of family caregivers of cancer patients. *Oncology* **68**(2–3): 107–114.

22. Davies B (2006). Supporting families in palliative care. In: Ferrell BR and Coyle N (ed.). *Textbook of Palliative Nursing*. New York: Oxford University Press. 545–560.

23. Wong RS, Franssen E, Szumacher E, Connolly R, Evans M, Page B, Chow E, Hayter C, Harth T, Andersson L, Pope J and Danjoux C (2002). What do patients living with advanced cancer and their carers want to know? *Support Care Cancer* **10**: 408–415.

24. Singer PA, Martin DK and Kelner M. Quality end-of-life care: patients' perspectives. *The Journal of the American Medical Association* **281**: 163–168.

25. Curtis JR, Patrick DL, Shannon SE, Treece PD, Engelberg RA and Rubenfeld GD (2001). The family conference as a focus to improve communication about end-of-life care in the intensive care unit: opportunities for improvement. *Critical Care Medicine* **29**(Supplement 2): N26–33.

26. King DA and Quill T. Working with families in palliative care: one size does not fill all. *Journal of Palliative Medicine* **9**(3): 704–715.

27. Lautrette A, Ciroldi M, Ksibi H and Azoulay E. End-of-life family conferences: rooted in evidence. *Critical Care Medicine* **34**(Supplement 11): S364–S372.

28. McDonagh JR, Elliott TB, Engleberg RA, Treece PD, Shannon SE, Ruben feld GD, Patrictc DL and Curtis JR (2004). Family satisfaction with family conferences about end-of-life care in the intensive care unit: Increased proportion of family speech is associated with increased satisfaction. *Critical Care Medicine* **32**(7): 1484–1488.

29. Curtis JR, Engelberg RA, Wenrich MD Melsen EL, Shannon SE, Treece PD, Tonelli MR, Patrick DL, Robins LS, McGrath BB, and Rubenfeld GD (2002). Studying communication about end-of-life care during the family conference: development of a framework. *Journal of Critical Care* **17**(3): 147–160.

30. Glajchen M (2004). The emerging role and needs of family caregivers in cancer care. *Journal of Supportive Oncology* **2**(2): 145–155.

31. Oncology Nursing Society (2007). Caregiver Strain and Burden. Accessed on September 1, 2007 <http://www.ons.org/outcomes/volume2/caregiver.shtml>

32. Martire LM, Lustig AP, Schulz R, Miller GE and Helgeson VS (2004). Is it beneficial to involve a family member? A meta-analysis of psychosocial interventions for chronic illness. *Health Psychology* **23**: 599–611.

33. Sorensen S, Pinquart M and Duberstein P. How effective are interventions with caregivers? An updated meta-analysis. *Gerontologist* **42**: 356–372.

34. Dubrof J, Ebenstein H, Dodd SJ and Epstein I (2006). Caregivers and professionals partnership caregiver resource center: assessing a hospital support programme for family caregivers. *Journal of Palliative Medicine* **9**(1): 196–205.

Chapter 9

Family caregiving in the home

Kelli Stajduhar and Robin Cohen

Introduction

It is increasingly evident that family members play an important role in the provision of home healthcare. Programmes to support patients and their carers continue to expand worldwide, as more patients wish to spend their dying days at home (1). An essential component to enable this wish to be fulfilled is the availability of a family carer who is willing and able to take on the responsibility for care of the patient at home (2). Research has confirmed there are numerous risks to carers when they assume the caregiving role, including sleep deprivation (3), depression and anxiety (4), and economic consequences related to the out-of-pocket costs (1, 5). Despite the risks, many family members continue to provide palliative care at home because of a desire to do so and/or because cutbacks in the healthcare system are placing more responsibilities on family members (6, 7). Clinicians working with dying patients and their families therefore require knowledge about how to best support home-based carers. This chapter provides a synthesis of the literature on the impact to family members when they provide care to an individual dying at home and makes recommendations about strategies that might help in supporting family carers in their roles.

Setting the context: factors influencing dying at home

A number of conditions need to be in place to most effectively support dying at home. Foremost, there needs to be a desire on the part of the patient, to be cared for at home (2). Population surveys have established that the majority of people would prefer to be cared for at home and to die at home (8). At the same time, one of the consistently reported predictors of dying at home is the availability of a carer (9, 10). Many carers agree to provide care willingly, whereas others do so out of a sense of duty or obligation (7). What is clear, however, is that the family member's desire to provide home care is required to affect the desired outcome (2).

Other factors to support family caregiving include adequate support from the healthcare system (7, 11), ideally with 24-hour access to service (12, 13), the availability of more than one carer, especially if the carer is elderly and if the patient has been sick for several weeks or months (2, 14), and having adequate financial resources, even when the state pays for healthcare (15). The patient's functional status is a significant factor in location of care (16, 17), as well as pain and other intractable symptoms, which often necessitate hospitalization (18). Therefore, access to specialized home palliative care services, such as symptom management, has been found to increase the likelihood of people dying at home (19, 20).

The number of hospital beds available in a community has also been found to influence the location of dying (21). That is, the more hospital beds available, the more people die in hospital. This information, however, should not be interpreted as people inappropriately dying in hospital. It is possible that patients may spend most of their time at home but desire or need to spend their last days in hospital. Alternatively, when hospital beds are available and adequate home care services are not available, people who would like to die at home may have to go to hospital to receive the healthcare they need.

Profile on family carers in the home and the people they care for

Studies show the average age of people who die at home, and those who care for them, is about 60 (22–26), though some studies report age ranges for patients in the seventies (23, 26); however, the importance of the patient's and carer's age is unclear (11, 19, 27).

In general, studies indicate that males are more likely to die at home and, accordingly, the majority of carers are women, since most carers are the spouse (19, 22–26). Estimates suggest that 68–77 per cent of carers are female (28, 29), though the numbers of male carers may be increasing due to a variety of social demographic factors (30, 31). Home care for the dying occurs more frequently when the patient lives with a spouse or partner (22, 24, 26). However, when patients have a non-cancer diagnosis, support from children is more important than the presence of a spouse (19). When the patient is female, their care is provided predominately by their daughters or daughters-in-law (26).

Few studies report the education levels of family carers. Studies investigating the relationship between socioeconomic status, education levels and home-based palliative care, show that cancer patients who have higher education or who live in higher socioeconomic neighbourhoods are most likely to die at home (32–34). Approximately one-third of carers are employed while caregiving (23), and many of them stop working temporarily or decrease their paid work to provide home care (23, 24). Grande *et al.* (1998) reported that individuals with a cancer diagnosis and a higher socioeconomic status were more likely to utilize specialized and intensive home care and die at home (19). This relationship with socioeconomic status was not apparent among the non-cancer palliative population.

Finally, some research suggests dying at home occurs more often for people with a cancer diagnosis than for people with a non-cancer diagnosis (26); however, Fried *et al.* (1999) did not find significant differences between these groups (27). For non-cancer diagnoses, Grande *et al.* (1998) reported that dying at home was more prevalent among patients in the UK who had heart disease and other vascular diseases than for individuals with cerebrovascular disease, pneumonia and influenza (19). In the same review, the authors also found that patients with gastrointestinal and genitourinary cancers were more likely to die at home than those with haematological cancers. By contrast, Gomes and Higginson (2006) found that a diagnosis related to non-solid tumours was most strongly associated with dying at home (11).

The roles of home-based palliative carers

In addition to their usual roles, there are new roles that carers take on, including roles that were previously those of the patient. This creates the potential for extra physical, emotional and social workload, in addition to time-management pressures. The situation can be complicated by the fact that in many cultures, roles are strongly defined as belonging to people in a certain position within the family, within the community, of a certain gender or in other ways. If carers do not fall within the category of people who are accepted in a role they must now take on, a layer of emotional and social complexity may be added. These different community and family cultures must interact closely with the healthcare system, itself a culture containing many sub-cultures (35).

There are many ways to identify the various roles of carers; here, we list only some of them. It must be remembered that in most cases all roles related to maintaining the household, including childcare, eldercare, pet care and, in some cases, employment are, sooner or later, required to be fulfilled by the carer.

- ◆ Physical care (35):
  - help with activities of daily living, including intimate tasks such as bathing and toileting;
  - wound prevention and management (turning, applying moisturizers/barrier creams);
  - re-positioning for comfort; lifting and transferring the patient.

- Symptom control (24, 35, 36):
  - often more than one symptom at a time is being managed;
  - constant assessment;
  - treatment including preparing medications, giving medications, distraction, heat, massage and others;
  - re-assessment, including whether professional help is required;
  - proxy reporter to the healthcare team, regarding the patient's symptom and well-being.

- Emotional support for the patient (35):
  - without constant in-patient support from the palliative care team, the patient's emotional needs must be satisfied by the carers;
  - when there is only one carer, this role can be difficult to fulfill;
  - carers have the advantage of knowing the patient; however, they also have their own emotional needs;
  - there is potential for harm where relationships between patient and carer are strained.

- Spokesperson, advocate and proxy decision maker roles:
  - carers who take on roles as spokesperson for the patient and perhaps the family (37), as proxy decision-maker (35, 37) and patient advocate (35, 38) may not be comfortable with the role;
  - some carers need to act as a buffer between the patient and other family members, such as children (38), particularly in relation to information sharing;
  - the balance between autonomy and safety can be difficult for some carers, particularly when the patient is at risk (38, 39).

- Practical and social support:
  - carers at home have an important role in preparing meals (35), attending to laundry and ensuring recreational and social activities are appropriate;
  - carers are often the liaison between the patient and other family and friends (38, 40);
  - management of social gatherings can often place the family carer in conflict with those from whom support is needed;
  - organizing the social calendar can be an exhausting and unfamiliar role for some carers.

- Coordinator of care:
  - managing appointments and healthcare provision (35), as well as keeping records of tests and reporting same to the healthcare team, are common carer tasks (35, 38);
  - pre-death and post-death planning, including funeral arrangements can be burdensome, especially for those unfamiliar with the processes;
  - although help may be available, ultimately much of the planning is left to the carer, who may be already being emotionally and physically vulnerable.

Given all these roles, it is easy to understand that carers are often strained and stressed. They experience what many people call burdens. However, depending on their attitude towards caring, they may not perceive these roles as a burden and may, in fact, find caregiving beneficial. Many carers experience both benefits and burdens.

Benefits, demands and known health outcomes of palliative caregiving

Much research has focused on the benefits, demands and health outcomes of palliative caregiving. Benefits include the sense of life-enrichment and accomplishment in fulfilling the wishes of the dying person (7, 24), opportunities to find meaning in the situation, to share intimate times with the dying person and to give something back to the person they are caring for (7). The 'home' constitutes a site where people feel most comfortable and where they are at liberty to be themselves (41). As such, at-home caregiving promotes a sense of freedom and control that is not accorded in institutional settings, and helps sustain relationships with family and friends (42). At least four conditions seem to contribute to a positive caregiving experience in the home (7, 43, 44):

- the decision for home care was negotiated between the patient and carer;
- the carer felt their needs were given equal consideration to those of the patient;
- carers felt respected for their caregiving knowledge and contributions to the healthcare system; and
- they felt they had adequately met the patient's needs.

Along with the benefits, carers also experience a number of demands, identified (above) in the various roles undertaken by carers. Physical demands are rivalled by psychosocial demands, including feelings of isolation, helplessness, anger, anxiety, resentment, guilt and a sense of inadequacy (39, 45). Social demands, including restrictions on time and freedom, uncertainty about the timing and manner of death, and difficulties with decision-making, are also commonly experienced by carers (6, 46). Many carers are overwhelmed by the complexity and amount of information required, putting them at risk for mental fatigue and burnout (39, 47). In addition, a loss of privacy in the home is common (7, 24, 48). Visitors, including families from 'out of town', numerous clinicians and home health aides, can erode the intimate times that carer and patient need together before the patient dies. Privacy can also be compromised by other factors such as having a hospital bed in the living room. Many carers also bear the strain and grief themselves rather than burdening the patient (38, 39).

Issues of financial hardship are evident in over 25 per cent of all carers (39, 45, 49). While some countries have adopted palliative benefits programmes providing partial financial aid to families in palliative care (50), at present such programmes are not universal, nor are they adequate.

The physical, psychosocial and economic demands placed on at-home carers have been linked to negative health outcomes, leaving them at risk for physical and mental illness (45, 51–53), weight loss subsequent to reduced appetite (48, 53), depression and anxiety (4). The risk of mortality for carers experiencing emotional and mental strain is increased by 63 per cent compared to non-carer controls matched by age and sex (54). According to reports of hospice care in the US, this increased risk is reduced if the carers receive palliative care at home (55).

Clearly, the benefits, demands and health outcomes associated with caregiving at home can influence the quality of life of carers. For this reason, understanding the needs of at-home carers and the strategies that may effectively support them is of utmost importance.

The needs of home-based palliative carers

Carers' needs that, according to the literature, must be satisfied in order to prevent problems occurring, are summarized below.

+ Physical:
  - strength to transfer the patient from bed to chair, and to lift and turn the patient in bed (40, 45);
  - adequate sleep (36, 49, 51, 53, 56);
  - appetizing food and protected time and atmosphere to eat properly;

- safety and security in the home, for both the patient and the carer;
- practical support with, for example, providing care to the patient, transportation of the patient, special meal preparation, doing extra laundry, etc. (36, 38, 45);
- education regarding safe procedures for caring for the patient; for example, lifting, transferring, changing bed sheets, hygienic practices, etc. (35, 38, 45).

- ◆ Psychosocial:
  - psychologically adapt to providing intimate care for the patient, which may be especially difficult for children of the opposite sex caring for a parent (35, 48);
  - recognition for their efforts and experience by family and friends (7);
  - supports to prevent social isolation (36, 39, 40);
  - assistance in dealing with past strongly negative experiences with the patient; for example, abuse;
  - conflict resolution, where family or patient's quality of life is impaired;
  - privacy with spouse and children if the patient is neither of these (24);
  - prevention and/or early treatment for depression and anxiety;
  - time to adapt to the role of carer—since the role is often changing rapidly, this should be considered an ongoing process, with extra help available as the carer adjusts to new circumstances (37).

- ◆ Cognitive:
  - assistance in preparing for complex cognitive tasks, such as organizing healthcare, patient treatments at home, complex medication administration;
  - mental breaks and respite from the illness, and, for some, from the patient (51, 58);
  - recognition that cognitive problems can arise from extreme fatigue (48).

- ◆ Financial—here we have listed some common costs created by the caregiving situation (7, 40, 45, 56, 57, 59), which may or may not be covered by the state, depending on the country in which one lives:
  - medical, nursing, physiotherapy, home healthcare aides and other care as needed in the home;
  - medications;
  - modifications to the home required for patient mobility and/or safety;

- equipment such as mobility aids, commode, hospital bed, etc.;
- clothes that fit a thinner body;
- diapers;
- extra bed sheets;
- parking at medical appointments or other transportation costs (48);
- adjusting to temporary loss of own income (45, 56) and the patient's income.

◆ Formal/Informal support:
  - acknowledging the carer's primary concern that they will suffer if the patient is suffering (36, 48, 56);
  - acknowledging that carers who evaluate the patient's healthcare as worse are more often depressed (29);
  - effective communication and continuity of care both from within the healthcare system and from family and friends;
  - helping the carer to ask for help, and how to organize help most effectively

Carer needs are, of course, individual and require careful assessment. First, it is clear that most carers do not view themselves as legitimate care recipients (44, 45). Meeting the needs of the patients they are caring for is their top priority (56). Most carers will resist any attempt to help them if they perceive that this will take attention or resources away from the patient. Therefore, carers must be reassured that everything possible is being done for the patient, and that any care they receive is, indirectly, likely to benefit the patient. For example, if patients' hospitalization due to carers' burnout can be prevented, patients might be able to stay at home longer, or even to die at home, thereby fulfilling their wish. Preventing disabling anxiety and depression in home carers will also help the patient as relationships are an important determinant of palliative care patient quality of life (60). Second, carer needs change over time and must be frequently re-assessed by a professional healthcarer with specialized training in palliative care from one or more of various professions (e.g. medicine; nursing; occupational therapy; physiotherapy; psychology; social work).

Table 9.1, taken from King and Quill (2006), provides a useful prompt for assessing family needs and roles (37).

Ethical issues and caregiving in the home

Several ethical issues arise related to caregiving in the home; a brief overview is given here and the interested reader is referred to Arras (61) for greater detail.

Table 9.1 Questions to assess family needs and roles

Question	Targeted family function	Purpose
Tell me the story of (patient's) illness … e.g., How diagnosed?, What happened next?	Communication	Open communication Assessing family perspective
How did each of you learn about/respond to the news of the diagnosis? Is there anyone important to (patient) who does not know?	Communication, attachment bonds	Identify patterns of communication, assess strength of attachment bonds Increase communication
What is your relationship with (patient) like? (if patient unable to participate)	Attachment bonds	Assess strength of attachment bonds
What was (patient) like before he/she got sick? What do you think (patient) would want under these circumstances? (if patient unable to participate)	Communication, attachment bonds	Increase communication, assess and reinforce bonds of attachment, create shared vision of patient's values and preferences
How are big decisions made in your family? Does anyone take the lead in … decision-making, caregiving?	Problem-solving/ decision-making	Identify patterns of decision-making, identify family roles
We all want what is best for (patient), but it is natural to have some areas of agreement/ disagreement as to what should be done. What things do you all agree should be done for (patient)? What are your areas of disagreement? (If patient unable to participate: What do you think (patient) would want?)	Problem-solving/ decision-making	Identify common ground among family members, explore differences of opinion, remind family of need to focus on patient's preferences and values

King DA and Quill T (2006). Working with families in palliative care: One size does not fit all. *J Palliat Med* **9**, 704–715. Reproduced with permission.

The first ethical question that arises from patients' stated preference to die at home in comfort (8) is: Who decides that care at the end of life should be given at home, in any individual case? If there is a lack of institutional health-care resources, either because of a shortage or because of cost required to the family, then it is the state that in fact makes the 'decision' by limiting options. Similarly, if excellent institutional resources are available, but support at home is negligible, then, except in cases that are straightforward, staying home in comfort is not a real option (7). Therefore, the question that needs to be addressed is: How much of the care required by a person at the end of life should be provided by the state, and how much is the responsibility of the family? (35).

When resources permit a true choice of either being cared for at home or in an institution, should the carer be part of a decision-making process? If it is the patient's home, does he or she have a right to determine the location of care regardless of carer constraints or other factors? If the patient has such a right, is it absolute or can it be constrained by the need to consider others' needs and expectations? What factors might impinge on the safety of a person living alone who might be a hazard to themselves, their carers or others? Fortunately, the decision about location of care can usually be made on the basis of comprehensive information, together with appropriate review, if and when the situation of either the patient or the carer changes (7).

In addition to the patient and the carer, others will be affected by the decision of location of care; for example, others living in the same house as both the patient and the carer. Grown children living on their own may also be affected. The traditional nuclear family, consisting of a mother and father and children who are a product of their marriage (whether biological or adopted) represents a diminishing part of the social landscape in many countries. Other scenarios might include the following: a new spouse and relationships with the patient's children from a previous marriage, the role of the former spouse in the patient's life, relationships with other family members, the presence of a lover, and access for others who want to visit during a stressful time. While sometimes all of the various families and friends connected to the patient get along well, in many cases important emotional issues will arise that are heightened in the home situation rather than on more neutral ground, where visits can be staggered and the patient can have more control, if desired.

Strategies to support home-based palliative carers

Because carers often focus all their attention on the patient, thereby neglecting their own health (24, 36, 44, 53), they may not be perceived as needing support by the healthcare system (62). Strategies are therefore needed to maximize the benefits of caregiving and minimize the negative health outcomes.

Strategies to support carers' preferences and needs

Carers' perceptions of, and response to, their role vary (7, 44); strategies are needed to ensure carers' preferences and needs are considered in addition to those of the patient. Consideration of expectations and constraints ought to be a part of any discussions about home-based palliative care, including the positive aspects of caregiving as well as the likely physical and psychosocial strains, the possibility of having to forgo employment and other pursuits outside the home, supports available from the healthcare system, and the impact of healthcare provider visits on family privacy. If carers are excluded from decision-making, it is likely to increase their frustration, isolation, and distress (63).

Healthcare workers can also support carers by acknowledging that caregiving is not always a clear choice—they should not feel obligated or pressured (4, 7) and they have the right to change their minds. The decision should be negotiated and re-negotiated between the patient and the carer. This should be initiated early in the disease trajectory to prevent carers from making unrealistic promises, to alert patients and carers that intentions to care may be influenced over time as the disease progresses and/or the patient becomes more debilitated. Clinicians may need to help facilitate discussions between the carer and patient, as even though terminal illness can make the relationship between carer and patient closer, it may also become strained (24, 58), making such sensitive conversations difficult.

Strategies to help carers continue to care if they wish to do so

Carers have reported they need someone to talk to (6) but have difficulty expressing their needs (64). When clinicians develop collaborative relationships with carers they are better able to cope with their demands and feel a sense of purpose in their role. Careful listening to, and empathy with, the carer is important, as well as a perception that carers are known by the clinicians involved. Emanuel and colleagues (2000) found that carers who reported that their physician had listened to their concerns and opinions about the patient's illness were less likely to be depressed (49) and the more effective the emotional support the less prone they were to fatigue and burnout (39). Importantly, carers need to feel reassured that the care they are giving at home is equal to the quality of care in the hospital (38, 56), that everything possible is being done and that they are respected for their knowledge of the patient and the patient's specific circumstances (7, 40, 57). Ideally, arrangements should be made to speak with the carer without the patient being present, to enable the carer to be candid about expressing their needs (24, 39).

A number of more pragmatic strategies can help carers to continue in their role; these include the need to remain healthy themselves, the need to adapt to the fact that their family member is dying (37) and the time needed to rest and replenish their energy so they can clearly think through the many complex decisions that their role entails. Clinicians can help carers work toward caring for themselves by identifying family goals. What do they hope for? What are their expectations of their experience, of clinicians and of the healthcare system? What is achievable and realistic to accomplish? Unrealistic expectations should be discouraged; however, hope should not be bluntly destroyed, for example, by statistics that are unlikely to be meaningful on an individual basis (47). Clinicians can also help carers achieve their goals by finding out which aspects of care they are comfortable with, and the situations for which they need further advice, education, support or referral to another agency.

Research suggests that carers feel ill prepared for the level of responsibility, the unpredictable nature of the work they are undertaking, and the physical and psychological impact of their role (24). They want to understand (7):

+ how the patient's disease will progress;
+ the health services available to support them; and
+ the pros and cons of providing care at home.

Preparatory, individualized information should be given in the right amount and at the right time so that information does not become burdensome (6); for example, information about the disease, symptoms, treatment, death and what will happen following the death (7, 36, 58). Such information helps the carer to manage problems as they arise. Information may be made available through written material, via telephone 24 hours a day 7 days a week (35), or at an internet site where reliable information is available in a way that is easy to find., such as the Canadian Virtual Hospice (www.virtualhospice.ca).

Prevention of social isolation is also important (36, 39, 40). Extended family and friends can be a good source of support but organization of visitors should be such that they come at the best time for the patient and carer. Visitors all at once can be overwhelming, while one at a time can mean visitors all day (58). Clinicians can help carers manage these situations by encouraging the development of house rules and expectations that will help everyone live together during a stressful period. When face-to-face visiting is not an option, carers can be encouraged to stay connected to others by telephone or by individual and/or group email (40). On-line support groups with carers going through similar situations may also be helpful for those who have limited time for more active engagement.

The limited literature on family carer interventions (for an in-depth review, see Harding and Higginson 2003) suggests there may be specific interventions that are feasible and acceptable to use with carers, but much of the research in this area is limited by a lack of focus on effectiveness and methodological inconsistencies and shortcomings (65, 66). Nevertheless, there is a small body of research suggesting that specific interventions may contribute to reductions in burden and stress, increased confidence, problem-solving and satisfaction with care (65). Respite services and particular services conceptualized as respite, like massage therapy, have been shown to decrease levels of emotional and physical stress in a small sample of carers (67, 68). Specialized services such as palliative nursing care up to 24 hours daily (69) or hospice care (70) have been shown to enhance carers' satisfaction with care and reduce anxiety (70). A review of the literature on palliative care teams showed that, in general, they led to increases in satisfaction with care, decreased hospitalization, decreases in costs of care (one study) and increased or maintenance of quality of life (71). These studies, however, did not solely focus on carers. As Ingleton and colleagues point out, the views of carers are frequently sought, but as proxies for patients rather than in their own right (66).

More recently, evaluation of a group intervention aimed to address the informational needs of carers of palliative care patients at home suggests that the carers found the group to be supportive and increased their knowledge (72). A brief intervention designed to improve the problem-solving abilities of carers of people with advanced cancer found an increase in positive problem-solving strategies, confidence in the ability to provide care and a decrease in emotional tension (73).

Strategies to improve healthcare systems to support carers in their roles

The healthcare system and its providers play a crucial role in supporting palliative carers; however, improvements are still needed to enhance the quality of healthcare provided to families at the end of life (44). In most Westernized countries, the delivery of palliative care in the home is seen as a way of creating a more normal environment for care to occur and to address the lack of available in-patient palliative beds (1). Such moves are welcomed because, with the exception of specialized palliative care wards, in-patient care has been characterized by carers as depersonalized and highly problematic (44).

Although palliative home care is often seen as the 'gold standard', the reality is that not all families are able to achieve a home death or allow the patient to remain at home for lengthy periods before they die. In such cases, consideration should be given to expanding alternate care settings, such as free-standing hospices or long-term palliative care units, so that carers who can no longer continue to care, are provided with legitimate options. For those patients who must be in an in-patient setting, efforts to continually improve hospital care are needed.

Respite care has often been proposed as a way of helping carers get a break from the caregiving situation. However, careful assessment is required to ensure the type of respite meets the carer's needs (51, 65, 66). Many carers report that what they need is a mental break from being a carer, where, for a period of time, their life does not revolve around the patient's illness, or where they can spend time with a spouse or other significant other, without needing to give care (24, 49). Allowing the carer to define what respite might mean for them is the best approach, providing the potential for individual needs to be met.

One of the biggest challenges home carers face within the healthcare system is discontinuity of care (7); numerous studies have highlighted problems with continuity of care at the end life (40). Strategies to enhance continuity include those that ensure:

- Care between home, out-patient clinics and hospital is well-coordinated (7, 36, 40, 57, 58).

- Information and communication systems are in place that minimize the number of times that carers have to repeat the same information to clinicians.

- The carer is given the required information to manage the system, or someone is assigned to help the carer manage the system (patient navigator). This includes knowing, in advance of need, what services are available under what conditions (36, 38, 57).

- Home care services are arranged for maximum consistency of personnel attending each patient/carer dyad (7, 24, 40, 57).

Future research and clinical priorities

At this point we know much about the average carer in Western societies, but there are few studies testing interventions to help them with these known needs. Rigorous testing of existing interventions and services, development and testing of new ones, and discovering which works best for whom, represent some of the priorities for future research. Testing the effectiveness of interventions includes evaluating both the costs and the savings. Savings may be obtained through reduced hospitalization of the patient, reduced use of healthcare during bereavement and, perhaps, fewer days of work lost during bereavement if the carer is employed. Benefits to the carer should be measured not only while caring but also in the bereavement period. To date, studies of the effect of palliative care and hospice teams on carers at home suggest a small improvement in carer satisfaction with the care provided. However, study limitations are numerous and the true effectiveness of such services is not yet known (71).

Health service research is also needed to determine how to best integrate care for the carer into the system, which is presently not designed to address their needs. Should a separate dossier be opened for the carer, or should they be part of the patient's dossier? How should the reimbursement system for clinicians or services be changed to allow them to charge for their time spent caring for the carer?

More research is required regarding access to care for those who are not part of the mainstream culture or who are marginalized. This includes, for example, assisting those whose cultural background requires different forms of care than those represented in current studies, the clash in expectations between an immigrant population and their children born in a new country, assistance for carers of people who have no home and for those who live in rural and remote areas.

We recognize that, in non-Western countries, and all places where palliative care is not well developed (they are not always one and the same), caregiving at home may be very different from what is described in this chapter. Research into the experience of these carers, and how to best help them, is almost completely lacking.

Finally, few Government policies exist to support carers in maintaining their own physical, mental, social, spiritual and financial health. The strengths and weaknesses of the studies that do exist should be identified and their application by other countries considered. Additional policies will be needed to deal with some of the ethical issues that arise and to optimize the carer's as well as the patient's quality of life.

Conclusion

Family carers play a critical role in maintaining terminally ill patients comfortably at home. However, they require education and care to do so effectively, while avoiding jeopardizing their own health. More research is required, as well as acting on existing evidence to change the healthcare system and Government policies. While caring for a family member at the end of life will always be difficult, the appropriate effort of society to support carers will increase the chances that the experience is, on the whole, more positive, and does not threaten the well-being of the carer.

Key learning points

+ The family carer's desire to provide home care needs to be established and regularly reviewed in the light of family goals.

+ Other support services for the family carer, e.g. financial, educational and in-patient hospital care, need to be readily available.

+ The benefits and burdens of family caregiving need to be carefully assessed, together with the impact of cultural factors.

+ Support for family carers needs to be carefully targeted to their unique, and sometimes changing, circumstances.

+ Ethical issues require sensitive attention, as well as the impact of family caregiving on other family members.

+ Policies are needed which support carers in maintaining their own health throughout the caregiving experience.

Recommended reading and resources

Aoun SM, Kristjanson LJ, Currow DC and Hudson PL (2005). Caregiving for the terminally ill: At what cost? *Palliat Med* **19**, 551–555.

Arras JD (1995). *Bringing the Hospital Home*. Baltimore: Johns Hopkins University Press.

Canadian Virtual Hospice (www.virtualhospice.ca)

Harding R and Higginson IJ (2003). What is the best way to help carers in cancer and palliative care? A systematic literature review of interventions and their effectiveness. *Palliat Med* **17**, 63–74.

Houts, PS pioneered the COPE technique. Information can be found at:

www.apos-society.org APOS's *Quick Reference for Oncology Clinicians: The Psychiatric and Psychological Dimensions of Cancer Symptom Management* features the COPE model.

Hudson P (2004). Positive aspects and challenges associated with caring for a dying relative at home. *Int J Palliat Nurs* **10**, 58–65.

Macmillan K, Peden J, Hopkinson J and Hycha D (2005). *A Carer's Guide: a Handbook About End of Life Care*. The Military and Hospitaller Order of St. Lazarus of Jerusalem and Canadian Hospice Palliative Care Association.

Stajduhar K and Davies B (1998). Death at home: Challenges for families and directions for the future. *J Palliat Care* **14**, 8–14.

Stajduhar KI (2003). Examining the perspectives of family members involved in the delivery of palliative care at home. *J Palliat Care* **19**, 27–35.

References

1. Stajduhar KI and Davies B (1998). Palliative care at home: Reflections on HIV/AIDS family caregiving experiences. *Journal of Palliative Care* 14: 14–22.

2. Cantwell P, Turco S, Brenneis C, Hanson J, Neumann CM and Bruera E (2000). Predictors of home death in palliative care cancer patients. *Journal of Palliative Care* 16: 23–28.

3. Carter PA (2003). Family carers' sleep loss and depression over time. *Cancer Nursing* 26: 253–259.

4. Ramirez A, Addington-Hall J and Richards M (1998). ABC of palliative care: the carers. *British Medical Journal* 316: 208–211.

5. Farber SJ, Egnew TR, Herman-Bertsch JL, Taylor TR and Guldin GE (2003). Issues in end-of-life care: Patient, carer, and clinician perceptions. *Journal of Palliative Medicine* 6: 19–31.

6. Wennman-Larsen A and Tishelman C (2002). Advanced home care for cancer patients at the end of life: A qualitative study of hopes and expectations of family carers. *Scandinavian Journal of Caring Sciences* 16: 240–247.

7. Stajduhar KI (2003). Examining the perspectives of family members involved in the delivery of palliative care at home. *Journal of Palliative Care* 19: 27–35.

8. Higginson IJ and Sen-Gupta GJA (2000). Place of care in advanced cancer: A qualitative systematic literature review of patient preferences. *Journal of Palliative Medicine* 3: 287–300.

9. Pritchard RS, Fisher ES, Teno JM, Sharp SM, Reding DJ, Knous WA, Wenniberg JE and Lynn J (1998). Influences of patient preferences and local health system characteristics on the place of death. *Journal of the American Geriatrics Society* 46: 1242–1250.

10. Tang ST (2003). Determinants of hospice home care use among terminally ill cancer patients. *Nursing Research* 52: 217–225.

11. Gomes B and Higginson IJ (2006). Factors influencing death at home in terminally ill patients with cancer: systematic review. *British Medical Journal* 332: 515–521.

12. Grady A (2003). Practice development. Hospice at home 2: evaluating a crisis intervention service. *International Journal of Palliative Nursing* 9: 326–335.

13. Travers E (2002). Hospice at home 1: the development of a crisis intervention service. *International Journal of Palliative Medicine* 8: 162–168.

14. Wilson DM (2000). End-of-life care preferences of Canadian senior citizens with caregiving experience. *Journal of Advanced Nursing* 31: 1416–1421.

15. Dudgeon DJ and Kristjanson L (1995). Home versus hospital death: assessment of preferences and clinical challenges. *Canadian Medical Association Journal* 152: 337–340.

16. Fainsinger RL, Demoissac D, Cole J, Mead-Wood K and Lee E (2000). Home versus hospice inpatient care: Discharge characteristics of palliative care patients in an acute care hospital. *Journal of Palliative Care* 16: 29–34.

17. Karlsen S and Addington-Hall J (1998). How do cancer patients who die at home differ from those who die elsewhere? *Journal of Palliative Medicine* 12: 279–286.

18. Evans WG, Cutson TM, Steinhauser KE and Tulsky JA (2006). Is there no place like home? Carers recall reasons for and experience upon transfer from home hospice to inpatient facilities. *Journal of Palliative Medicine* 9: 100–110.

19. Grande GE, Addington-Hall JM and Todd CJ (1998). Place of death and access to home care services: Are certain patient groups at a disadvantage? *Social Science and Medicine* **47**: 565–579.

20. King G, Mackenzie J, Smith H and Clark D (2000). Dying at home: evaluation of a hospice rapid-response service. *International Journal of Palliative Nursing* **6**: 280–287.

21. Gallo WT, Baker MJ and Bradley EH (2001). Factors associated with home versus institutional death among cancer patients in Connecticut. *Journal of American Geriatrics Society* **49**: 771–777.

22. Carlsson ME and Rollison B (2003). A comparison of patients dying at home and patients dying at a hospice: Sociodemographic factors and carers' experiences. *Palliative and Supportive Care* **1**: 33–39.

23. Ferrario SR, Cardillo V, Vicario F, Balzarini E and Zotti AM (2004). Advanced cancer at home: Caregiving and bereavement. *Palliative Medicine* **18**: 129–136.

24. Hudson P (2004). Positive aspects and challenges associated with caring for a dying relative at home. *International Journal of Palliative Nursing* **10**: 58–65.

25. Hudson P (2005). A psycho-educational intervention for family carers of patients receiving palliative care: a randomized controlled trial. *Journal of Pain and Symptom Management* **30**: 329–341.

26. Visser G, Klinkenberg M, Broese van Groenou MI, Willems DL, Knipscheer CPM and Deeg DJH (2004). The end of life: Informal care for dying older people and its relationship to place of death. *Palliative Medicine* **18**: 468–477.

27. Fried TR, Pollack DM, Drickamer MA and Tinetti ME (1999). Who dies at home? Determinants of site of death for community-based long-term care patients. *Journal of the American Geriatrics Society* **47**: 25–29.

28. Gill P, Kaur JS, Rummans T, Novotny PJ and Sloan JA (2003). The hospice patient's primary carer: What is their quality of life? *Journal of Psychosomatic Research* **55**: 445–451.

29. Fleming DA, Sheppard VB, Mangan PA, Taylor KL, Tallarico M, Adams I, Ingham J (2006). Caregiving at the end of life: perceptions of health quality among patients and carers. *Journal of Pain and Symptom Management* **31**: 407–420.

30. Kramer BJ and Thompson EH (ed.) (2000). *Men as Carers: Theory, Research and Service Implications*. New York, NY: Springer Publishing.

31. Spillman BC and Pezzin LE (2000). Potential and active family carers: changing networks and the 'sandwich generation'. *The Milbank Quarterly* **78**: 347–374.

32. Costantini M, Camoirano E, Madeddu L, Bruzzi P, Verganelli E and Henriquet F (1993). Palliative home care and place of death among cancer patients: a population-based study. *Palliative Medicine* **7**: 323–331.

33. Gilbar O and Steiner M (1996). When death comes: where should patients die? *The Hospice Journal* **11**: 31–48.

34. Seale C, Addington-Hall J and McCarthy M (1997). Awareness of dying: prevalence, causes and consequences. *Social Science and Medicine* **45**: 477–484.

35. Canadian Hospice Palliative Care Association (2004). *The Role of Informal Carers in Hospice Palliative and End-of-life Care in Canada: a Discussion of the Legal, Ethical and Moral Challenges*. Ottawa, ON: Canadian Hospice Palliative Care Association.

36. Aoun SM, Kristjanson LJ, Currow DC and Hudson PL (2005). Caregiving for the terminally ill: at what cost? *Palliative Medicine* **19**: 551–555.

37. King DA and Quill T (2006). Working with families in palliative care: one size does not fit all. *Journal of Palliative Medicine* **9**: 704–715.

38. Mangan PA, Taylor KL, Yabroff KR, Fleming DA and Ingham JM (2003). Caregiving near the end of life: Unmet needs and potential solutions. *Palliative and Supportive Care* 1: 247–259.

39. Proot IM, Abu-Saad HH, Crebolder HFJM, Goldsteen M, Luker KA and Widdershoven GAM (2003). Vulnerability of family carers in terminal palliative care at home: balancing between burden and capacity. *Scandinavian Journal of Caring Sciences* 17: 113–121.

40. Jo S, Brazil K, Lohfeld L and Willison K (2007). Caregiving at the end of life: Perspectives from spousal carers and care recipients. *Palliative and Supportive Care* 5: 11–17.

41. Ruddick W (1995). Transforming homes and hospital. In: Arras JD (ed.). *Bringing the Hospital Home.* Baltimore: Johns Hopkins University Press, 369–380.

42. Davies B, Chekryn Reimer J, Brown P and Martens N (1995). *Fading Away: the Experience of Transition in Families with Terminal Illness.* New York: Baywood Publishing.

43. Cohen SR, Frisch S, Deschamps M, Penrod J, Plante H, Bellavance M and Lauzon N (2001). *Evaluation of the MUHC-CLSC Project to Develop an Integrated Continuum of Palliative Care Services.* Report submitted to Health Canada Health Policy and Communications Branch April, 2001.

44. Stajduhar KI and Davies B (2005). Variations in and factors influencing family members' decisions for palliative home care. *Palliative Medicine* 19: 21–32

45. Rabow MW, Hauser JM and Adams J (2004). Supporting family carers at the end of life. *Journal of the American Medical Association* 291: 483–491.

46. Loke AY, Liu CF and Szeto Y (2003). The difficulties faced by informal carers of patients with terminal cancer in Hong Kong and the available social support. *Cancer Nursing* 26: 276–283.

47. Rose KE (1999). A qualitative analysis of the information needs of informal carers of terminally ill cancer patients. *Journal of Clinical Nursing* 8: 81–88.

48. Cohen SR, Bunston T and Leis AM (1998). Domains relevant to the quality of life of family carers of palliative care patients with cancer. 12th International Congress on Care of the Terminally Ill, Montreal, September 1998. *Journal of Palliative Care* 14: 105.

49. Emanuel EJ, Fairclough DL, Slutsman J and Emanuel LL (2000). Understanding economic and other burdens of terminal illness: the experience of patients and their carers. *Annals of Internal Medicine* 132: 451–459.

50. Williams A, Crooks V, Stajduhar KI, Allan D and Cohen R (2006). Canada's Compassionate Care Benefit: Views of family carers in chronic illness. *International Journal of Palliative Nursing* 12: 438–445.

51. Strang VR, Koop PM and Peden J (2002). The experience of respite during home-based family caregiving for persons with advanced cancer. *Journal of Palliative Care* 18: 97–104.

52. Grbich C, Parker D and Maddocks I (2001). The emotions and coping strategies of carers of family members with terminal cancer. *Journal of Palliative Care* 17: 30–36.

53. Denham SA (1999). Part 2: Family health during and after death of a family member. *Journal of Family Nursing* 5: 160–183.

54. Schulz R and Beach SR (1999). Caregiving as a risk factor for mortality: the carer health effects study. *Journal of the American Medical Association* 282: 2215–2219.

55. Christakis N and Iwashyna T (2003). The health impact of health care on families: a matched cohort study of hospice use by decedents and mortality outcomes in surviving widowed spouses. *Social Science Medicine* 57: 465–475.

56. Leis AM, Kristjanson L, Koop PM and Laizner A (1997). Family health and the palliative care trajectory: a cancer research agenda. *Cancer Prevention and Control* 1: 352–360.

57. Canadian Hospice Palliative Care Association (2006). *The Pan-Canadian Gold Standard for Palliative Home Care: Towards Equitable Access to High-Quality Hospice Palliative and End-of-life Care at Home.* Ottawa, ON: Canadian Hospice Palliative Care Association.

58. Hudson PL (2006). How well do family carers cope after caring for a relative with advanced disease and how can health professionals enhance their support? *Journal of Palliative Medicine* **9**: 694–703.

59. Grunfeld E, Coyle D, Whelan T, Clinch J, Reyno L, Earle CC, Willan A, Viola R, Coristine M, Janz T, Glossop R (2004). Family carer burden: Results of a longitudinal study of breast cancer patients and their principle carers. *Canadian Medical Association Journal* **170**: 1795–1801.

60. Cohen SR (2003). Assessing quality of life in the terminally ill. In: Portenoy RK and Bruera E (ed.). *Issues in Palliative Care Research.* New York: Oxford University Press, 231–242.

61. Arras JD (1995). *Bringing the Hospital Home.* Baltimore: Johns Hopkins University Press.

62. Northouse LL, Mood D, Templin T, Mellon S and George T (2000). Couples' patterns of adjustment to colon cancer. *Social Science and Medicine* **50**: 271–284.

63. Rose LE (1997). Caring for carers: perceptions of social support. *Journal of Psychosocial Nursing and Mental Health Services* **35**: 17–23.

64. Payne S, Smith P and Dean S (1999). Identifying the concerns of informal carers in palliative care. *Palliative Medicine* **13**: 37–44.

65. Harding R and Higginson, IJ (2003). What is the best way to help carers in cancer and palliative care: a systematic literature review of interventions and their effectiveness. *Palliative Medicine* **17**: 63–74.

66. Ingleton C, Payne S, Nolan M and Carey I (2003). Respite in palliative care: a review and discussion of the literature. *Palliative Medicine* **17**: 567–575.

67. Clark D, Ferguson C and Nelson C (2000). Macmillan carers schemes in England: results of a multicentre evaluation. *Palliative Medicine* **14**: 129–139.

68. McDonald G (1998). Massage as a respite intervention for primary carers. *The American Journal of Hospice and Palliative Care* **14**: 43–37.

69. Grande GE, Todd CJ, Barclay SIG and Farquhar MC (2000). A randomised controlled trial of a hospital at home service for the terminally ill. *Palliative Medicine* **14**: 375–385.

70. Kane RL, lkein SJ, Bernstein L, Kane RL, Klein SJ, Bernstein L, Rothenberg R and Wales J (1985). Hospice role in alleviating the emotional stress of terminal patients and their families. *Medical Care* **23**: 189–197.

71. Higginson IJ, Finlay IG, Goodwin DM, Hood K, Edwards AGK, Cook A, Douglas HR and Normand CE (2003). Is there evidence that palliative care teams alter end-of-life experiences of patients and their carers? *Journal of Pain and Symptom Management* **25**: 150–168.

72. Harding R, Higginson J, George R, Robinson V and Taylor L (2004). Evaluation of a sort-term group intervention for informal carers of patients attending a home palliative care service. *Journal of Pain and Symptom Management* **27**: 396–408.

73. Cameron J, Shin J, Williams D and Stewart D (2004). A brief problem-solving intervention for family carers to individuals with advanced cancer. *Journal of Psychosomatic Research* **57**: 137–143.

Chapter 10

Family and palliative care in care homes for older people

Mike Nolan and Rosalie Hudson

A strong message is the interdependence of staff, residents and family members, and any attempts to promote a positive culture within the care home setting needs to nurture these important relationships.

(1, p.61)

Introduction

Countries throughout the world are now promoting a policy of 'ageing in place'; the goal being to enable older people to live and, if possible, to die in an environment of their choice. The majority of older people continue to live, if not always to die, within the community, either independently or with the support of family carers. However, a significant minority require support in a care home setting and consequently growing numbers of older people are now dying in care homes. It is estimated that one-fifth of older people currently die in a care home (1, 2), representing approximately 100 000 deaths per year in the UK (3). It is widely accepted that this figure will rise (1, 4); for example, from 20 per cent of deaths to 40 per cent of deaths by 2020 in the US (5), with Seymour *et al.* (6) arguing that in the future the majority of people over the age of 85 are likely to die in a care home. Clearly then ensuring a 'good' death in such settings is essential.

It must therefore be a cause for concern that a major review of the literature on dying in care homes, conducted by the Social Care Institute for Excellence (SCIE) in the UK, concluded that there is a lack of standards for terminal care in care homes, planning for a resident death is rarely undertaken and that, even when plans exist, they are often poorly implemented (4). Despite the fact that residents often anticipate dying and tend to demonstrate a 'calm acceptance' of the fact (5), issues to do with death usually remain 'hidden and denied' by staff (1). To compound matters, staff primarily focus on the 'technical' aspects of dying (7), to the relative neglect of the spiritual, social and psychological needs of residents and their families (4). While there has been relatively little research on the end-of-life preferences of residents, it is clear from the available literature that:

- residents are often aware they are likely to die in the care home;
- they want to mark the death of fellow residents and to receive adequate bereavement support themselves; and
- they are critical of attempts to hide or fail to mention the death of fellow residents (4).

It therefore seems that overall the quality of death and dying in care homes leaves much to be desired, and that for too many residents death remains 'cold, lonely and painful' (5).

In this chapter we argue that, if the situation is to improve, then at least two things need to happen:

- there should be a more widespread adoption of a palliative care philosophy within care homes; and
- staff and families should work together in an equal and active partnership.

The barriers to achieving these two aims will be explored, and it is suggested that the application of a 'relationship-centred' (8–10) approach may provide a potential solution. The evolution of relationship-centred care (8) and the 'senses framework' (9–12) will be described, and their potential use in relation to a palliative care model in care homes explored.

A palliative care philosophy

Whilst the importance of 'orchestrating' a good death in care homes is recognized (13), it is also realized that this cannot be separated from the care practices and cultures that exist within a given setting (1). Too often a consideration of dying is confined to the terminal phase (14), and several authors now argue that there is a need to extend the vision and move towards a palliative care approach (1, 4, 15–17).

In the palliative care approach, dying is seen more as a process rather than as an event, having an extended trajectory in many cases (1). Consequently, a palliative care model focuses as much on living as it does on dying (14, 16) and thereby helps to create a culture of care that values both (2). Furthermore, such a model does not just attend to the needs of residents, but also actively includes those of the family (5, 14, 17) and, as we will argue later, should also attend to the needs of staff. The benefits of adopting a palliative care approach have been demonstrated. Using an action-research approach,

Hockley *et al.* (2) introduced a palliative care model into several care homes in Scotland and found that subsequently:

- death and dying were less likely to be treated as peripheral issues;
- there was better communication both within the homes and with outside agencies;
- the care assistants' role in ensuring a good death was more highly valued; and
- there were more meaningful conversations between staff, residents and relatives.

Several other authors extol the virtues of adopting a philosophy that embodies the principles of palliative care (13, 16, 18, 19) with, for example, Shega *et al.* (19) suggesting that, if there is to be excellence in dementia care, then a palliative care approach needs to be applied from the time of diagnosis. In the evidence-based *Guidelines for a Palliative Approach in Residential Aged Care* (17), the chapter on advanced dementia states:

> Symptoms of people with dementia were compared to the symptoms of people with cancer and it was found that people dying from dementia have symptoms and healthcare needs comparable to those dying from cancer.

The guidelines also emphasize the responsibility of the aged care team in facilitating family involvement and providing family support in the context of advanced dementia (17). The evidence, based on a systematic literature review, clearly shows the benefits of a palliative approach, both for the resident's quality of life and the family's satisfaction (17).

However, the issues involved in death and dying in care homes are often complex and, following a detailed review of the literature, Nicholson (1) identified three main themes that need to be addressed, if the tenets of palliative care are to be more widely applied. These were:

- the need to integrate living and dying within care homes;
- the importance of encouraging an open and supportive approach; and
- more efforts to promote the type of supportive environment needed to help residents, families and staff to work with continuing loss.

Notwithstanding the far greater recognition now afforded to the introduction of a palliative care approach within care homes, several formidable barriers need to be addressed. Travis *et al.* (20) identified four obstacles to palliation and end-of-life care in long-term care facilities: (1) failure to recognize treatment futility; (2) lack of communication among decision makers; (3) no agreement on a course for end-of-life care; and (4) failure to implement a timely plan of care.

Similarly, Hockley *et al.* (2) see the barriers as cultural, institutional and clinical. Culturally, a medical model approach to ageing continues to predominate in most Western societies (5), so that open discussion about dying is still a relatively rare event (21). The overall result is 'closed discussions' (2), and there is often a failure to recognize when a curative/restorative model is no longer appropriate and a palliative approach is required (4). As Hockley *et al.* (2) note, this tends to result in a clinical environment that does not acknowledge dying; something that is reinforced by several institutional barriers, particularly a lack of sufficient time and too few staff with the necessary skills and competence. The situation is not helped by the fact that care homes are often isolated from specialized palliative care support (2), indicated by a lack of systematic involvement of outside help (4). The input provided is limited and reactive, focusing primarily on the needs of people with cancer (4).

In Australia, the guidelines referred to above are based on the fact that almost every resident in an aged care facility has a life-threatening illness, with many having several co-morbidities. In accordance with the World Health Organization definition of palliative care, all these residents therefore meet the criteria for a palliative approach. The guidelines call for an attitudinal change, encouraging the application of the philosophy and principals of palliative care for all residents and their families, including open discussion of death and dying (17). Factors that inhibit this philosophical and practical shift are, however, fully acknowledged in the guidelines. Such factors include the wide diversity in aged care facilities, the range of skills and training levels of staff, the high incidence of dementia, and fragmented medical oversight. The aim of the guidelines is to build on the strengths of those aged care facilities that already provide excellent end-of-life care to residents and their families, and to encourage equal access to this approach for all other residents and families. This includes the promotion of active partnership with specialist palliative care services that can provide assistance with issues such as complex symptom management, education for aged care workers and family counselling. The guidelines include a comprehensive chapter on family support, highlighting the need for involving the family at every level of the resident's care, providing open communication and advocating regular, formally constructed meetings with every family. At present, however, it is not known how many aged care facilities are adopting this 'new' palliative approach and further research is needed to identify the benefits, particularly for families.

Overall, therefore, while the adoption of a palliative care model within care homes is widely promoted, formidable barriers to its more widespread use remain to be addressed. Ronch (22) argues that the situation is unlikely to improve until we move beyond an emphasis on policies and procedures and create a culture and environment within care homes that values and promotes personal growth for both residents and staff. Such an environment has been termed an 'enriched' environment of care (10, 23), and we will consider how it might be created shortly. However, a palliative care approach also requires that due attention is given to the needs of family carers and it is to this important component of care that we now turn.

Creating partnerships with family carers

The importance of staff in care homes creating positive partnerships with family carers is increasingly recognized (24–26), and this is particularly so when their relative is dying. Unfortunately, relatively little is known about the needs of carers at this time, and while a supportive environment is seen as essential (1), the social, spiritual and psychological needs of families are often overlooked (4).

Families often want to play an active role, and many wish to 'midwife' the death (27). However, their involvement may not be encouraged and staff are often reluctant to discuss the families' palliative care needs (4). Sander and Russell (13) suggest that staff need to give families a greater sense of control, paying attention both to what they say and what they might not say. Consequently, the quality of relationships between families and staff is a central issue (28), particularly around the time of the death, as this can bring about profound changes to the families' role (29). Unfortunately, because of the lack of transparency and open discussions between families and staff (28), carers often find it difficult to get involved and do not know what is expected of them (21). Therefore, rather than creating partnerships that are nurtured within a supportive and ongoing relationship (1, 28), conflict is often the dominant pattern of interaction between staff and families at this crucial stage (5). In large part this may reflect the type of relationships that have developed with families over time. Tensions between staff and relatives in care homes have been described for some time; for example, families who wish to play an active role can be seen as interfering (30, 31). Such tension leads to the rapid development of competitive and fraught relationships between families and staff (32, 36).

In exploring the types of relationship that can develop between relatives and staff, Davies (37) identified four broad categories:

- Partnership care ('working together'): this is based on reciprocal relationships between staff and relatives with clearly established responsibilities and opportunities for the family *carer* to remain involved.

- Substitutive care ('getting on with it'): here relatives perceive gaps and deficiencies in care, and attempt to fill these gaps themselves.

- Submissive care ('putting up with it'): submissive care is most likely to develop when care staff attempt to take control of the older person's care and relatives feel unable to challenge this, sometimes for fear of reprisals.

- Confrontational care ('battling it out'): where family *carers* perceive no alternative to constantly registering complaints about care standards on behalf of their relative (37).

Davies' findings are reinforced by those of Haesler *et al.* (36) who found 'when nurses do not value the role of the family, competitive relationships can develop' and when nurses want to maintain all control over resident care, 'family members do not feel staff are open to receiving information about the resident' (36). In these and other extensive findings from the literature regarding staff–family relationships in the residential aged care setting, Haesler *et al.* (36) found that family carers 'have always held an ambiguous position in the health system', being variously described as 'hidden patients, servants, visitors, workers, health team members, partners in care, advocates and protectors, resources, a problem, intruders, disrupters and superceded {sic} carers'. They also found significant evidence of the failure to address the needs of the family, arising from ineffective communication, as well as obstructive institutional rules and protocols.

It is now clear that positive relational dynamics are essential to creating good partnerships, and that the best partnerships exist when all parties within caring relationships are able to work together and appreciate each other's perspective.

Building a relationship of trust based on partnerships is part of the standards for care homes in some countries, such as Australia (38). Hudson and O'Connor (26) argue that such relationships need to be established from the time of admission, or even earlier; for example, in a pre-admission discussion and/or in an information brochure, where a partnership philosophy can be described (26). First impressions are often lasting, and how staff and families interact over time is likely to have a significant impact throughout the caring trajectory; this becomes even more important in the context of death and dying. Family support is likely to be optimized if:

- the care team acknowledges, welcomes, and affirms the family's involvement;
- the family is involved (if they wish) in assisting with the person's physical-care needs;

- the care team understands that families might come under stress and might need to withdraw from their caring role; and
- families receive clear communication and are given opportunities for discussion (17).

Apart from the opportunity to be involved in discussion about the resident's care, families found the following palliative approach interventions to be particularly helpful:

- access to 24-hour medical and nursing advice;
- use of family conferences for information sharing;
- attention by the aged care team to the resident as a 'whole person'; and
- comprehensive pain management and comfort measures (17).

Mirroring these findings, Sandberg *et al.* (24) concluded that family carers placing a relative in a care home enter a 'new world' and that staff need to demonstrate 'empathic' awareness from the outset. This involves staff:

- being sensitive to the difficult nature of the placement decision and the conflicting emotions that carers may experience;
- encouraging families to discuss their feelings openly;
- being aware of the lack of preparation for the placement, and families' potentially limited understanding of the nature and philosophy of care homes;
- helping families to gain a better understanding of the new environment;
- being aware of most families' desire to remain involved in care, and of their wish to impart their knowledge of their relative to staff;
- being proactive in initiating dialogue and of creating a first impression that makes carers feel welcome and involves their participation;
- encouraging carers to remain involved in care if they wish, or to 'let' go of their responsibilities, if appropriate;
- recognizing the potential for conflict and being aware of the fact that apparent complaints may well be a sign of carers' own mixed emotions;
- actively facilitating compromise and negotiation to prevent or resolve conflict; and
- recognizing that it takes time for families to 'trust' staff to provide good care for their relative.

Such early investment can create the type of relationships that enable staff and families to deal openly and honestly with the often difficult decisions that arise around the time of death. As Hudson and O'Connor (26) contend, each family deals with a forthcoming death in a unique way that is in large part determined by their prior relationship with the dying person. Consequently, there is no 'correct' way to react; therefore systems, such as family conferences, need to be established that facilitate the exploration of families' diverse views and responses (26). A well planned meeting with a resident's family can establish, for example, what kind of information (if any) the family would like about the resident's care and how the information is to be conveyed. Such a meeting can also elicit whether or not the family is seeking help with end-of-life treatment decisions, and whether they need assistance in communicating with each other and with the resident. Some families also welcome practical guidance about how to support the resident through the dying process. Lopez (39) found that, in this respect, nurses can act as 'knowledgeable guides for family members'. However, if staff are to adequately support families, they require education and support themselves; such support can be enhanced by effective liaison with external agencies as well as by sensitive managers (26).

It is also widely acknowledged that those who work in aged care are not necessarily skilled in conducting effective family meetings, or in dealing with complex family issues, especially where conflict is evident. Here, a multidisciplinary approach is advocated (17), together with strong partnerships with palliative care specialists or other agencies, who might have more experience in these matters. The proactive role of management is an essential component in sustaining and nurturing these partnerships (17, 26). Caring partnerships go beyond procedures and protocols to a philosophy that values every member's contribution.

As Kitwood (40) cogently argued, staff are unlikely to be able to promote optimal care for residents if their own needs are not attended to, and this is particularly so when dealing with death and dying.

Attending to the needs of staff

The impact of death on the living is often underestimated, and this is especially so for staff who may have to deal with multiple losses, often without adequate support (4). For example, the need to support staff in hospices is well recognized, but this is less so in care homes (13), with staff often feeling that their own needs for self-care are neglected (41). Therefore, while forming a close relationship between residents and staff that 'enriched and provided meaning to their work, it led to feelings of loss and grief upon the death of residents' (41), with such feelings often being suppressed and unaddressed (41).

Lopez (39) found that the suffering of families of nursing home residents had a significant impact on the nurses; indicating the need for the suffering of staff to be acknowledged and addressed. Staff need help to work with loss and to feel valued and supported (1); this requires an atmosphere in which candour and open discussion are the norm (42). This is particularly important for unqualified staff who often feel that their detailed knowledge of residents is not appreciated (41), yet they often lack the confidence to actively share such knowledge with senior staff (4). Consequently, they feel undervalued and may be particularly vulnerable to emotional distress (2). It therefore seems evident that the most effective teams will be those who recognize and encourage the input of all staff. However, achieving this is difficult in a sector where staff turnover is often high, the pay is grossly inadequate and many care staff may not have English as a first language.

Training for staff is essential for the development of effective teams (26). However, such training is often largely informal and random, instead of being part of a more consistent and coherent strategy (4). Staff need the opportunity to have their assumptions and beliefs about dying explored, with ongoing mentorship, supervision and adequate time to reflect and share their experiences (1, 2). The role of positive leadership in creating this sort of environment is essential (1). Even in an environment of limited time resources, a culture of listening and support can be fostered.

Following an extensive consideration of the literature, Nicholson (1) concluded that the introduction of a palliative care approach in care homes requires recognition of the multiple and complex needs of residents, staff and families and that all these groups need adequate and ongoing support. This requires an approach that fully acknowledges and seeks to attend to the interdependencies that exist within care home settings. One such approach is that of relationship-centred care (8), underpinned by the 'senses framework' (9–12).

Relationship-centred care and the senses framework

The term 'relationship-centred care' was first coined following a major review of the healthcare system in the US in the early 1990s (8). The taskforce considered that the major future health challenges facing society will be as a result of chronic illness, yet most healthcare systems are designed to deal with acute conditions. They argued that there was a need to create an approach that recognized the interdependencies that exist in the face of chronic illness and that addressing these interdependencies means attending to the relationships that develop (8):

> The phrase 'relationship-centred care' captures the importance of the interactions among people as the foundation of any therapeutic or teaching activity. Further,

relationships are critical to the care provided by nearly all practitioners and a sense of satisfaction and positive outcomes for patients and practitioners. Although relationships are a prerequisite to effective care and teaching, there has been little formal acknowledgement of their importance, and few formal efforts to help students and practitioners learn to develop effective relationships in healthcare.

Concurrently, work in the UK was being undertaken to elaborate both upon the nature of family care and the interactions between staff and families, especially in long-term caring contexts (11, 43, 44). Work in long-term settings with older people, such as care homes or long-stay wards, has traditionally lacked a clear sense of purpose, often being referred to as 'aimless residual care' (45) or 'good geriatric care' (46). The suggestion is that staff in such environments do not so much 'burn out' due to the rapidly changing challenges they face, but rather 'rust out' because of the unstimulating nature of their work (47), and the lack of any 'therapeutic reciprocity' in their relationship with older people (48). This attitude is reinforced when residents and their families are seen as mere *recipients* of care, rather than active agents in a caring partnership. A pervasive culture of *custodial* care also does little to provide a stimulating environment for staff, residents and families. By contrast, a creative community allows all partners to learn from one another. A vibrant, non-threatening environment also provides opportunities for joy and laughter, hope and optimism, even within a context of death and dying. This leads to important questions such as, what kind of attitudes will contribute to such a transformation and what factors would enhance such relationship-centred care?

Based on a consideration of the available literature, and a number of studies of family care (43, 44, 49), Nolan (11) argues that a positive environment of care could be achieved if staff set about creating 'six senses' for residents in care home settings. These were a sense of:

- ◆ security
- ◆ belonging
- ◆ continuity
- ◆ purpose
- ◆ fulfilment
- ◆ significance

However, Nolan also believed that if staff were to create these senses for others, then they also needed to experience the senses themselves. Staff need to feel safe, to feel they belong and to feel there is a clear sense of purpose and significance to their work. Subsequently, the senses have been further developed and tested in a range of contexts and settings for older people, including acute hospital environments (12) and community settings (50); their relevance to both family carers and students learning to work with older people has also been explored (10, 23). Over this period the senses too evolved, with a sense of achievement replacing a sense of fulfilment. The senses as they are currently defined are captured in Box 10.1.

A particular advantage of the senses framework is that it prompts consideration of the important components of care from the perspectives of older people, family members and staff working with them. Furthermore, through linking the experiences of older people, their families and staff, the senses framework has the potential to promote understanding of the experience of others, thus enhancing communication and the ability to work in partnership (10). Studies have highlighted the role that the senses play in helping to create an 'enriched' environment of care (9, 10, 23). Such 'enriched' environments ensure that the senses are met for all individuals/groups in a given care context, including, for example, residents/patients, staff, family carers and students. Our argument here is that the senses can be applied to a care home setting in order to create an 'enriched' environment that promotes a palliative care philosophy and potentially transforms the existing culture. However, while the senses were initially developed for general application in care homes, their foundation needs further work and elaboration within the context of a palliative approach to care.

Transforming the culture of care homes

Stone (52) argues that 'culture change' has become the 'buzzword' for the twenty-first century and that nowhere is it more apparent than in the care home sector. Fundamentally there is the need for a 'paradigm' shift in the way that 'care homes' are perceived (22, 53), both within the sector and, more generally, within society. Gibson and Barsade (54) highlight the need to question current underlying values, beliefs and assumptions about the way the world works, and to challenge the distinctions between, for example, 'cure vs care' and 'costs vs quality'. Such debates appear essential. However, in terms of the day-to-day reality of living and working in a care home, Tobin (55) believes that this will require a change to the 'fabric of the caring milieu' so that its essential humanity comes to the fore. Thus, as Ronch (22) notes, '… the mutual and complementary needs of residents and staff to grow are synergised, and the quality of life of the ageing and their carers is optimised'.

Although we favour transformation of the caring milieu through addressing attitudes, culture and promoting a philosophy of partnership, the evidence also points to the need for institutional changes that promote such synergy.

Box 10.1 The six senses in the context of caring relationships

A sense of security

- For older people: Attention to essential physiological and psychological needs, to feel safe and free from threat, harm, pain and discomfort. To receive competent and sensitive care.

- For staff: To feel free from physical threat, rebuke or censure. To have secure conditions of employment. To have the emotional demands of work recognized and to work within a supportive but challenging culture.

- For family carers: To feel confident in knowledge and ability to provide good care (51) without detriment to personal well-being. To have adequate support networks and timely help when required. To be able to relinquish care when appropriate.

A sense of continuity

- For older people: Recognition and value of personal biography; skilful use of knowledge of the past to help contextualise present and future. Seamless, consistent care delivered within an established relationship by known people.

- For staff: Positive experience of work with older people from an early stage of career, exposure to good role models and environments of care. Expectations and standards of care communicated clearly and consistently.

- For family carers: To maintain shared pleasures/pursuits with the older person. To be able to provide competent standards of care, whether delivered by self or others, to ensure that personal standards of care are maintained by others, to maintain involvement in care across care environments as desired/appropriate.

A sense of belonging

- For older people: Opportunities to maintain and/or form meaningful and reciprocal relationships, to feel part of a community or group as desired.

- For staff: To feel part of a team with a recognized and valued contribution, to belong to a peer group, a community of gerontological practitioners.

Box 10.1 The six senses in the context of caring relationships *(continued)*

♦ For family carers: To be able to maintain/improve valued relationships, to be able to confide in trusted individuals to feel that 'you're not in this alone'.

A sense of purpose

♦ For older people: Opportunities to engage in purposeful activity facilitating the constructive passage of time; to be able to identify and pursue goals and challenges, to exercise discretionary choice.

♦ For staff: To have a sense of therapeutic direction, a clear set of goals to which to aspire.

♦ For family carers: To maintain the dignity and integrity, well-being and 'personhood' of the care recipient, to pursue (re)constructive/reciprocal care (44).

A sense of achievement

♦ For older people: Opportunities to meet meaningful and valued goals, to feel satisfied with one's efforts, to make a recognized and valued contribution, to make progress towards therapeutic goals as appropriate.

♦ For staff: To be able to provide good care, to feel satisfied with one's efforts, to contribute towards therapeutic goals as appropriate, to use skills and ability to the full.

♦ For family carers: To feel that you have provided the best possible care, to know 'you've done your best', to meet challenges successfully, to develop new skills and abilities.

A sense of significance

♦ For older people: To feel recognized and valued as a person of worth, that one's actions and existence are of importance, that you 'matter'.

♦ For staff: To feel that gerontological practice is valued and important, that your work and efforts 'matter'.

♦ For family carers: To feel that one's caring efforts are valued and appreciated, to experience an enhanced sense of self.

Adapted from Davies *et al.* (12), Nolan (11) and Nolan *et al.* (9).

Partnerships with families do not arise from a vacuum; they need to be carefully negotiated, nurtured and sustained. While inclusion of the family has always been a hallmark of palliative care, the benefits of such partnerships have not been fully appreciated in aged care. One way of promoting the required culture change is to systematically build into the admission procedures a well-prepared orientation programme, together with a formal meeting with each resident and family, as soon as practicable after the resident's admission. Regarding orientation, families welcome practical advice, such as the layout of the residence, and an opportunity to discuss their ongoing caring role. Including the family in the initial assessment process helps to establish important factors such as:

* Who is the main spokesperson for the family?
* What kind of involvement do particular family members wish to have in the resident's care? (This, of course, allows for families to state they wish to have minimal or no involvement.)
* What knowledge and personal experience does the family wish to contribute about the resident, especially in the context of a resident's advanced dementia?
* Does the family have particular support needs, e.g. in managing ongoing visiting and so on?
* What kind of information does the family want or need, and in what form?
* Would the family benefit from any particular support services available from other agencies?
* What does the family understand about the resident's current diagnosis, condition and relevant treatments?
* Does the family understand the relevant communication channels, so they can make comments in the most effective manner?
* Does the family understand the goals of a palliative approach in maximizing quality of life through appropriate physical symptom management, as well as psychosocial and spiritual support?

In order to ascertain this information, best practice guidelines now advise a family meeting is the most appropriate forum for this exchange, provided the meeting is held in conversational style rather than an interrogation. 'Family meetings help plan interventions and set goals so that an older person, family members and the multidisciplinary team are all striving for the same outcomes' (56). Continual involvement of the family, both informally and in subsequent meetings, provides for the monitoring of family carer stress, affirms the value of family caregivers' contribution and allows for relevant information and discussion concerning the resident's changing needs (17). The initial meeting sets the scene for subsequent meetings, providing families with confidence and hope in a climate of open communication and trust. In situations where the resident has no family, other options need to be carefully explored.

As we have shown, a palliative approach has much to offer those suffering from chronic, life-threatening illness and their families, where the illness trajectory can be much longer than, for example, in people dying from cancer. While we acknowledge the time constraints, and staffing resource deficiencies in residential aged care, we also believe that well-planned, efficiently conducted family meetings can actually save time (26). However, time has other connotations for family members, who may be involved in supporting their relative for many months, if not years. During this time, a partnership culture can grow and develop with each family, for the ultimate benefit and satisfaction of the family and the resident who is dying (17).

One of the benefits of this partnership approach is a frank and continuous discussion about prognostication. In this population, where many residents have several life-threatening illnesses, including dementia, it is difficult to predict when death will occur. Glare *et al.* (57) have shown it is more difficult to give an indication of prognosis where co-morbidities are present than it is for a patient with cancer. This means exercising caution when discussing the issue of prognosis with family members, either by overestimating survival or by inappropriately predicting imminent death. However, health professionals in this context also require the skills to recognize the signs of imminent death, so they can appropriately prepare families wherever possible (17). Families also need to be advised that in some situations the resident might make an entirely unpredicted recovery, even when death seems imminent. The key issue here is support for families, underpinned by relevant information and open communication. When a resident's dying phase seems more protracted than the family had expected, it might be time for a review of goals to determine the family's understanding of symptom relief and/or expectations of a cure. On the other hand, families need also to be aware that in the context of co-morbidities and increasing frailty, death can occur unexpectedly. Rather than trying to estimate the length of the dying phase, health professionals can convey their support by building trusting relationships with families, so that concerns can be addressed at any stage of the resident's journey towards death. By fostering family partnerships the pervasive attitude of hopelessness and despair, so often evident in this context, can be transformed.

For a number of years the UK Government has been seeking to modernize the way in which health and social care are delivered and has introduced a series of radical reforms in order to do so. The results of a recent major programme of research has concluded that, if such modernization is achieved, there is a need to move away from an over-reliance on 'transactional' approaches to change, which focus on regulation and legislation, towards a transformational model that fully recognizes the interdependencies and relationships needed for successful and sustained improvements. Transactional models tend to result in 'compliant' behaviour motivated by fear of sanction, whereas transformational ways of working generate commitment to a set of core values (58).

The core values implicit in a palliative care model in care homes are, we feel, the appropriate ones. However, as demonstrated throughout this chapter, considerable barriers remain to be overcome. The adoption of relationship-centred care has the potential to create the type of enriched environment needed for progress to be made. Key issues therefore become:

- How can we create the senses for residents, relatives and staff that will help them to address openly and honestly the multiple losses they face?
- How do we ensure that all groups feel 'safe' to talk about death and dying rather than leaving such issues unspoken and unexplored?
- How do we create 'communities' where all groups feel that they 'belong'?
- How do we foster continuity of experience that acknowledges who the dying person is now largely dependent on who he or she has been?
- Most importantly of all, how do we ensure that death is accorded the same significance as life, and that enabling a 'good death' creates as much a positive sense of purpose and achievement as do other aspects of the culture of the care home?

The studies we have cited provide some important indicators, but fundamentally it is about a full appreciation and valuing of the role that everyone plays in 'enriching' the environment of care at the end of life.

As we have argued throughout this chapter, the values underpinning a palliative care approach and the senses framework, if suitably adapted to care homes, could do much to transform the ways in which the balance between living and dying is achieved.

Priority research, clinical and policy issues

In the light of this discussion on a partnership approach in care homes the following issues are identified as warranting further exploration:

- formulation of family satisfaction surveys to identify strengths and gaps in the service provided;

- development of policies for family meetings to be initiated for every resident as soon as possible after admission, with regular follow-up meetings, as required;
- formulation of clear policies to mark the death of a resident and relevant support for other residents, staff and bereaved families;
- development of policies for creative partnerships with palliative care specialists;
- further work on the relevance of the 'senses framework' and the factors needed to create the senses within a palliative care context for residents, relatives and staff;
- research into family carers' needs and expectations, including the kind of information and support they require; and
- guidelines for a palliative approach for every resident in a care home.

Key learning points

- Care homes can foster an attitude of partnership by regular, routine, well-planned meetings with family members, rather than waiting until a crisis occurs.
- Staff can learn from family members, particularly when the family have been the main caregivers prior to the resident's admission to the care home.
- Preparation for the resident's death, together with open communication and support for families should be a continuous process from admission, rather than being left until the resident's final hours or days of life.
- The support needs of staff need to be addressed create an enriched environment for relatives and residents.

Recommended reading and resources

Addington-Hall J and Higginson I (ed.) (2001). *Palliative Care for Non-cancer Patients.* Oxford: Oxford University Press.

Aged Care Standards and Accreditation Agency at:
http://www.accreditation.org.au/AccreditationStandards

Hudson R (2002). Creating caring communities. *ACHSE Health Manager* (Autumn): 5–9.

Katz J and Homeroom C et al. (1999). Understanding palliative care in residential and nursing homes. *International Journal of Palliative Nursing* 5(2): 58–64.

My Home Life at: http://www.myhomelife.org.uk

Nay R (1996). Nursing home entry: meaning making by relatives. *Australian Journal on Ageing* 15(3): 123–126.

Nay R (1997). Relatives' experiences of nursing home life: characterised by tension. *Australian Journal on Ageing* 16(1): 24–29.

Social Care Institute for Excellence at: http://ww.scie.org.uk

Terminal Care in Care Homes: Research Briefing 10 at: http://www.scie.org.uk/publications/briefings/briefing 10/index asp

Training resources for the guidelines for a palliative approach in residential aged care at:http://ww.pallcare.org.au

Training resources for the guidelines for a palliative approach in residential aged care at: http://ww.pallcare.org.au

References

1. Nicholson L (2006). End-of-life care. In: Owen T and the National Care Homes Research and Development Forum (ed.). *My Home Life: Quality of Life in Care Homes*. London: Help the Aged, 118–128.

2. Hockley J, Dewar B and Watson J (2004). *Developing Quality End of Life Care in Eight Independent Nursing Homes through the Implementation of an Integrated Care Pathway for the Last Days of Life*—Phase III, Executive Summary. St Columba's Hospice Bridges Initiative Project.

3. Seymour J, Witherspoon R, Gott M, Ross H, Payne S and Owen T (2005). *End-of-life Care: Promoting Comfort, Choice and Well-being for Older People*. London: Policy Press.

4. SCIE Terminal Care in Care Homes: Research Briefing 10 (2005). *http://www.scie.org.uk/publications/briefings/briefing 10/index asp* (accessed 20/7/07).

5. Forbes S (2001). This is Heaven's waiting room: end of life in one nursing home. *Journal of Gerontological Nursing* 27(11): 37–45.

6. Seymour J, Clark D, Floor K and Philp I (2001). Palliative care and geriatric medicine: shared concerns, shared challenges. *Palliative Medicine* 15: 269–270.

7. Katz JS, Sidell M and Komaromy C (2000). Death in homes: bereavement needs of residents, relatives and staff. *International Journal of Palliative Nursing* 6(6): 274–279.

8. Tresolini CP and the Pew-Fetzer Task Force Health Professions Education and Relationship-Centred Care (1994). *A Report of the Pew-Fetzer Task Force on Advancing Psychosocial Education*. San Francisco: Pew Health Professions Commission.

9. Nolan MR, Davies S and Grant G (ed.) (2001). *Working with Older People and their Families: Key Issues in Policy and Practice*. Buckingham: Open University Press.

10. Nolan MR, Brown J, Davies S, Nolan J and Keady J (2006). *The Senses Framework: Improving Care for Older People Through a Relationship-centred Approach. Getting Research into Practice (GRIP) Series*, No. 2. Sheffield: University of Sheffield.

11. Nolan MR (1997). *Health and Social Care: What the Future Holds for Nursing*. Keynote address at Third Royal College of Nursing Older Person European Conference and Exhibition, Harrogate.

12. Davies S, Nolan MR, Brown J and Wilson F (1999). *Dignity on the Ward: Promoting Excellence in Care*. London: Help the Aged.

13. Sander R and Russell P (2001). Care for dying people in nursing homes. *Nursing Older People* 13(2): 21–24.

14. National Council for Palliative Care (2005). *Improving Palliative Care Provision for Older People in Care Homes. Focus on Care Homes*. London: NCOP.

15. Davies S and Seymour J (2002). Historical and policy contexts. In: Hockley J and Clark D (ed.). *Palliative Care for Older People in Care Homes*. Buckingham: Open University Press, 4–33.

16. Nolan MR, Lundh U, Grant G and Keady J (ed.) (2003). *Partnerships in Family Care: Understanding the Caregiving Career.* Maidenhead: Open University Press.

17. Commonwealth of Australia (2006). *Guidelines for a Palliative Approach in Residential Aged Care: enhanced version May 2006.* Canberra: Australian Government Department of Health and Ageing.

18. Hudson R and Richmond J (2000). *Living, Dying, Caring: Life and Death in a Nursing Home.* Melbourne: Ausmed Publications.

19. Shega JW, Levin A, Hougham D and Cox-Heeley D (2003). Palliative Excellence in Alzheimer Care Efforts (PEACE): a programme description. *Journal of Palliative Medicine* **6**(2): 315–320.

20. Travis S, Bernard M, Dixon S, McAuley W, Loving G and McClanahan L (2002). Obstacles to palliation and end-of-life care in long-term care facility. *The Gerontologist* **42**(3): 343–349.

21. Caron CD, Griffith J and Arcand M (2005). End-of-life decision making in dementia: the perspective of family caregivers. *Dementia: the International Journal of Social Research and Practice* **4**(1): 113–136.

22. Ronch JL (2004). Changing institutional culture: can we re-value the nursing home? *Journal of Gerontological Social Work* **43**(1): 61–82.

23. Brown J (2006). Student nurses' experience of learning to care for older people in enriched environments: a constructivist inquiry. Unpublished PhD thesis. University of Sheffield.

24. Sandberg J, Lundh U and Nolan M (2001). Placing a spouse in a care-home: the importance of keeping. *Journal of Clinical Nursing* **10**(3): 406–411.

25. Davies S (2003). Creating community: the basis for caring partnerships in nursing homes. In: Nolan MR, Grant G, Keady J and Lundh U (ed.). *Partnerships in Family Care: Understanding the Caregiving Career.* Maidenhead: Open University Press.

26. Hudson R and O'Connor M (2007). *Palliative Care and Aged Care: a Guide to Practice.* Melbourne: Ausmed Publications.

27. Brown M-A and Stetz K (1999). The labor of caregiving: a theoretical model of caregiving during potentially fatal illness. *Qualitative Health Research* **9**(2): 182–197.

28. Caron CD, Griffith J and Arcand M (2005). Decision making at the end of life in dementia: how family caregivers perceive their interactions with healthcare providers in long-term-care settings. *The Journal of Applied Gerontology* **22**: 1–17.

29. Hudson P, Aranda S and Kristjanson L (2004). Meeting the supportive needs of family carers in palliative care: challenges for health professionals. *Journal of Palliative Medicine* **7**(1): 19–25.

30. Robinson CA and Thorne S (1984). Strengthening family interference. *Journal of Advanced Nursing* **9**: 597–602.

31. Darbyshire P (1987). Ask the family. *Nursing Times* **83**(37): 23–25.

32. Ehrenfield M, Bergman R and Alpert R (1997). Family and staff involvement in tending dementia patients in nursing homes. *Journal of Clinical Nursing* **6**: 505–506.

33. Nay R (1997). Relatives' experiences of nursing home life: characterised by tension. *Australian Journal on Ageing* **16**(1): 24–29.

34. Pillemer K, Hegerman C, Albright B and Henderson C (1998). Building bridges between families and nursing home staff. *Gerontologist* **38**(4): 499–503.

35. Hertzberg A and Ekman EL (2000). We, not us and them? Views on the relationship and interaction between staff and relatives of elderly people living permanently in nursing homes. *Journal of Advanced Nursing* **31**(3): 614–622.

36. Haesler E, Bauer M and Nay R (2006). Factors associated with constructive staff-family relationships in the care of older adults in the institutional setting. *International Journal of Evidence Based Healthcare* **4**: 288–336.

37. Davies S (2001). Relatives' experiences of nursing home entry: a constructivist inquiry. Unpublished PhD thesis. University of Sheffield.

38. Aged Care Standards and Accreditation Agency at: http://www.accreditation.org.au/ AccreditationStandards

39. Lopez R (2007). Suffering and dying nursing home residents: nurses' perceptions of the role of family members. *Journal of Hospice and Palliative Nursing* **19**(3): 141–149.

40. Kitwood T (1997). *Dementia Reconsidered: the Person Comes First*. Buckingham: Open University Press.

41. Ersek M, Kraybill BM and Hansberry J (2000). Assessing the educational needs and concerns of nursing home staff regarding end-of-life care. *Journal of Gerontological Nursing* **26**(10): 16–26.

42. Vallis J and Boyd K (2002). Ethics and end-of-life decision-making. In: Hockley J and Clark D (ed.). *Palliative Care for Older People in Care Homes*. Milton Keynes: Open University Press, 120–137.

43. Nolan MR and Grant G (1992). *Regular Respite: An Evaluation of a Hospital Rota Bed Scheme for Elderly People*. Age Concern Institute of Gerontology Research Papers Series No. 6. London: Ace Books.

44. Nolan MR, Grant G and Keady J (1996). *Understanding Family Care: a Multidimensional Model of Caring and Coping*. Buckingham: Open University Press.

45. Evers HK (1981). Multidisciplinary teams in geriatric wards: myth or reality. *Journal of Advanced Nursing* **6**: 205–214.

46. Reed J and Bond B (1991). Nurses' assessments of elderly patients in hospital. *International Journal of Nursing Studies* **28**(1): 45–54.

47. Pennington RE and Pierce WL (1985). Observations of empathy in nursing home staff: a predictive study. *International Journal of Ageing and Human Development* **21**(4): 281–290.

48. Marck P (1990). Therapeutic reciprocity: a caring phenomenon. *Advances in Nursing Science* **13**(1): 49–59.

49. Nolan MR (1991). Timeshare beds: a pluralistic evaluation of rota bed systems in continuing care hospitals. Unpublished PhD Thesis. University of Wales, Bangor.

50. Nolan MR, Davies S, Brown J, Keady J and Nolan J (2002). *Longitudinal Study of the Effectiveness of Educational Preparation to Meet the Needs of Older People and Carers: The AGEIN Project*. London: English National Board.

51. Schumacher *et al.* (1998)

52. Stone RL (2003). Selecting a model of choosing your own culture. *Journal of Social Work in Long-Term Care* **2**(3/4): 411–422.

53. Dixon DL (2003). Successfully surviving culture change. *Journal of Social Work in Long-Term Care* **2**(3/4): 423–438.

54. Gibson DE and Barsade SG (2003). Managing organizational culture change: the case of long-term care. *Journal of Social Work in Long-Term Care* **2**(1/2): 11–34.

55. Tobin SS (2003). The historical context of 'humanistic' culture change in long-term care. *Journal of Social Work in Long-Term Care* **2**(1/2): 53–64.

56. Griffith J, Brosnan M, Lacey K, Keeling S and Wilkinson T (2004). Family meetings—a qualitative exploration of improving care planning with older people and their families. *Age and Ageing* **33**(6): 577–581.

57. Glare PJ, Virik K, Jones M, Hudson M, Eychmuller S, Simes J and Christakis NA (2003). A systematic review of physicians' survival predictions in terminally ill cancer patients. *British Medical Journal* **327**(7408): 195–197.

58. Newman J and Hughes M (2007). *Modernising Adult Social Care: What's Working?* London: Department of Health.

Chapter 11

Family carers of children confronting life-threatening illnesses

Sharon De Graves and Jenny Hynson

Introduction

Children with life-threatening illnesses form a unique population. Their healthcare needs and the impact on their carers are complex and intertwined with those of normal childhood and parenting. It is difficult to accept a diagnosis of a life-threatening illness in a child and the often uncertain disease trajectory places considerable stress on the family unit. A child's death is seen to disturb the natural order of life and presents ongoing and multifaceted challenges for bereavement. Indeed, the diagnosis of life-threatening illness in a child inexorably transforms their family's life (1).

Central to the care of children with life-threatening illnesses is the notion that the unit of care is the child and family; family being defined as 'those who provide physical, psychological, spiritual and social comfort to the child, regardless of genetic relationship' (2). The concept of family is, therefore, very broad and inclusive of two-parent families, single-parent families, blended families, families with adopted children, foster families, extended families, families where grandparents/relatives are sole carers and families where siblings are the carers. The make-up of different families has financial, cultural and social implications for their ability to adapt to and cope with life-threatening illnesses.

For the purposes of this discussion, childhood will be defined as encompassing the perinatal period, infancy, early and middle years, and adolescence. It is a socially constructed phase of life that is influenced by cultural, ethnic, spiritual, socio-economic and familial forces. Childhood is a time of rapid physical, psychological, emotional and spiritual development and from the tiniest newborn to the adolescent, children cannot be seen as 'little adults'.

Just as concepts of childhood are context-dependent, so too is the experience of life-threatening illnesses in children. In developing countries, for example, the types of life-threatening illnesses that affect children are different to those living in more developed societies. Sadly, children in these countries may die from conditions considered curable in circumstances where sophisticated and expensive treatments are available. Further, there may be challenges accessing appropriate care and support, and the family carer may even be a sibling if the children have been orphaned by Human Immunodeficiency Virus (HIV) in Africa or war in the Middle East.

Little is known about the influence of ethnicity and culture on the experience of life-threatening illnesses in childhood. However, there is some evidence that significant differences exist in how childhood illness is interpreted, lived and communicated (3, 4). The context in which the child and family live is a key determinant of what constitutes appropriate care and support.

The aim of this chapter is to highlight the particular needs of family carers of children confronting life-threatening illnesses. It begins with an overview of the nature of the various conditions that affect children, before moving on to an exploration of the issues facing those caring for children with such illnesses. Case examples will be used to illustrate key points. Considerations relating to various care settings, strategies to support family carers and bereavement will be discussed.

The nature of life-threatening illnesses in childhood

Throughout this chapter, the term 'life-threatening illness' will refer to any condition for which there is little prospect of cure and from which an affected individual is likely to die during childhood (5, 6). It is important to remember that most of the world's children live in underdeveloped countries, where infant and child mortality rates are high as a result of malnutrition and poor sanitation. In developed countries, however, neurodegenerative conditions, chromosomal abnormalities, congenital anomalies and malignancies account for the majority of life-threatening illnesses (7). Available epidemiological data are limited but recent estimates suggest that, in such countries, 16 per 10 000 children and adolescents aged 0–19 years are likely to die from a non-malignant life-threatening condition (8).

Although the individual circumstances of each child and family are unique, the illnesses from which they suffer can be thought of in four broad categories (5):

1. Conditions where curative treatment is available but may fail (e.g. cancer, organ failure).

2. Conditions where premature death is inevitable but where intensive therapy can prolong and enhance quality of life (e.g. cystic fibrosis, HIV infection).

3. Progressive conditions for which no curative treatment exists (e.g. Tay Sachs disease, certain mucopolysaccharidoses).

4. Irreversible conditions that are not themselves progressive but predispose the child to premature death as a result of respiratory complications, seizure disorders and other associated complications (e.g. severe cerebral palsy or congenital anomalies).

The way in which a life-threatening illness unfolds has significant implications for family carers. For the majority of children with cancer, for example, treatment is at least a possibility and the initial focus of care is on curing their condition. Relapse or failure to achieve remission may raise concern but it can be very difficult to predict the outcome for individuals given that some children with poor prognostic indicators survive, while others with seemingly better prognoses die (9). Families and health professionals may find it very difficult to abandon the hope for a cure in this context.

Families of children with conditions such as cystic fibrosis experience a different course. They know that premature death is inevitable and the focus of care is on helping the child to enjoy as long and good a life as possible. Toward the end stage of the illness, the child is likely to suffer episodes of life-threatening respiratory failure but it can be very difficult to predict which of these will be the terminal event. In circumstances where the child has survived episodes of severe illness, families often find it hard to believe that death is imminent and may struggle with decisions to withdraw treatment (10).

The course of many life-threatening conditions is long and unpredictable. Neurodegenerative conditions, in particular, progress over months to years and often result in significant levels of disability. Limited mobility and communication are common as are seizures, respiratory complications, musculoskeletal problems and pressure sores. For some children, there is a slow and inexorable decline towards death. For others, the illness course is characterized by multiple relapses and remissions, and it may be very difficult to predict when the child might die (11). Families must somehow construct a life in the face of this chronic uncertainty.

Children with static encephalopathies are susceptible to a range of complications that heighten their susceptibility to premature death. In many ways, their illness course is similar to that of children with neurodegenerative conditions (12).

Although a diverse range of life-threatening conditions affect children, prognostic uncertainty is a feature that is common to almost all. This uncertainty may relate to the question of whether or not the child will ultimately survive the illness or it may concern expectations about when the child will die. This creates a series of tensions for family carers. On the one hand, they wish to exhaust all possible curative options. On the other, there is a need to avoid unnecessary suffering for the child. Further, there is a desire to sustain hope, whilst simultaneously dealing with the reality of the child's likely demise.

Principles of paediatric palliative care

Although most of the existing evidence relates to adult patients with cancer, palliative care offers a framework for approaching the provision of care to children with life-threatening illnesses. The World Health Organization defines palliative care for children as 'the active total care of the child's body, mind and spirit, and also involves giving support to the family. It begins when illness is diagnosed and continues regardless of whether or not a child receives treatment directed at the disease' (13). Outdated notions of palliative care that present cure and palliation as mutually exclusive options have been replaced by more inclusive models that promote the integration of palliative care and curative or life-promoting efforts from diagnosis (2, 5, 12–17). These more recent definitions and models of palliative care recognize the specific challenges of providing comprehensive care to children with life-threatening illnesses, notably the impact of chronicity and uncertainty.

A number of position statements on paediatric palliative care have been produced and provide general principles to guide those caring for children with life-threatening illnesses (2, 5, 7, 13). These include:

- Paediatric palliative care should aim to improve the child and family's quality of life by proactively addressing the full range of physical, emotional, psychological, social and spiritual issues that accompany life-threatening illnesses.

- Palliative care should start when a child is diagnosed with a life-threatening illness and continue throughout the disease trajectory. It can be integrated with ongoing efforts to cure or modify disease.

- It is important that, wherever possible, the child and family are cared for in the place of their choice.

- Care should be responsive to the unique needs of the child and family.

- Care should be planned and coordinated to enhance continuity across time and care settings.

- Families must be able to access appropriate clinical, financial and practical support (including respite care).

- Bereavement support is a key consideration.

Parents and carers seek honest information about the illness and its prognosis but they also need to maintain hope. They frequently want to take responsibility for the child's care but do need the assistance of others. Supporting family carers requires the careful negotiation of these tensions. Information needs to be sensitively provided but in a way that allows some hope. Guidance and leadership are required to ensure that the desperate pursuit of cure does not impose suffering on the child. Support must be provided in a way that allows carers to maintain a central role. Above all, it is the human connection between health professional and parent or carer that is of greatest importance. The provision of compassionate care allows parents to see that their child's life is valued and meaningful to others. It also facilitates trust, continuity and emotional support (18, 19).

Caring for children with life-threatening illnesses

Children have distinctive needs

The issues faced by children with life-threatening illnesses and their family carers differ from those faced by adults. The following dimensions require consideration:

- ◆ Childhood death in developed countries is now relatively rare. This has changed societal expectations surrounding childhood death and has affected community reactions when a child dies. Friends, relatives and acquaintances may distance themselves from the situation for fear of saying or doing the wrong thing.
- ◆ Developmental factors influence the child and family's illness experience including:
  - the child's cognitive and emotional understanding of illness and death;
  - the child's experience of, and ability to describe, symptoms;
  - communication;
  - the process of decision-making: from infancy parents act as the main decision-makers regarding treatment but as the child develops and reaches their adolescent years, it is important they become increasingly involved in decisions concerning their treatment;
  - physiologic and pharmacokinetic considerations: health professionals must be mindful of how medications are metabolized, distributed and excreted at various ages (20).
- ◆ The family carer role is different where a child is affected by life-threatening illnesses:
  - parents or others tend to be more involved in the provision of care;
  - parents are surrogate decision-makers;
  - a parent's fundamental role—to nurture and protect—is challenged by life-threatening illness;

- the chronicity of childhood life-threatening illnesses places a tremendous burden of care on families;
- parents who are carriers of genetic conditions may feel a sense of responsibility for their child's illness.

◆ The impact on other family members:
  - siblings can experience both negative (stress) and positive (resilience) reactions to having a brother or sister with a life-threatening illness (21);
  - grandparents can experience feelings of guilt and helplessness as they watch their child in distress and their grandchild facing death—this can be seen as 'double grief'.

◆ Medical advances have resulted in more treatment options later in the disease trajectory, thus blurring the boundaries between cure-focused therapy and palliation. For children with potentially curable illnesses, there is often a continued hope for survival that may be difficult for families and health professionals to relinquish, even when death seems imminent (9, 22).

Meeting the needs of children

Family carers of children with life-threatening illnesses will need support and information to help them understand their child's awareness of their illness and to respond to any questions the child may ask. A child's cognitive and emotional understanding of illness and death is related to their developmental age, individual circumstances (including religion and culture) and life experience. Importantly, children who have experienced bereavement or who have a life-threatening illness have been shown to have a greater awareness and understanding of their illness than other children their age (23, 24). Consequently, knowledge of theories of cognitive development can only provide a general guide as to how individual children might understand their situation. Some important considerations for those supporting children of various ages are as follows:

◆ Children younger than 18 months have little understanding of their illness but have strong emotional reactions to hospitalization, pain and separation from family carers (25).

◆ Pre-schoolers are characterized by a tendency to egocentricity and magical thinking (25). They may believe they have caused illness or death with their own actions or thoughts, and may view illness, pain or death as punishment (24, 25). It is important that explanations are simple and factual, and care should be taken to correct misconceptions that may cause feelings of guilt and anxiety.

- School-age children are less self-centred and more social. By the age of seven, most children have an understanding of four basic concepts about death: that death is irreversible (irreversibility); that death means the cessation of all bodily functions (finality); that all living things ultimately die (universality); and that death is caused by illness, age or trauma (causality) (25). Given the considerable variability between individuals, care should be taken to establish each child's level of understanding, rather than operating on assumptions.

- Adolescents have different informational and support needs from younger children. Their need for privacy, autonomy and control is challenged by the restrictions imposed by life-threatening illnesses, and they may strive for normalcy, acceptance and independence (26). Adolescents often seek support from their peer group rather than from their parents. Normal risk-taking behaviour may manifest as non-adherence to treatment regimens.

While the principles of good communication, such as establishing a level of understanding and soliciting opinions and wishes, apply equally to children, there are a number of issues that require specific consideration (26):

- Observation of non-verbal communication (e.g. crying, withdrawal, aggression, clinginess and a flaccid or stiff body) is especially important in younger children or children with communication or learning difficulties, and can be integral to establishing their physical and emotional needs.

- Play or art therapy can be a useful communication aid and provides a medium through which to address the child's concerns and anxieties.

- It can be normal for a child, and especially an adolescent, to express a range of emotions in response to stress and illness, including fear, shame, resentment, denial, hostility and bravado (26).

- Family carers will be able to provide valuable information regarding how a child normally communicates and their normal responses to stress and illness.

- Children are known to protect their parents from distress by denying or minimizing symptoms, avoiding difficult conversations and maintaining a positive or courageous demeanour (23). This may mean that their physical, emotional, psychological and spiritual issues are not recognized and addressed.

The impact of life-threatening illnesses on the family

When a child is diagnosed with a life-threatening illness, parents are confronted with their greatest fear. Initial reactions can include shock, disbelief, anger, guilt, despair and a sense of loss for the child that they had known and hoped for (27). Indeed, life-threatening illnesses involve multiple losses (12): parents face the loss of the well child, the loss of that child's future and, ultimately, the death of the child. In addition, they must confront the loss of their hopes and dreams, the loss of the lifestyle they knew and the loss of their identity as the parent of a well child. Throughout the illness continuum, grief reactions first experienced at diagnosis can re-surface at critical junctures, such as disease progression, relapse or clinical deterioration (27).

Much of the impact of life-threatening illnesses in childhood centres on uncertainty. Cohen (1) states that '[t]o live with a child who has a life-threatening, chronic illness is to live with sustained uncertainty'. Just as grief reactions are heightened at diagnosis and critical junctures, so too is uncertainty. While the threat of deterioration and loss is always present, uncertainty surrounds the timing of such an event (28). Parents or carers must deal with what has been termed 'certain death at an unknown time' (11). They know their child will die but do not know when, since the course of many life-threatening illnesses involves multiple relapses and remissions, and children may appear close to death on a number of occasions. Triggers of heightened uncertainty include routine medical appointments, changes in symptoms, comments made by health professionals, changes in the therapeutic regimen and evidence of disease progression (28). Meleski (29) has identified the five most difficult transition times and stressors for families of children with chronic illnesses as diagnosis, family reorganization, tasks related to the management of chronic illness, developmental milestones and changes in the course of illness. Understanding potential triggers of uncertainty, and the resultant distress families experience, assists in the development of services that meet their needs at all stages of disease (27).

Case vignette 1: child with a malignant condition

Jack was diagnosed with acute lymphoblastic leukaemia when he was 4 years old. His family were devastated. They had recently moved to the city and were far away from close family and friends. Jack's grandparents came to stay for the first 2 months of his treatment to help look after his two younger siblings. When they left, Jack's family felt isolated, as they concentrated on providing care to Jack and caring for his siblings. The cancer ward's social worker helped the family make links in the community and establish a support network for the family. Jack underwent 2 years of standard chemotherapy. He lost his hair, had trouble maintaining weight and developed anticipatory nausea when arriving at the hospital. Bringing him in for treatment caused his parents great anguish as they watched the medications they hoped would save him result in so much pain and suffering. During his treatment, Jack experienced two life-threatening septic episodes, one of which resulted in an admission to the intensive care unit. Never had his parents felt so helpless and fearful. Jack survived only to relapse six months later. Although his parents were worried that Jack would not survive, they maintained a positive approach. Jack now required a bone marrow transplant

(BMT). His younger brother was found to be a match and Jack had his transplant when he was 7 years old. His parents were concerned about the impact on Jack's younger brother and sought advice surrounding how to minimize any feelings of responsibility for Jack's recovery. Eight months after his transplant Jack has once again relapsed and is having treatment with the hope that his cancer will go into remission again and he can have another BMT. His family is aware that his chances of cure are dramatically reduced but remain focused on the hope for cure.

The experience described in the above case vignette reflects the often unpredictable trajectory of childhood cancer, where little certainty surrounds which, if any, deterioration will result in death. Families have often faced many crises over the course of the child's illness, including the initial diagnosis, coping with the rigours of treatment, hospital admissions, relapses and sometimes bone marrow transplantation. At these times, the psychosocial needs of the entire family are increased. Fluctuating disease trajectories require a flexible response. While ongoing attempts may be made to cure or modify the underlying disease, palliative or supportive care must be provided simultaneously to ensure the child is as physically comfortable as possible, and that their emotional and spiritual needs are met. It is also important that the child and family's uncertainties, fears of treatment failure, anxieties and concerns are openly discussed and managed.

Life-threatening illnesses in childhood have far-reaching consequences. There can be a significant effect on family social activities due to illness, mobility issues or frequent and unexpected hospitalization (27). Consequently, families may find themselves isolated from important sources of support. In addition, many families experience financial stress due to the combined effects of reduced income and medical expenses, as well as the need to obtain equipment and modify the home environment (30). Perhaps more importantly, individual family members may find themselves coping with the challenge of life-threatening illness in different ways (31). One partner, for example, may find it helpful to talk about, and openly display, their emotions, while the other may prefer to deal with these alone. One partner may want to make plans and decisions ahead of time, while the other may prefer to take 'one day at a time'. Parents may need reassurance that there is no 'right way' to manage grief and uncertainty.

Implications for the parent or carer

Fundamental to being a parent is the role of protector and nurturer. This is threatened when a child is diagnosed with a life-threatening illness and parents may experience a sense of failure. These feelings may relate to their inability to protect the child from illness and death but they may also relate to the inability to prevent suffering. Some parents are required to make treatment decisions in which they must knowingly subject the child to considerable pain and suffering in the pursuit of a cure. The role of nurturer is also challenged by the progression of a disease over which parents have no control and parents may find feeding difficulties and weight loss especially hard to bear (12). For parents of children with genetic illnesses there may be an added sense of responsibility and guilt (32).

Parents who feel they have failed to protect their child from illness and death often become committed to ensuring their child's remaining life is as good as it possibly can be. Most parents and carers want to take responsibility for this and seek a system of care that can support them in their efforts. Caring for a child with a life-threatening illness, however, necessitates a large shift in roles within a family (29). Family members, especially mothers, need to extend and adapt their existing roles according to the child's disease trajectory and medical needs. Although the role of a parent naturally involves the provision of care to the child, the tasks involved in looking after a child with life-threatening illness may be much more complex and intense (5). Family carers must learn about their child's illness and the service system available to support them. They also need to administer medications and other treatments such as physiotherapy. Some are required to manage more complex tasks such as gastrostomy feeds, seizures and even the operation of ventilators. In addition, parents or carers must address the child's emotional and social needs. Even these needs are beyond the scope of 'normal' parenting. Few will have any knowledge of or experience with the concerns and emotional needs of a child facing life-threatening illness and death. At times, the care needs of a very sick child can seem overwhelming, especially when they are sustained over a long period or when parents are deprived of sleep. Many family carers are also responsible for the coordination of their child's care (27). This may involve the management of a sometimes bewildering array of individuals and agencies. These responsibilities and the associated stress are prone to increase at times of ill-health, disease progression and at the end of life, and have the potential to impact on family relationships. Open negotiation of roles and responsibilities within a family may help in maintaining family stability (29). The case described in the next vignette highlights some of the issues faced by families caring for a child with life-threatening illness.

Case vignette 2: child with a neurodegenerative condition

Manuel is a 12-year-old boy with adrenoleukodystrophy. His condition was diagnosed some years ago and he has progressively deteriorated over that time. He is now immobile, unable to communicate and requires nasogastric feeding. He also suffers constipation, seizures and appears to be in pain when moved. Manuel is completely dependent on his parents for all his care needs. He requires regular turning through the night and, due to his excessive secretions, he needs to be suctioned frequently, especially when he is unwell. Manuel's mother is his main carer but she has found it increasingly difficult to cope over the last year. Her husband has stopped working in an effort to help her at home. They have been struggling to find the equipment they need to care for him and only 4 hours of respite care is available to them fortnightly. Over the last 12 months, Manuel has been admitted to the intensive care unit at the children's hospital seven times with respiratory tract infections. His overall condition is deteriorating with each admission. The paediatrician has expressed the view that it may no longer be in Manuel's best interest to be treated in the intensive care unit. He has asked the family to think about this. Manuel's parents are distressed. On the one hand they want to have as much time with their child as possible and cannot bear the thought that he will die. On the other hand, they don't want him to suffer needlessly. Eventually they decide that the next respiratory illness will be managed at home where Manuel can spend time with his brothers and sisters, his parents and his dog. Manuel becomes unwell with pneumonia and dies peacefully at home. His parents are present and describe the moment of death as 'beautiful'. They are relieved that his suffering is over and treasure the hours they spend with him after death.

Implications for siblings

The considerable impact of life-threatening illness extends to the entire family. Siblings also experience grief and loss when a brother or sister is unwell. Research has found that adults repeatedly underestimate the effects of traumatic events on children (33). Siblings may feel the loss of the relationship with their brother or sister, as well as the physical and emotional loss of their parents as they care for their sick child. They may feel lonely, sad, isolated and displaced within their family, as they negotiate new and changing boundaries and responsibilities (27, 34). It is natural for siblings to envy the attention received by the sick child but they may struggle with feelings of guilt and remorse. They may also have misconceptions about the cause of their brother's or sister's illness, the nature of the illness, and the experience of hospital admission and treatment (27). Parental preoccupation with the sick child may mean they are unable to meet their healthy child's emotional needs. Further, a change in family dynamics often occurs and normal routines may be disrupted. This shift in dynamics, grief and uncertainty can result in distress for siblings and can manifest as difficult and challenging behaviour. Supportive interventions include assisting parents to provide information to all of their children, including the sibling, in the care of the sick child, and maintaining as much normality in family life as possible.

Family coping

Some family carers are better resourced to manage the challenges of caring for a child with a life-threatening illness than others (27). Variables include individual coping strategies, degree of family cohesion, intellectual ability, social supports, financial resources and spiritual beliefs and support. Identification of families at risk is essential to targeting interventions aimed at providing appropriate support (35).

Families use various strategies to cope with living with a child with a life-threatening illness. Hodgkinson and Lester (32) identified three main coping strategies utilized by mothers caring for children with cystic fibrosis: problem-focused, appraisal-focused and emotion-focused strategies. Problem-focused strategies involved support seeking and the identification of goals and rewards. Appraisal-focused coping involved adjusting to the situation and normalizing problems. Finally, emotion-focused strategies involved resigned acceptance and maintaining hope (32).

Uncertainty has been identified as a significant challenge for families caring for children with life-threatening illnesses. It has been said '[t]he management of uncertainty involves strategies to manipulate the known, the unknown and the unknowable' (1). In the specific circumstance of childhood cancer, living in the moment, maintaining normality, information seeking and sustaining hope, have been found to help families cope with the uncertainty of the illness (9). Exploring how families of children diagnosed with a range of chronic life-threatening illnesses live with sustained uncertainty, Cohen found that they must learn to manage six dimensions of daily life, including: time, social interaction, information, awareness, illness and the environment (1). Recognizing how families manage the stress of uncertainty is important to developing targeted interventions and programmes that support the family unit over time.

Supporting family carers

There is limited evidence regarding specific interventions that health professionals can use to support family carers of children with life-threatening illnesses. However, a number of organizations have produced standards of care to guide practice (2, 5, 7). In addition to the general principles outlined above, it is important to consider the following:

- Respect and support the family caregiver's central role in providing care to the child.
- Try to understand and respond to the caregiver's concerns. A priority for most families is to minimize the child's suffering, so managing symptoms effectively is critical. There will be a range of emotional, spiritual and psychological concerns but these will vary and are best understood by listening to the individual caregiver.

- Good communication is consistently cited by parents as a correlate of effective palliative care. Attention to the relationship between family and health professional builds trust and creates an environment in which communication is enhanced. Parents often seek honest information about their child's condition, prognosis and treatment, as well as the supports available to them and the physical changes that accompany dying. They may also need advice regarding how to address the sick child's questions and concerns. Information needs to be provided with sensitivity and compassion.

- Ensure practical supports are provided. While most carers want to remain responsible for their child's care, they need the necessary medicines, equipment, financial support and respite.

- Continuity and coordination. Caring for a child with a life-threatening illness requires the input of a number of individuals and agencies. It is crucial that these are coordinated. Appointing a key-worker can be a useful practical strategy.

- Compassion. The importance of compassion cannot be overstated. When their child is dying, parents greatly value 'simple acts of human kindness' (18). Compassion has intrinsic human value but it is also fundamental to trust and communication.

- The provision of bereavement support (see section on bereavement below).

Location of care

When thinking about where care should be provided, consideration should be given to the options and resources available, the child's medical needs, and the child and family's preferences. Over the course of a life-threatening illness it can be expected that a child will spend most of their time at home, some time in hospital and, in some countries, some time in a children's hospice. In this way, the care of a child with life-threatening illness is a dynamic process. Success is dependent on effective coordination between care providers and agencies across various locations, so that continuity and communication are enhanced (36). Where possible, care should be provided with minimal disturbance to normal home and school routines (37), although there may be times when hospital admission is unavoidable.

Home care

Medical and treatment advances have resulted in increased survival rates, improved quality of life and longer lifespans for children with life-threatening illnesses, and have also resulted in an increase in the number of children with complex needs who are cared for at home (38). There is evidence that home is the preferred place of care for many families (39, 40). Many parents see home as a place where they can promote family unity, create a sense of normality, exert greater control and improve their child's quality of life (18, 40–42). Although the majority of parents seek to take primary responsibility for caring for their child and see this as a natural extension of their role as parents, providing care in the home is challenging and time-consuming and can place stress on the family unit (41, 43). Boling (43) has demonstrated a relationship between the health of a chronically ill child and the health and quality of life of their family carers, with the latter decreasing as the child's disease severity increases. The provision of sufficient support to family carers during periods of home care is essential in order to combat feelings of abandonment, to detect physical or emotional stress, and to promote family coping (37).

Hospital

Children with life-threatening illnesses are likely to require frequent hospitalization due to acute illness, treatment or exacerbation of their condition. These episodes can be a source of increasing stress and demands on family carers (29). Carers of children with complex care needs can find hospital admissions particularly challenging (37). The following issues should be considered when caring for such children in the hospital setting:

- Family carers of children with life-threatening illnesses develop a unique knowledge of their child's condition, as well as expertise in symptom management, and can feel that this experience and understanding is not acknowledged or respected (44).

- Hospitalization may be the result of an exacerbation or progression of illness or a change in the therapeutic regimen. These have been shown to result in increased stress and uncertainty for family carers (28, 29).

- Family carers will be required to interact with a multidisciplinary team that may or may not be aware of their child's condition and individual care needs.

- Different approaches to care by different health professionals may give rise to confusion and mistrust.

- Parent carers of children with chronic illnesses have been shown to have a preference for high levels of participation and control in their child's care (including technical care) during hospitalization (38).

- Information sharing is important to families. There is an expectation that they will be kept informed and may become anxious when this does not occur (38).
- Siblings of a hospitalized child with a life-threatening illness find their parents are emotionally unavailable and preoccupied.

Hospice

The children's hospice movement began in the early 1980s in the UK with the opening of Helen House in 1982 (45). Since then there has been a growth in children's hospices. There are now 38 in the UK (46), and many other countries, including Australia, Poland, Canada and Germany, offer this option of care to children with life-threatening illnesses. Hospices offer respite and terminal care to children and families living with life-limiting, progressive illnesses in a community-based, home-like environment. In contrast to adult hospices, the paediatric equivalent tends to be utilized predominantly for respite care, rather than terminal care (8). This is a crucial role, however. Psychosocial support is integral to hospice care and extends across the disease continuum into bereavement (37).

Bereavement considerations for family carers whose child has died

The death of a child leaves you feeling helpless, guilty, powerless and broken.

(47 p.179).

The death of their child, the one person they were meant to protect, may be the most sorrowful experience known to parents. Parental grief is known to be especially severe, prolonged and prone to complication (48). Indeed, a large population-based study has demonstrated an increased mortality rate among bereaved parents (49). Enabling a child and family to gain a sense of control over the events, environment and circumstances of death may help them find some comfort in the turmoil. The health professional's role is not '… to tell them how they should think or behave, but to stay with them while they discover the answers within themselves' (47). Following a child's death, it is important that parents or carers know there is no right or wrong thing to do. Rather, they should be offered the opportunity to discuss their options and preferences (47).

Our understanding of grief has moved away from linear, stage-based models, towards grief work models (50). It is now understood that the relationship with the deceased child does not need to end but is instead transformed (50). Families of a child who has died face the challenge of redefining their world without that child. This new world is full of reminders of the child who has died and families are constantly confronted with their loss. This may be experienced most profoundly at anniversaries, birthdays and when important milestones (e.g. graduation, first job, marriage and childbirth) are reached by others within and close to the family.

Religious and cultural influences are important determinants of how families mourn the loss of a child. It is important, however, not to assume that carers from certain cultural groups will respond in stereotypical fashion. Individuals will vary in their beliefs and in how closely they follow traditions.

Conclusion

In summary, the diverse range of life-threatening conditions suffered by children, the uncertainty associated with many of these illnesses and the rapid developmental changes that occur throughout childhood, mean that a different approach is required to their care. The needs of the child and the needs of the family are inextricably linked and are strongly influenced by cultural factors. Despite this considerable diversity, family carers share a number of common needs. They must manage a complex array of physical and organizational tasks, whilst simultaneously attending to their own grief, the complex emotional needs of the sick child and the needs of their other children. At the same time, they may need to manage financial pressures, as well as the impact of the illness on relationships within the family. Many children with life-threatening illnesses are ill for months or years and great uncertainty often surrounds their prognosis. Those involved in caring for such families must be able to provide support through this period of chronicity and uncertainty, and into bereavement. Care needs will vary across time and according to the personal, social, financial and other resources available to the carers. Some carers are able to manage their child's illness relatively independently, while others require considerable assistance. Although parental grief can be especially severe and prolonged, some carers are able to reflect positively on the experience of caring for their very sick child.

Key learning points

+ Life-threatening illnesses affecting children are different to those affecting adults with a wider variety of diagnoses, many of which are characterized by chronicity and uncertainty.

- The developmental stage of the child influences their physical, emotional, psychological and spiritual needs.
- Children are dependent on family carers and health professionals to make decisions in their best interests and to provide care.
- Caring for a child with a life-threatening illness may seem to contradict the parenting role, which is to nurture and protect.
- Life-threatening illness affects the child, their parents/carers and siblings, their extended family and the broader community.
- Parental grief is especially severe and prone to complication.
- Family caregivers need a system of care that empowers them to maintain a central role as parent and decision-maker.

Recommended reading and resources

ACT (The Association for Children's Palliative Care). PaedPal Literature Search www.act.org.uk

American Academy of Pediatrics (2000). Palliative care for children. *Pediatrics* **106**: 351–357.

Association for Children with Life-threatening or Terminal Conditions and their Families and the Royal College of Paediatrics and Child Health (2003). *A Guide to the Development of Children's Palliative Care Service* (2nd edn). Report of a joint working party of the Association for Children with Life-threatening or Terminal Conditions and their Families and the Royal College of Paediatrics and Child Health. London: ACT.

Bluebond-Langner M (1978). *The Private World of Dying Children*. New Jersey: Princeton University Press.

EAPC task force (2007). IMPaCCT: standards for paediatric palliative care in Europe. *European Journal of Palliative Care* **14**: 109–114.

Goldman A, Hain R and Liben S (ed.) (2006). *Oxford Textbook of Palliative Care for Children*. Oxford: Oxford University Press.

Institute of Medicine (2003). *When Children Die: Improving Palliative and End-of-life Care for Children and their Families*. Washington DC: National Academies Press.

IPPC. *The initiative for pediatric palliative care*. www.ippcweb.org

Kuttner L (2004). *Making Every Moment Count* [film]. Canada: National Film Board of Canada and Stillwater Productions.

Mellonie B (2005). *Beginnings and Endings with Life Times in Between*. Australia: Penguin Books. Children's picture book recommended for children 4 years and older.

References

1. Cohen MH (1993). The unknown and the unknowable—managing sustained uncertainty. *Western Journal of Nursing Research* **15**(1): 77–96.
2. EAPC task force (2007). IMPaCCT: standards for paediatric palliative care in Europe. *European Journal of Palliative Care* **14**(3): 109–114.

3. Kolk AM, Schipper JL, Hanwald GJFP, Casari EF and Fantino AG (2000). The impact-on-family scale: a test of invariance across culture. *Journal of Pediatric Psychology* **25**(5): 323–329.

4. Thibodeaux AG and Deatrick JA (2007). Cultural influence on family management of children with cancer. *Journal of Pediatric Oncology Nursing* **24**(4): 227–233.

5. Association for Children with Life-threatening or Terminal Conditions and their Families and the Royal College of Paediatrics and Child Health (2003). *A Guide to the Development of Children's Palliative Care Service* (2nd edn). Report of a joint working party of the Association for Children with Life-threatening or Terminal Conditions and their Families and the Royal College of Paediatrics and Child Health. London: ACT.

6. Lenton S, Stallard P and Mastroyannopoulou K (2001). Prevalence and morbidity associated with non-malignant, life-threatening conditions in childhood. *Child: Care, Health and Development* **27**: 389–398.

7. American Academy of Pediatrics (2000). Palliative care for children. *Pediatrics* **106**: 351–357.

8. Craft A and Killen S (2007). *Palliative Care Services for Children and Young People in England*. An independent review for the Secretary of State for Health. Department of Health, London, United Kingdom.

9. De Graves S (2003). Living with hope and fear—the uncertainty of childhood cancer after relapse Unpublished PhD thesis. The University of Melbourne.

10. Robinson WM, Ravilly S, Berde C and Wohl ME (1997). End-of-life care in cystic fibrosis. *Pediatrics* **100**(2): 205–209.

11. Steele R (2000). Trajectory of certain death at an unknown time: children with neurodegenerative life-threatening illnesses. *Canadian Journal of Nursing Research* **32**: 49–67.

12. Hynson J (2006). The child's journey: transition form health to ill-health. In: Goldman A, Hain R and Liben S (ed.). *Oxford Textbook of Palliative Care for Children*. New York, USA: Oxford University Press, 14–27.

13. World Health Organization (2007). *Palliative Care* [online] (cited 2007 June 9). Available from: URL: www.who.int/cancer/palliative/definition/en

14. Goldman A and Heller K (2000). Integrating palliative and curative approaches in the care of children with life-threatening illnesses. *Journal of Palliative Medicine* **3**(3): 353–359.

15. Mack JW and Wolfe J (2006). Early integration of pediatric palliative care: for some children, palliative care starts at diagnosis. *Current Opinion in Pediatrics* **18**: 10–14.

16. Wolfe J, Grier HE, Klar N, Levin SB, Ellenbogen JM, Salem-Schatz S, Emanuel EJ and Weeks JC (2000). Symptoms and suffering at the end of life in children with cancer. *The New England Journal of Medicine* **342**(5): 326–333.

17. Himelstein BP, Hilden JM, Boldt AM and Weissman D (2004). Medical progress: pediatric palliative care. *The New England Journal of Medicine* **350**(17): 1752–1762.

18. Davies B, Deveau E, deVeber B, Howell D, Martinson I, Papadatou D, Pask E and Stevens M(1998). Experiences of mothers in five countries whose child died of cancer. *Cancer Nursing* **21**(5): 301–311.

19. Heller K and Solomon M (2005). Continuity of care and caring: what matters to parents of children with life-threatening conditions. *Journal of Pediatric Nursing* **20**: 335–346.

20. McGrath PA (1996). Development of the World Health Organization guidelines on cancer pain relief and palliative care in children. *Journal of Pain & Symptom Management* **12**(2): 87–92.

21. Fleitas J (2000). When Jack fell down… Jill came tumbling after: siblings in the web of illness and disability. *American Journal of Maternal and Child Nursing* **25**(5): 267–273.

22. Frager G (1996). Pediatric palliative care: building the model, bridging the gaps. *Journal of Palliative Care* **12**(3): 9–12.

23. Bluebond-Langner M (1978). *The Private World of Dying Children.* New Jersey: Princeton University Press.

24. Faulkner KW (1997). Dealing with death. Talking about death with a dying child. *American Journal of Nursing* **97**(6): 64.

25. Schonfeld DJ (1993). Talking with children about death. *Journal of pediatric healthcare* **7**(6): 269–274.

26. Down G and Simons J (2006). Communication. In: Goldman A, Hain R and Liben S (ed.). *Oxford Textbook of Palliative Care for Children.* New York, USA: Oxford University Press, 28–41.

27. Lewis M and Prescott H (2006). Impact of life-limiting illness on the family. In: Goldman A, Hain R and Liben S (ed.). *Oxford Textbook of Palliative Care for Children.* New York, USA: Oxford University Press, 154–78.

28. Cohen MH (1995). The triggers of heightened parental uncertainty in chronic life-threatening childhood illness. *Qualitative Health Research* **5**(1): 63–77.

29. Meleski DD (2002). Families with chronically ill children. *American Journal of Nursing* **102**(5): 47–54.

30. Dockerty J, Skegg D and Williams S (2003). Economic effects of childhood cancer on families. *Pediatric Child Health* **39**: 254–258.

31. Mastroyannopoulou K, Stallard P, Lewis M and Lenton S (1997). The impact of childhood non-malignant life-threatening illness on parents: gender differences and predictors parental adjustment. *Journal of Child Psychology and Psychiatry* **38**: 823–829.

32. Hodgkinson R and Lester H (2002). Stresses and coping strategies of mothers living with a child with cystic fibrosis: implications for nursing professionals. *Journal of Advanced Nursing* **394**: 377–383.

33. Yule W and Williams RM (1990) Post-traumatic stress reactions in children. *Journal of Traumatic Stress* **3**: 279–295.

34. Stallard P, Mastroyannopoulou K, Lewis M and Lenton S (1997). The siblings of children with life-threatening conditions. *Child Psychology and Psychiatry Review* **2**(1): 26–33.

35. Kazak A, Kassum-Adams N, Schneider S, Zelikovsky N, Alderfer MA and Rourke M (2006). An integrative model of pediatric medical traumatic stress. *Journal of Pediatric Psychology* **31**(4): 343–355.

36. Davies B (1996). Assessment of need for a children's hospice program. *Death Studies* **20**: 247–268.

37. Brook L, Vickers J and Barber M (2006) Place of care. In: Goldman A, Hain R and Liben S (ed.). *Oxford Textbook of Palliative Care for Children.* New York, USA: Oxford University Press, 533–548.

38. Balling K and McCubbin M (2001). Hospitalized children with chronic illness: parental caregiving needs and valuing parental expertise. *Journal of Pediatric Nursing* **16**(2): 110–119.

39. Liben S and Goldman A (1998). Home care for children with life-threatening illness. *Journal of Palliative Care* **14**(3): 33–38.

40. Vickers JL and Carlisle C (2000). Choices and control: parental experiences in pediatric terminal home care. *Journal of Pediatric Oncology Nursing* **17**(1): 12–21.

41. Dangel T, Fowler-Kerry S, Karwacki M and Bereda J (2000). An evaluation of a home palliative care programmeme. *Ambulatory Child Health* **6**(2): 101–114.

42. Papadatou D, Yeantopoulos J and Kosmidis KV (1996). Death of a child at home or hospital: experiences of Greek mothers. *Death Studies* **20**(3): 215–235.

43. Boling W (2005). The health of chronically ill children. lessons learned from assessing family caregiver quality of life. *Family Community Health* **28**(2): 176–183.

44. Burke S, Kaufamann E, Costello E and Dillon M (1991). Hazardous secrets and reluctantly taking charge: parenting a child with repeated hospitalisations. *Image: Journal of Nursing Scholarship* **23**: 39–45.

45. Dominica F (1982). Helen House a hospice for children. *Maternal Child Health*, 355–359.

46. Association of Children's Hospices (2004). *Children's Hospice Services: a Guide for Professionals*. Bristol, UK: Association of Children's Hospices.

47. Dominica F (2006). After the child's death: Family care. In: Goldman A, Hain R and Liben S (ed.). *Oxford Textbook of Palliative Care for Children*. New York, USA: Oxford University Press, 179–192.

48. Rando T (1983). An investigation into grief and adaptation in parents whose children have died of cancer. *Journal of Pediatric Psychology* **8**: 3–19.

49. Li J, Precht D, Mortensen P and Olsen J (2003). Mortality in parents after death of a child in Denmark: nationwide follow-up study. *Lancet* **361**: 363–7.

50. Davies B, Attig T and Towne M (2006). Bereavement. In: Goldman A, Hain R and Liben S (ed.). *Oxford Textbook of Palliative Care for Children*. New York, USA: Oxford University Press, 193–203.

Chapter 12

Family carers of people with advanced cancer

Donna Milne and Karen Quinn

Introduction

To fully appreciate the role that family carers of people with advanced cancer perform, and to comprehend the number of people that carry out this impor-tant role, it is necessary to examine some of the cancer incidence statistics from around the developed world. In Australia in 2006, the risk of being diagnosed with cancer before the age of 75 years was one in three for men and one in four for women; this translated into 106 000 new cases of cancer and, in the same year (2006), 39 200 people died from cancer (1). In Canada 39 per cent of women and 44 per cent of men will develop cancer in their lifetime and 44 per cent of new cancers will occur in people aged 70 years or more. In terms of mortality, one out of every four Canadians will die of cancer (2). The American Cancer Society estimates that in 2007 there will be 1 444 920 new cases of cancer diagnosed and 559 650 people will die of cancer. This translates into one of every four deaths in America being attributed to cancer (3). In England there were 233 600 new cases of cancer diagnosed and 125 600 deaths from cancer in 2004. In keeping with Australia, America and Canada, one in every three people in the UK will develop cancer in their lifetime and one in four deaths will result from cancer (4).

Such figures provide some insight into the large number of patients and families that are affected by cancer resulting in a significant burden on the national health systems of all these countries. The current method for reduc-ing the burden on health systems around the world seems to rely heavily on shifting the burden of care to family members. The question of sustainability of this approach has to be raised when consideration is given to other develop-ments in cancer care, such as longer survival times for patients with a cancer diagnosis and emerging availability of out-patient treatments, both of which have resulted in a move toward patients with advanced cancer being cared for at home (5–7). Most often, responsibility for the caregiving role at home is primarily undertaken by family members and friends, ideally complemented with practical advice and support from community nursing or palliative care services. While taking on this role can be seen as normative, or an expected family function (8), it is imperative that clinicians working with people with cancer and their family members understand the negative and positive outcomes for the family members providing the care.

This chapter provides details on the nature of advanced cancer, describes the complexity of the family carer role, as well as the impact such a role can have on the person in the role. In particular, the impact of the caregiving role is distinguished from the needs of the family carer. Both are discussed and then suggestions for interventions and supports to meet identified needs are described in light of best available evidence.

What is advanced cancer?

The term 'advanced cancer' refers to cancer that has spread from the site of origin to other parts of the body. The diagnosis of advanced cancer is commonly acknowledged as a critical point in the illness trajectory (9), as hope for a cure is dashed, and in fact such a development indicates a poor prognosis. Advanced cancer can be diagnosed following a disease-free period (recurrence) or during or immediately after the administration of anti-cancer treatments (progression). In reality, the diagnosis of advanced cancer requires the patient and family members to deal with the transition from receiving treatment with a curative intent to treatment with a palliative intent.

The profile of a family carer

Sometimes in a cancer setting, the family carer is not a 'family member' in the traditional sense such as someone related by blood or marriage; rather, the carer may be a close friend or distant relative who takes on the role and associated responsibility. Therefore, the literature on families needs to be considered in broad terms that cater for a vast range of definitions of the term 'family'. This literature suggests that change in one aspect of the family unit will result in changes to the entire unit and the effects of change are multidirectional; the impact of the illness on the family and the family's impact on the illness are interdependent (10). Therefore, the family cannot be viewed merely as the principal source of support; they must be seen as the unit that faces the disease.

It is difficult to obtain exact numbers of family carers in any country because so many people fulfil the role without recognition or registration with any formal body. Carers Australia estimates there are 2.6 million carers of people with a disability or chronic illness, including cancer, in Australia. In America the figure is thought to be closer to 50 million (11) and in the UK six million (12). These figures are inflated as they represent family carers of people with other illnesses, not only cancer. However, by looking at the numbers of people diagnosed with cancer in a given year in each of these countries, and presuming the vast majority have a least one family carer, it is easy to see that a reasonable percentage of the overall carer group will be caring for someone with a cancer diagnosis. Consideration should be given to the fact that some patients do not have a family carer at any stage during their illness.

Australian statistics demonstrate that most primary family carers are female, aged over 65 years; they care for someone in a similar age group and live in the same residence. American figures are similar with 30 per cent of carers aged over 65 years (3). In Australia, the relationship between family carer and the patient is predominantly that of a partner (43 per cent); 25 per cent are children and 21 per cent are parents (7). Canadian research demonstrates similar findings: 75–85 per cent of care given to patients with advanced cancer occurs at home and is provided by family members in an unpaid capacity (13).

Most clinicians prefer to think family carers are performing adequately in their role; an assumption that holds true as long as carer needs are not routinely or formally assessed. However, research has identified numerous factors that impact on the caregiving arrangement. Factors include an ageing population, increased number of women in the workforce, decreased birth rate, increased rate of relationship breakdown and geographical separation of family members. In addition, there is increased pressure on family members to take on the caring role because other options, such as care provided in an in-patient hospital setting, are declining (14). Therefore, the role of the family carer has to be assessed and appropriate supportive interventions developed and implemented that respond to the identified carer needs.

The role of the family carer

Caring for someone with advanced cancer is an evolving role, it is one that changes as the patient's condition deteriorates and they become increasingly dependent on others for all care. Added to the complexity of the role is the fact that many carers take on the caregiving role out of a sense of duty, family responsibility and/or expectation, or simply because there is no-one else to do it (7, 13). Not only is caregiving a new role for most, but it may also be the first time the carer has been exposed to dying and ultimately to death.

A further layer of complexity for family carers occurs when the newly assumed carer role is at odds with the original basis of the patient–carer relationship, which may have been that of spouse, child, parent, friend or other relative. Traversing the new path of carer, combined with the pre-existing family or friend relationship, can be fraught with challenges, particularly in situations where there may be complete role reversal.

Commonly family carers of people with advanced cancer find themselves fulfilling multiple roles including those of nurse, symptom assessor, care coordinator, mediator in family tensions and the link person between the patient and health providers (13). Often family tension, resulting from pre-existing issues, can be exacerbated as a result of the diagnosis of a life-limiting illness in a family member. Consequently families struggle with communication, intimacy and problem-solving abilities. The cumulative result of dysfunctional coping strategies may exhibit as excessive drinking, drug use or avoidance of issues; therefore, clinicians need to be alert to the way the family functions as a unit.

Responsibilities and activities undertaken by carers include the following: attending to the patient's personal care (including hygiene, feeding, mobilization), liaison with community and hospital services, providing transportation, providing emotional support, preparation of meals, attending to financial matters, and management and decision-making regarding medications and their administration, as well as providing increasingly complex strategies for cancer care and symptom management (7).

Not surprisingly, the time required to fulfil the multiple roles performed by a family carer can be equivalent to that of a full-time occupation but the entitlements are vastly different. Family carers are usually lacking in the preparation or training required to carry out the role effectively; they receive neither ongoing support nor monetary reward for the role (7, 15, 16).

The role of the family carer in an advanced cancer setting is undoubtedly very complex. Without the care provided by family carers, particularly in the latter stages of their illness, the patients' overall care and well-being would be sub-optimal (17). Often literature on family carers fails to distinguish clearly between carer needs and the impact the role has on the person performing the role. For the purpose of this chapter 'impact' refers to the outcome of the caregiving role on the carer and 'need' describes a condition deemed important by the carer but is unmet.

Impact of caring on the carer

Many family carers report the impact of caregiving as positive; it may include a sense of pride and satisfaction with having performed the role and providing invaluable practical care (7, 13, 18). In an Australian study, 60 per cent of carers reported valuing the opportunity to simply be with their relative/friend, to express love and share special times with that person (19). Importantly, positive outcomes such as contributing to patient comfort, respecting the patient's wishes and having quality time with the patient have been demonstrated to have a positive influence on bereavement outcomes for the family carer (6, 7).

Family carers also experience negative outcomes of their role, some of which are viewed as inevitable (20). Negative outcomes can be psychological, such as experiencing feelings of inadequacy (20), anger and resentment (21), and an increase in symptoms of depression and anxiety (22). One study of 893 carers (over half of whom were caring for someone with advanced cancer) found that 31.4 per cent of these carers demonstrated significant depressive symptoms if they were caring for someone with substantial care needs (23). Other studies suggest between 18 and 58 per cent of carers experience clinical levels of depression (24).

Australian data suggest younger female carers have higher levels of psychological distress, especially when the caregiving role is combined with being the patient's spouse (7). Carer distress, including psychological, physical and spiritual, is also more likely when the role is taken on because the patient has been diagnosed with cancer that has already advanced. Carers seem to experience less distress when they have time to adjust to their role and their own emotions regarding the diagnosis before the patient develops advanced cancer (25, 19).

Being a carer can impact physically on a person and result in poor sleep patterns (21), physical exhaustion and illness such as muscle pain, (22) hypertension and stress (26). Such physical problems, as well as the worsening of pre-existing medical conditions (27), are often problematic for carers who commonly fall into the older age bracket. Research has found that, unfortunately, carer health seems to deteriorate in line with the patient's deterioration and the decline continues into bereavement (28).

Carer outcomes can also be influenced by the patient's age. Caring for younger patients or caring in an environment of limited social support and networks increases the risk of distress for the carer (21). Carers of all ages can also experience decreased opportunities for socializing, personal relationships and time to themselves (8), all of which result in an overall decrease in the carer's quality of life (29).

Other factors identified by research that contribute to negative caregiving outcomes include fulfilling the role of family carer for extended periods of time (16, 30) and caring for someone who has multiple symptoms or poor physical functioning (13). Carer factors that contribute to negative caregiving outcomes include limited education, which is thought to limit the carers' ability to cope with distress, and financial worries due to loss of income while performing the caregiving role (7).

The role of family carer impacts on the physical and psychological health of the person in the role. Consequently family carers have many unmet needs that clinicians should be aware of so that, when support is available and desired by the carer, it can be provided. The next section provides an overview of family carer needs that have been identified through research.

Carer needs

Many of the major research studies into the needs of family carers of people with cancer were completed in the 1980s and 1990s (29, 31–34). Few new studies seeking to identify carer needs have been conducted since then; instead the focus has shifted to identifying appropriate, acceptable and sustainable ways of meeting carer needs. A brief review of carers' needs is provided here and is followed by a discussion of interventions and supports for family carers.

A need refers to a condition that is important to the respondent and is not being currently satisfied by their environment (33). In the literature carer needs are commonly discussed within six categories: informational, psychological, patient care, personal, spiritual and household. These categories reflect an holistic approach to the assessment process and in turn are useful in informing supportive interventions developed for the carer. These categories have been used for the brief overview of needs provided here and are carried over into the discussions about carer assessment.

Despite the fact that carer needs have been identified and reported by numerous researchers, it is important to keep in mind that carers are often very reluctant to admit to their own needs and may need encouragement to do so. This problem occurs when carers prioritize the patient's wishes before their own, when they feel embarrassed about having needs, when they worry about being perceived as inadequate or not coping, or when they feel that identifying their own needs will take services away from the patient. If this reluctance to report needs is not identified and addressed, then the carer may experience negative outcomes (13, 20, 35).

Informational needs of family carers

Regardless of when advanced cancer is diagnosed, patients and carers want information. Many studies report a high incidence of informational needs amongst family carers. Unsatisfied informational needs commonly relate to treatment side-effects, what will happen in the future, symptoms of the disease, availability of community resources, patient comfort and the state of the patient's illness (9, 28, 33). The identification of informational needs is important because providing carers with information allows them to understand the expected course of the illness, thereby relieving some of their uncertainty, as well as enabling them to provide the required care (18). Jones' 1993 study (34) of UK carers found that only 62 per cent of the 181 carers of cancer patients who died at home had received sufficient information. It is important to remember two important points about the provision of information. First, carers are listening to and processing the information for themselves, as well as for the patient. Concurrently, carers are required to support the patient who is hearing the same information. Second, it is common for carers to want more information than the patient especially around care at the end of life (36). This situation needs to be handled sensitively by the clinician.

Psychological needs of family carers

The psychological needs of carers commonly manifest as anxiety and depression. An Australian study found that one-third of spousal and 25 per cent of off-spring carers were clinically depressed, suggesting a significant level of psychological support needs (37). Psychological needs are commonly linked with the level of information about the disease, treatment options and prognosis provided by clinicians; therefore, the better informed the carer is, the better they cope psychologically (38). Others suggest psychological needs are closely linked with appraising the caregiving situation as stressful, being anxious about the future (39) and having few opportunities to discuss fears (40). Similarly, when the carer's health is poor or the patient is experiencing significant symptoms, the carer's psychological needs increase (30). However, one study (22) found that, even though carers experienced their own psychological problems, one in five did not want professional support to deal with these issues.

Family carer needs related to patient care

Most carers want their family members to be comfortable and well cared for; however, managing physical care can be very demanding. In an early study of 83 family carers (40), researchers found that assistance with physical care was an unmet need for 31 per cent of the sample. Another study, conducted 10 years later, of the needs of 76 carers of people with advanced cancer being cared for at home, still found that carers wanted assistance to learn about the physical care and signs that were important to be aware of (25 per cent), as well as how to deal with the patient's pain (21 per cent) (22).

Personal needs of family carers

Personal needs of family carers are significant; they include difficulty in sleeping, difficulty in maintaining their own health and difficulty in having time to themselves. However, uncovering personal needs of carers often presents the greatest challenge for clinicians. Payne *et al.* (39) suggest it is difficult for family carers to admit to their own needs unless they are specifically asked about themselves and in a setting away from the patient.

Spiritual needs of family carers

The data on spiritual needs of family carers is sparse. However, studies that do ask about spiritual needs suggest that some family carers have a need to develop or continue a relationship with God (32). The lack of information on this category of needs may indicate that spiritual needs are not important to carers and consequently do not feature in results, or they are not important to researchers and are not investigated. Alternatively, finding culturally and secularly appropriate ways of framing questions to measure this category may be difficult, with 'spiritual' often being equated with 'religious'.

Household needs of family carers

A review of the literature on household needs suggests that this category of needs is generally less important to carers than other needs, such as information or psychological needs. One study reported that carers found managing the household and finances, or managing the environment, as very demanding and some resorted to rostering family and friends to provide assistance (17). While this study focused on carers of persons with cancer and AIDS at home, it is reasonable to assume that the same issues and problems arise for carers when the patient is hospitalized. Perhaps carers view household needs as they do personal needs; that is, less significant than needs directly impacting on the patient.

This review has served to highlight the range of unmet needs family carers might experience. While clinicians may uncover various kinds of unmet carer needs they also have to be aware that not all carers want assistance to meet these needs. A study of the needs of 76 carers of people with advanced cancer being cared for at home found that on average carers had two or three definite problems with up to 17 being described as 'somewhat of a problem'. Carers, however, were only requesting additional support for four to five of the less significant problems (22). Not only is it important for clinicians to meet carer needs in terms of maintaining their health so they can continue in the role, but when needs are met prior to the death of the patient, bereavement outcomes tend to be better (41).

Identifying carer needs through comprehensive assessment

Navigating a path that meets the needs of both the carer and the patient can be challenging, but must be made a priority focus for future planning. One way of meeting this challenge is by legitimizing carer needs through comprehensive needs assessment conducted at pertinent points in the illness. This approach is in keeping with the World Health Organization's inclusion of the health and well-being of the family members caring for patients receiving palliative care (42).

While a systematic approach to the assessment of carer needs seems to be important in identifying those at greatest risk of distress, it appears to rarely occur in practice. This can partially be explained by the fact that many clinicians are concerned that if carer needs are identified, they may not be able to be met within the confines of available resources (22). Another explanation is that clinicians find it difficult to identify an assessment tool that is acceptable to carers and manageable within the constraints of their already busy workload. While many assessment tools can be found in the literature, not all meet the criteria of acceptability and manageability. The two need assessment tools presented here meet one or both criteria; they were designed specifically for use with family carers of people with cancer and may be useful starting points for those interested in pursuing formal assessment of carer needs.

The Home Carer Needs Survey (HCNS) was developed in 1990 (33) to identify the important but unsatisfied needs of home-based carers caring for people with cancer. The survey consists of 89 needs statements that assess six need domains, including informational, psychological, patient care, spiritual, household and personal. Carers are given the option of indicating needs that are not personally applicable, making the tool appropriate for a wide range of carers. Scores are transformed according to specific criteria to produce a barrier needs score, which indicates the carer's perception of both the importance of the specified need and the level of satisfaction of the need. While the tool is comprehensive in terms of possible needs, its length is unappealing to carers, and the need to transform scores is unappealing to the clinician. Despite these limitations it has been found to be very useful in identifying needs of family carers at various points in the patient's illness (33, 35).

Problems and Needs in Palliative Care questionnaire-carer form (PNPC-c) was developed in the Netherlands (43) to provide a comprehensive list of problems experienced by carers, as well as identifying their perceived subsequent needs for care. The tool was designed to provide structure to a consultation with a general practitioner, following its completion by the family carer. The tool has 67 items covering the domains of taking care of the patient, their own physical symptoms, their relationship with the patient, autonomy, social support, psychological, spiritual, financial and administrative issues, and activities of daily living, problems in consultations and over-riding problems in the quality of care. There is also a miscellaneous section that addresses issues such as leaving the patient alone, patient denial and taking time off work. Carers are asked to indicate whether or not they felt the issue is a problem for them and then whether they need professional support to deal with it. The authors believe this needs assessment is useful because it was designed as a need assessment as opposed to a research instrument, and because it does not merely identify a large number of unmet needs that can seem unmanageable to the clinician; instead, it identifies a few specific needs that require professional attention (22).

Another clinically useful, simple to use, reliable and well-validated Australian-designed instrument is the Family Inventory of Needs (FIN) (44). The FIN was designed to measure the importance of family carer needs, as well as identifying how well the family feels the needs have been met. It asks about symptoms, information requirements and psychological needs. The FIN consists of 20 items that are rated from 0 to 10 in terms of importance, and then the respondent indicates whether the need is met or unmet. This measure of needs provides a shorter alternative to the other measures already described.

There is no disputing the importance of accurate assessment of family carer needs; however, it remains an area where further input is required from both researchers and clinicians. Even though assessment of carer needs requires further development, there are still a number of interventions, some having been tested more rigorously than others, which are of use to the clinician.

Interventions to support carers of patients with cancer

Despite widespread acknowledgement that carers are pivotal to providing care and contributing to the optimal quality of life for a patient with advanced cancer, there is surprisingly limited research regarding interventions to best provide support to carers. The following discussion provides a summary of available family carer interventions that may assist clinicians in supporting carers.

Practical Information

Carers are very often intimately involved and active participants in the illness journey with the patient. They therefore have an ongoing need for information, which may differ in content to that of the patient (38). It is important that information sharing is conducted with consistency, preferably by one clinician, trusted and respected by the carer, rather than by multiple people (19). Carers have identified they require advice and assistance to address four key information areas of caregiving:

(1) how best to provide and ensure patient physical comfort;

(2) general information about caring for their relative/friend and what to expect as their relative approaches the dying phase;

(3) practical care needs, including access to equipment and resources; and

(4) emotional support for themselves (5).

Carers value information if it is timely, reinforced and delivered in a method suited to their learning style. This provides carers with strategies for an approach to care, as well as contingency plans well in advance of needing them. Providing information in a variety of modalities, including verbal, written, audio and timed appropriately has potential to reduce anxiety and empower carers in their role (17).

When preparing written carer resources, consideration should be given to the target audience, ensuring information can be understood by the majority of people, regardless of age or caregiving experience. An Australian publication, which is evidence-based and prepared specifically for carers of palliative care patients, provides a reference point for carers (45). Information includes suggestions regarding the caregiving role, practical caring advice, self-care and care as the patient's death approaches.

A recently developed programme, Caregiving at Life's End (CGLE) (46), a train-the-trainer workshop for carers, was designed to provide practical assistance to carers. The programme consists of five sessions, and includes take-home resources for the carers, discussion questions, self-directed activities, quality of life activities with multimedia options to evoke participation and discussion. Programme content included modules such as the experience of caregiving, self-care, life affairs, relationships with the community and experience of love of self and love of others. Benefits for carers who completed the programme included improved confidence in delivering practical care, improved closure experiences and positive attitude to the caregiving experience.

Programmes that promote carer problem-solving skills are beginning to emerge. Allen et al. (47) refer to an as yet unpublished study aimed at providing carers with problem-solving skills. The Creativity, Optimism, Planning and Expert information (COPE) study is targeted at teaching carers' strategies and providing information to manage three common symptoms: pain, constipation and dyspnoea. However, COPE study results are not yet available.

The Care Integration Team (CIT) is an intervention (unpublished) that combines problem-solving skills with social support, meaning-centred therapy or both (47). The programme consists of four weekly home visits focused on symptom management, communication with hospice staff, carer self-care and anticipatory grief.

Communication

Evidence suggests that once patients are referred to palliative care services, their carers value the opportunity for open and honest communication (7). There are several key competencies essential for clinicians to impart information effectively. These include a demonstrable effective communication style, exceptional listening skills and the ability to convey information to the carer in a way that is comprehensible (9, 30). One positive way clinicians can provide help to carers is to encourage them to be proactive in communicating with treating doctors, nurses, hospitals and community services. A study by Rabow (48), found that clinicians who spend even a short time listening to carer concerns can help decrease that carer's risk of depression.

One method of facilitating communication with the carer is a family meeting (49). A family meeting can have multiple purposes, including the sharing of information and concerns, clarifying the goals of care for the patient, discussing diagnosis, treatment, prognosis and developing a plan of care for the patient (49). Further research is required to establish when and how family meetings should be conducted to maximize usefulness.

Advance care directives

Carers often find themselves, particularly toward the end of the patient's life, making decisions on behalf of the patient; a situation for which they feel ill prepared. The carer's burden can be eased by the health professional and the carer working with the patient, while they are able to inform their carer and health professional about their wishes (47). Engaging patients and their carers in discussion about planning for the future needs of the patient has potential to promote identification of issues and the opportunity for clarification (47). Whilst an advance care plan can provide a communication framework for the carer, it often requires revisiting over time as situations change.

Psychosocial care

As previously discussed, there may be a reticence on the part of the carer to declare or acknowledge his/her own needs ahead of the patient's (26, 41), primarily because they do not want to deflect focus from the patient or because they prioritize the patient's needs ahead of their own. However, the reality is that carers have as much, if not more, need for emotional support during the dying phase of the patient's illness (25).

Hope has been described as a psychosocial and spiritual strategy implemented by carers to deal with their caregiving experience (50). Given that hope is a dynamic phenomenon involving spirituality, relationships, goal-setting and cognitive reframing, carer interventions that nurture hope can be effective.

Recent pilot research of the Living with Hope Program (LWHP) (50) suggested carers found value in journaling their caregiving experiences (with prompts to guide entries), providing both a way of recording events and an opportunity for self-reflection. The programme would benefit from continued evaluation with larger sample sizes.

Self-care

Evidence to recommend ways of encouraging carers to acknowledge and meet their need for self-care are scant in the existing literature. However, care for the carers is obliquely referred to in reference to carer-support programmes. Suggestions include accessing volunteers to sit with the patient to provide the carer with valuable 'time out', allocating time with a member of the care team for the carer to share their concerns, and inviting other members of the family and friends to contribute to the care.

Evidence suggests that carers who continue social activities while committed to the caregiving role have better psychological outcomes, with reduced risk of depression and increased life satisfaction (47).

Specialist palliative care services

Referral to community palliative care services provides carers with access to a range of clinicians, skilled in assessing and responding to needs. Carers report satisfaction with a single point of contact, once referral to a palliative care service has been made. They repeatedly report their satisfaction with community palliative care services and value the knowledge and skill of the clinicians involved (25).

Day hospices evolved in response to community-based palliative care services, providing a valuable link between the community and inpatient facilities (51). Day hospices can provide an opportunity for both the patient and the carer to have some respite from each other, with the carer secure in the knowledge that the patient is being cared for. Day hospice models primarily are based on either a social or biomedical model, often dependent on availability of resources to the service (52).

Specialist in-patient palliative care services (hospices) practise holistic care delivered by a multidisciplinary team, providing assessment and care to both the patient and their carers (53). Carers report the opportunity to access respite services of an in-patient palliative care service provides them with support and relieves them from the stress and physical fatigue associated with the caring role (54). However, it should be recognized that access is often limited and confined to a set time-frame, simply due to limitations of the hospices to meet the need within their available resources.

Box 12.1 provides a summary of carer interventions, which could translate into the development of carer education and support processes to better provide them with strategies for their role. However, there is an urgent need to conduct research into exploring ways of ensuring the carer's needs are assessed and appropriate management plans are made available.

Box 12.1 Summary of carer interventions

Information:

- On both patient disease and practical care.
- Provided often, and in appropriate language.
- Given via multiple modalities: verbal, written, video.
- Ensure consistency of contact with health professionals.
- Provide opportunities for discussion with medical staff.
- About services available, how to access and when.
- About what to expect as death approaches.
- About what to do after the patient has died.

Practical skills education on:

- Giving medication.
- Providing personal care to the patient.
- Ensuring patient comfort.
- Accessing equipment.

Social support

Provide:

- Opportunities for social contact.
- Contact with caregivers in similar situations.

> **Box 12.1 Summary of carer Interventions** *(continued)*
>
> - Time to continue activities of enjoyment.
> - Financial guidance and support.
> - Option of respite, either formally in hospice care or by volunteers, family and friends.
>
> ### Personal health
>
> Encourage:
>
> - Self-care priority to prevent negative events.
> - Attention to own healthy nutrition requirements.
> - Attention to personal relationships.
> - Regular medical check-up.
>
> ### Emotional support:
>
> - Provided either formally by health professionals or informally by friends and family.
> - To explore concerns over imminent death of patient.
> - To develop a trusting relationship with health professionals.

Carers who receive appropriate professional support or interventions, especially for day-to-day issues, report fewer unmet needs and better bereavement outcomes in the first 6–12 months after the death of the patient, than those carers who do not seek help (55). Additionally, providing carers with practical advice and resources has the potential to enhance their problem-solving strategies and sense of control over their situation (19).

Conclusion

While palliative care promotes the patient and the family as the unit of care, from diagnosis into bereavement, there are gaps in adequately meeting and delivering the ideal. Healthcare providers and the community will increasingly be reliant on unpaid, ill-prepared people to take on the caregiving role for people with advanced cancer. Our ageing population suggests that responsibility for caregiving will fall to an ever-decreasing pool of people, influenced by several factors. These factors include declining global birth rates, changing societal attitudes to caring for ageing family members, more women choosing to pursue careers, increasing geographical distances between family members and the financial burden of forsaking paid employment to commit to the caregiving role. To that end, Governments should be encouraged to proactively develop realistic financial support packages to provide for carers whilst they are providing care, particularly if they are required to temporarily relinquish their paid employment.

Carer unmet needs are evident from the existing literature; however, interventions and management strategies to better meet their needs are urgently required. In the meantime, empowering carers with information, resources, skills and strategies to enable them to fulfil the role has potential to improve both the care of the patient and the well-being of the carer.

Key learning points

◆ As distinct from other caregiving roles, the outcome of providing care for someone with advanced cancer is the unavoidable and sometimes rapid deterioration and then death of the individual.

◆ Family carers are reluctant to admit to their own needs, let alone seek help. Therefore, the needs of carers have to be assessed systematically at key points during the illness and away from the person they are caring for. Carers need to be reassured that it is acceptable and in fact expected, that they will have legitimate unmet needs that will be contributing to the burden of the caregiving role. Appropriate supports and interventions specifically designed to address carer needs can then be provided.

◆ Family carers benefit from targeted interventions to support them in their caregiving role. Interventions are strongly reliant on the effective communication skills of the clinician/s, provision of information in a variety of ways (written, oral, video) and information being repeated, as required.

◆ Family carers require support to identify the positive aspects of caring, acknowledge their own needs and factor in some time for self-care. They value advice regarding community services and resources available to them, including utilizing the services of volunteers and respite care.

Recommended reading and resources

Carers Australia: http://www.carersaustralia.com.au/

Carers UK. *The Voice of Carers*: http://www.carersuk.org/Home

Girgis A, Johnson C, Currow D, Waller A, Kritjanson L, Mitchell G *et al.* (2006). *Palliative Care Needs Assessment Guidelines*. Available from: The Centre for Health Research and Psycho-oncology, Newcastle, NSW or from the website: http://health.gov.au/internet/wcms/publishing.nsf/Content/palliativecare-needs-assess-guide-1

Hileman JW, Lackey NR and Hassanein RS (1992). Identifying the needs of home carers of patients with cancer. *Oncology Nursing Forum* **19**(5): 771–777.

Hudson PL, Aranda S and Hayman-White K (2005). A psycho-educational intervention for family carers of patients receiving palliative care: a randomized controlled trial. *Journal of Pain and Symptom Management* **30**(4): 329–341.

Kristjanson LJ (1999). Families of palliative care patients: a model for care. In: Aranda S and O'Connor M (ed.). *Palliative Care Nursing: a Guide to Practice.* Ausmed Publications: Melbourne.

Kurtz M, Krutz J, Given C and Given B (2005). A randomised controlled trial of patient/carer symptom control intervention: Effects on depressive symptomatology of carers of cancer patients. *Journal of Pain and Symptom Management* **30**(2): 112–122.

National Caregivers Library: http://www.caregiverslibrary.org/

National Family Carers Association USA: http://www.nfcacares.org/

National Institute for health and Clinical Excellence (NICE) http://www.nice.org.uk/page/publicinfo

References

1. AIHW (Australian Institute of Health and Welfare) and AACR (Australian Association of Cancer Registries) (2007). *Cancer in Australia: an Overview, 2006. Cancer Series* No. 37, Cat. No. CAN 32. Canberra: AIHW.

2. Canadian Cancer Society (2007). *Canadian Cancer Statistics 2007.* National Cancer Institute of Canada, Toronto Canada.

3. American Cancer Society (2007). *Cancer Facts and Figures 2007.* Atlanta: American Cancer Society.

4. National Statistics Online (accessed 08/07/07). http://www.statistics.gov.uk/default.asp

5. Aoun S, Kristjanson L, Currow D and Hudson P (2005). Caregiving for the terminally ill: at what cost? *Palliative Medicine* **19**: 551–555.

6. Hudson P (2006). How well do family caregivers cope after caring for a relative with advanced disease and how can health professionals enhance their support? *Journal of Palliative Medicine* **9**(3): 694–703.

7. Girgis A, Johnson C, Aoun S and Currow D (2006). Challenges experience by informal caregivers in cancer. *Cancer Forum* **30**(1): 21–25.

8. Schofield HL, Herrman HE and Bloch S (1997). A profile of Australian family caregivers: diversity of roles and circumstances. *Australian and New Zealand Journal of Public Health.* **21**(1): 59–66.

9. Schofield P, Carey M, Love A, Nehill C and Wein S (2006). 'Would you like to talk about your future treatment options?' discussing the transition from curative cancer treatment to palliative care. *Palliative Medicine* **20**: 397–406.

10. Wright LM and Leahey M (1989). *Nurses and Families: a Guide to Family Assessment and Intervention.* Philadelphia: FA Davis Company.

11. National Family Caregivers Association USA. http://www.nfcacares.org/who_are_family_caregivers/care_giving_statistics.cfm

12. Carers UK. *The Voice of Carers.* http://www.carersuk.org/Aboutus/Whoarecarers

13. Stajduhar K (2003). Examining the perspectives of family members involved in the delivery of palliative care at home. *Journal of Palliative Care* **19**(1): 27–35.

14. National Centre for Social and Economic Modelling (2004). *Who's Going to Care? Informal Care and an Ageing Population.* Report prepared for Caregivers Australia. Canberra: University of Canberra.

15. Hayman JA, Langa KM, Kabeto MU, Katz SJ, DeMonner SM, Chernew ME *et al.* (2001). Estimating the cost of informal caregiving for elderly patients with cancer. *J Clin Oncol* **19**(13): 3219–3225.

16. Kim Y, Baker F, Spillers R and Wellisch D (2006). Psychological adjustment of cancer caregivers with multiple roles. *Psycho-Oncology* **15**: 795–804.

17. Stetz K and Brown M (1997) Taking care: caregiving to persons with Cancer and AIDS. *Cancer Nursing* **20**(1): 12–22.

18. Grbich C, Parker D and Maddocks I (2000). Communication and information needs of care-givers of adult family members at diagnosis and during treatment of terminal cancer. *Progress in Palliative Care* **8**(6): 345–349.

19. Hudson P, Aranda S and Kristjanson L (2004). Information provision for palliative care families *European Journal of Palliative Care* **11**(4): 153–157.

20. Ramirez A, Addington-Hall J and Richards M (1998). ABC of palliative care: the caregivers. *BMJ* **316**(7126): 208–211.

21. Andershed B (2006). Relatives in end of life care—art 1: a systematic review of the literature the five last years, January 1999–February 2004. *Journal of Clinical Nursing* **15**: 1158–1169.

22. Osse B, Vernooij-Dassen M, Schade E and Grol, R. (2006). Problems experienced by the informal caregivers of cancer patients and their needs for support. *Cancer Nursing* **29**(5): 378–388.

23. Emanuel E, Fairclough D, Slutsman J and Emanuel L (2000). Understanding economic and other burdens of terminal illness: the experience of patients and their caregivers. *Annals of Internal Medicine* **132**(6): 451–459.

24. Kurtz M, Kurtz J, Given C and Given B (2005). A randominsed, controlled trial of a patient/caregiver symptom control intervention: effects on depressive symptomatology of caregivers of cancer patients. *Journal of Pain and Symptom Management* **30**(2): 112–122.

25. Harding R and Higginson I (2003). What is the best way to help caregivers in cancer and palliative care? A systematic literature review of interventions and their effective-ness *Palliative Medicine* **17**: 63–74.

26. Briggs H and Fisher D (2000). *Warning—Caring is a Health Hazard.* Canberra: Carers Association of Australia.

27. Haley WE, LaMonde LA, Han B, Narramore S and Schonwetter R (2001). Family caregiving in hospice: Effects on psychological and health functioning among spousal caregivers of hospice patients with lung cancer and dementia. *Hosp J* **15**(4): 1–18.

28. Kristjanson LK, Sloan JA, Dudgeon D and Adaskin E (1996). Family members' percep-tions of palliative cancer care: predictors of family functioning and family members' health. *Journal of Palliative Care* **12**(4): 10–20.

29. Kershaw T, Northouse L, Kritpracha C, Schafenacker A and Mood D (2004). Coping strategies and quality of life in women with advanced breast cancer and their family caregivers. *Psychological Health* **19**: 139–155.

30. Grov E, Fossa S, Sorebo O and Dahl A (2006). Primary caregivers of cancer patients in the palliative phase: a path analysis of variables influencing their burden. *Social Sciences and Medicine* **63**: 2429–2439.

31. Tringali CA (1986). The needs of family members of cancer patients. *Oncol Nurs Forum* **14**(4): 65–70.

32. Wingate AL and Lackey NR (1989). A description of the needs of noninstitutionalized cancer patients and their primary caregivers. *Cancer Nursing* **12**(4): 216–225.

33. Hileman JW, Lackey NR and Hassanein RS (1992). Identifying the needs of home caregivers of patients with cancer. *Oncology Nursing Forum* **19**(5): 771–777.

34. Jones RVH, Hansford J, Fiske J (1993). Death from cancer at home: the carers' perspective. *BMJ* **306**: 249–250.

35. Milne DJ (1999). When cancer won't go away: the needs and experiences of family caregivers. Unpublished Masters Thesis. The University of Melbourne.

36. Butow PN, Maclean M, Dunn SM, Tattersall MH and Boyer MJ (1997). The dynamics of change: cancer patients' preferences for information, involvement and support. *Ann Oncol.* **8**: 857–863.

37. Kissane DW, Bloch S, Burns WI *et al.* (1994). Psychological morbidity in the families of patients with cancer *Psychoncology* **3**: 47–56.

38. Morris S and Thomas C (2002). The need to know: informal carers and information. *European Journal of Palliative Care* **11**: 183–187.

39. Payne S, Large S, Jarrett N and Turner P (2000). Written information given to patients and families by palliative care units: a national survey. *The Lancet* **355**(9217): 1792.

40. Hinds C (1985). The needs of families who care for patients with cancer at home: are we meeting them? *Journal of Advanced Cancer* **10**: 575–581.

41. Kissane DW (2004). Bereavement. In: Doyle D, Hanks G, Cherny N and Calman K (ed.). *Oxford Textbook of Palliative Medicine* (3rd edn). New York: Oxford University Press, 1137–1151.

42. Sepulveda C, Marlin A, Yoshida T and Ullrich A (2002). Palliative care: the World Health Organization's global perspective. *Journal of Pain and Symptom Management* **24**(2): 91–96.

43. Osse B, Vernooij-Dassen M, Schade E and Grol R (2004). Towards a new clinical tool for needs assessment in palliative care of cancer patients; the PNPC instrument. *The Journal of Pain and Symptom Management* **28**(4): 329–341.

44. Kristjanson LJ, Atwood J and Degner LF (1995). Validity and reliability of the Family Inventory of Needs (FIN): measuring the care needs of families of advanced cancer patients. *Journal of Nursing Measurement* **3**(5): 109–126.

45. Hudson P (2004). *Supporting the Person Who Needs Palliative Care: a Guide for Family and Friends.* Melbourne: Palliative Care Victoria.

46. Kwak J, Salmon J, Acquaviva K, Brandt K and Egan A (2007). Benefits of training family caregivers on experiences of closure during end-of-life care *Journal of Pain and Symptom Management* **33**(4): 434–445.

47. Allen R, Haley W, Roff L, Schmid B and Bergman E (2005). Responding to the needs of caregivers near the end of life: enhancing benefits and minimizing burdens. In: Werth J and Blevins D (ed.). *Psychosocial Issues Near the End of Life.* Washington: American Psychological Association, 183–201.

48. Rabow MW, Hauser JM and Adams J (2004). Supporting family caregivers at the end of life: 'They don't know what they don't know'. *JAMA* **291**: 483–491.

49. Moneymaker K (2005). The family conference. *Journal of Palliative Medicine* **8**(1): 157.

50. Duggleby W, Wright K, Williams A, Degner L, Cammer A and Hotslander L (2007). Developing a living with hope programme for caregivers of family members with advanced cancer. *Journal of Palliative Care* **23**(1): 24–31.

51. Spencer D and Daniels L (1998). Day hospice care—a review of the literature. *Palliative Medicine* **12**: 219–229.

52. Corr C and Corr D (1992). Adult hospice day care. *Death Studies* **16**: 155–171.

53. Centre to Advance Palliative Care website: www.capc.org

54. Skilbeck J, Payne S, Ingleton M, Nolan M, Carey I and Hanson A (2005). An exploration of family carers' experience of respite services in one specialist palliative care unit. *Palliative Medicine* **19**: 610–618.

55. Abernathy AP, Fazekas BS, Luszcz M and Currow DC (2005). *Specialised Palliative Care Services Improve Caregiver Outcomes*. 8th Australian Palliative Care Conference, 30 Aug 2005, Sydney Australia.

Chapter 13

Family carers of people with advanced organ failure and neurodegenerative disorders

Janice Brown and Julia Addington-Hall

Introduction

Hospice and specialist palliative care provision in the United Kingdom is focused almost entirely on the care of people with advanced cancer, and of their families before and in bereavement: in 2004–05, only 5 per cent of patients receiving in-patient care or home care from a hospice had a diagnosis other than cancer, and 11 per cent of patients receiving support from hospital palliative care teams (1). The needs of people with diagnoses other than cancer for physical, psychological, social and spiritual support in the last weeks and months of life is, however, increasing recognized, and the need for palliative care to be provided equitably, based on need not diagnosis, emphasized (2, 3). Some countries already provide care for many patients who die from causes other than cancer: in the USA, for example, the proportion of hospice patients in 2005 who had a diagnosis other than cancer was 54 per cent. Although important questions remain about appropriate and cost-effective models of palliative care provision beyond cancer (2), palliative care provision beyond cancer is likely to grow. Further impetus for this comes from the ageing profile of the population in developed countries and the associated increase in the numbers of people living with, and dying from, chronic organ failure and progressive degenerative conditions.

An important aspect of developing appropriate palliative care provision beyond cancer is to begin to understand the needs and experiences of family carers in these conditions and the evidence on effective interventions to support them. This will enable an informed debate about whether, to what extent and for whom palliative care has a role in addressing the needs of family carers of people with diagnoses other than cancer. This debate is essential: palliative care is not alone in recognizing the importance of understanding the social context in which patients live, in espousing concern for families as well as for patients, in identifying the essential contribution family carers make to sustaining care in the community, and in (at least sometimes) attempting to support them in their role. It may be that the appropriate knowledge, expertise and skills to support family carers beyond cancer already exists in, for example, family practice, healthcare of older people, rehabilitation services or within social care. This chapter, therefore, considers the evidence about what is known about the needs and experiences of family carers of people with neurodegenerative disorders (multiple sclerosis, motor neurone disease, Parkinson's disease and Huntington's disease), and with organ failure (chronic heart failure and chronic obstructive pulmonary disease). It looks specifically at the evidence for effective interventions to support these carers. It begins in each case by providing information about the epidemiology and nature of each condition, to enable the reader to begin to debate whether the disorder raises specific issues for family carers which might lie within the remit of palliative care and, if so, what these might be. Of the four neurodegenerative conditions, only one (MND) currently has relatively good access to hospice and specialist palliative care services in the UK at least, although there is not universal access or a consistent model of care (4). Appropriate palliative care provision for people with MS (5), PD (6) and HD (7) is under discussion internationally, but relatively few patients and families currently receive care. Similarly, the debate about palliative care needs (if not actual provision) in heart failure is more advanced than in COPD or in other conditions such as chronic kidney or liver failure (where both the debate and the evidence on carers' experiences are so limited that there is insufficient evidence to include these conditions in this chapter). As will be seen below, these conditions differ in important ways including age of onset, duration of illness and symptoms, which means that together they illustrate many aspects of the debate about the appropriate role of palliative care in supporting family carers beyond cancer.

Neurodegenerative disorders

Multiple sclerosis

Multiple sclerosis (MS) is a neurological condition with a chronic and often fluctuating time course, which can be highly disabling: it is the most common cause of non-traumatic disability in young adults. Its prevalence in Europe is estimated to be 83 per 100 1000 (8). MS is believed to affect over 2 million people world-wide, including approximately 300 000 people in the USA and 85 000 in the UK (9). Prevalence is estimated to be highest in the 35 to

64-year-old age group (8) and is higher in women, with a female: male ratio of 2:1 (10). MS is characterized by signs of neurological dysfunction, such as limb weakness, visual and sensory disturbance, gait problems, and bladder and bowel problems. Changes in cognitive function may also occur. Episodes of neurological dysfunction may initially be followed by recovery, but irreversible neurological deterioration will occur over time as a result of acute exacerbations or relapses, leading to increasing disability. MS is classified into four major types based on clinical presentation: remitting relapsing MS; secondary progressive disease; primary progressive disease; progressive relapsing disease (10). Over 80 per cent of cases are remitting relapsing or secondary progressive disease, with the latter developing on from the former over time, characterized by progressive deterioration and increasing disability. On average, people with MS live with the condition for 30 to 45 years after initial diagnosis (8). Recent evidence suggests that MS is associated with an elevated risk of death, with life-expectancy in one Austrian study, 15 years less than in the general population (8).

A key feature of MS is the slow deterioration of physical abilities over time. The impact of increased functional disability on the quality of life of the person with MS is compounded by the fact that many experience significant fatigue: a community survey found that 25 per cent reported that their activities were often or always limited by fatigue (11). Depression is also common, with the lifetime prevalence estimated to be about 50 per cent and annual prevalence 20 per cent (12). Almost a third of early MS patients (on average 2.6 years disease duration) have been found to have cognitive deficits (13) compared with half of an out-patient sample (14). Sexual dysfunction is also common, affecting over 70 per cent, with a significant increase in the number and severity of problems over time (15). A study of symptom prevalence and severity in severe MS found that patients had a mean of nine symptoms, six of which (problems using legs, problems using arms, fatigue, spasms, pain and feeling sleepy) affected more than half of the sample. The authors concluded that many symptoms were as common and as severe in these patients as those experienced by patients with advanced cancer (16).

McKeown et al. (17) conducted a systematic review in which they reviewed 24 studies addressing the needs and experiences of family carers in MS. The studies had methodological limitations but the review demonstrated that caring for people with MS has a far-ranging effect on all aspects of carers' lives, their physical and mental health and well-being, finances, social life and overall quality of life. Given the impact on the lives of people with MS themselves, reported above, and their increasing need for care, this is not surprising. Impact on overall quality of life was particularly associated with age, with those between 50 and 59 at greatest risk, and income, with those with low income showing the greatest effects. Those spouses who had been caring for longer and who cared for longer each day, were also particularly at risk of impaired quality of life, as were those caring for a person with MS with an increased severity of symptoms or an unstable disease course. Evidence on impact on health was difficult to interpret, as declining health over time might be attributable to increasing age, but one small study reported an association between increased dependency in care recipients and reduced engagement in health-promoting behaviours amongst family carers, which would substantiate such a relationship (18). Further evidence comes from the fact that three-quarters of carers report that their own health was the most likely reason for them being unable to continue caring. Evidence that MS can have a detrimental effect on family carers' psychological wellbeing was found to be particularly robust, with functional disability, the progressive nature of MS and the resultant uncertainty about the future being found to be particularly related to carer stress. Cognitive impairment has been reported to be a source of stress, as have depression and anxiety: these have a contribution to carer stress over and above that of functional disability (19).

The systematic review found evidence of the impact of caring in MS on the carers' social lives and finances (17). They note, however, that similar findings have been reported for carers of cancer patients and in other chronic conditions. One difference may, however, be that there is some evidence in the MS literature that carers' financial state worsens as the number of years they provide care increases (17). The progressive nature of MS results in increasing dependency and increased costs resulting from, for example, need for paid assistance, adaptations and aids (20). It may also result in increasing difficulty for MS carers to remain in employment (17), resulting not only in loss of income but also in a loss of skills for the workplace and social isolation (21). The latter may be particularly important given the beneficial effects of social support on health, family life and depression (17), and evidence that MS carers have reduced levels of social support compared with the general population (22). Hunt (23) advocates that more attention should be given to gender differences in caring. This is particularly relevant in MS as it affects more women than men, which, together with its age profile, probably means more men are carers than is usual in the carer population as a whole, although exact figures are unknown. Wives of men with MS report higher levels of social support and more resources than husbands.

There is currently no evidence of effective interventions to promote wellbeing of MS carers (24). On the basis of their systematic review, McKeown et al. (17) conclude that family carers in MS need encouragement to look after their own health, to access sources of social support and (given evidence that less than half use community services or support) to access these services. The importance of improving service provision is highlighted in a study of the experiences of people with severe MS and their family carers, which identified a lack of continuity and co-ordination of care, and a lack of information about services, aids and appliances, and welfare benefits: the overarching theme that emerged from this qualitative study is of people with MS and their carers having to struggle to get their needs met (25).

It is important to recognize, however, that the emphasis to date of the literature on family carers in MS has been on the negative impact of caregiving. This is an issue in the literature on family carers in general, which has tended to identify negative aspects of caring, although there is increased interest and acknowledgement of positive aspects of the role (26), which is important to avoid socializing carers to only expect burden. Positive aspects of the caring role that have been identified include caregiver esteem, satisfactions and finding meaning. Pakenham (27, 28) has investigated how MS carers find benefit and meaning in their experience. From qualitative research, he identified seven benefit themes: gaining insight into illness/hardship, personal growth, life priorities/goals, appreciation of life, caregiving specific benefits, greater appreciation of health and interpersonal benefits. Carer benefit finding impacted positively on life satisfaction, positive mood and adjustment of the carer and the person with MS. A greater understanding of how carers find meaning and benefit in the face of often long-term, arduous caring commitments would inform the development of appropriate interventions.

Motor neurone disease

Motor neurone disease (MND) (or amyotrophic lateral sclerosis, ALS) is a rare neurodegenerative condition characterized by progressive muscle weakness, paralysis and eventual respiratory failure. It has a low global incidence of MND of 1.5 to 2.5 per 100 000 people a year (29), with approximately 5000 people estimated to be living with MND in the UK at any one time. In population-based studies in Europe, 22 per cent die within a year of diagnosis, 44 per cent within 2 years and 68 per cent within 4 years (29). Prognosis depends on patient age and on the type of MND. Three principal types have been identified (30): amyotrophic lateral sclerosis (ALS), progressive bulbar palsy (PBP) and progressive muscular atrophy (PMA). More recently, progressive lateral sclerosis (PLS) has been identified. Although each type has a unique presentation, symptoms may merge over time. Although MND has been thought to affect more men than women, recent studies suggest that this is not (or is no longer) the case (29). Most people diagnosed with MND are aged over 40, with peak incidence in the late 60s and early 70s.

People with MND may present with weakness in legs, hands or shoulders with some signs of atrophy of muscles or with speech and swallowing difficulties. These initial symptoms and signs progress to severe disability and death. As the disease progresses they, and their family carers, face multiple losses: the loss of mobility, the use of their hands, the ability to communicate, the ability to swallow and, eventually, the ability to breathe unaided (31). As a consequence, they may also face decisions about whether or not to have medical interventions, such as a percutaneous endoscopic gastrostomy tube (PEGs) to enable artificial nutrition, non-invasive ventilation (NIV) or tracheostomy ventilation to overcome the effects of increasing respiratory weakness, and, if so, when to start—and when to stop—these interventions. Although there is growing research evidence of cognitive impairments in MND (32) one of its key features is that the intellect of the person with MND usually remains essentially intact in the face of rapid changing and disabling circumstances. Rates of clinical depression of only about 10 per cent have, however, been reported (33), lower than in people with MS or Parkinson's Disease (34), although hopelessness and end-of-life concerns are more common (35) and may be related to the prominence of people with MND in debates about assisted suicide and euthanasia (36).

Mockford et al. (37) have reviewed the literature on the impact of caring on family carers in MND and their experiences of service provision. The research evidence is limited but demonstrates a negative impact of caring on the physical and mental health of many family carers. The impact is increased as the number of hours the carer spends caring increases and as the patient's health declines, with evidence of ill health, even when outside services were also providing high levels of care, and with the introduction of tracheostomy ventilation (which also impacts negatively on life satisfaction). Compared with the caregivers of Alzheimer's disease, MS and post-stroke patients, Krivickas et al. (38) suggest caregivers of people with MND have an even greater physical and emotional burden because of the much more rapid progression of this disease and its severely disabling final stages. The fact that the person with MND normally remains intellectually intact may also create specific challenges for carers in that they are watching the physical and social decline of their loved one who is watching with them. However, the unimpaired intellect of the patient may increase the motivation of the carers to care as they can continue a relationship with them to some extent and understand that the patient can understand them at all times, even if this is not always possible to reciprocate. As in MS, carers' depression levels were found to be associated with patients' depression levels, and probably with increased functional impairment. Anxiety was common. Carers experience disturbed sleep as they need to turn the person with MND in bed, which leads to increased fatigue and little energy for other activities, impacting on their physical and mental health (37).

Chronic sadness was identified as an issue for family carers who grieve continually as the person with MND becomes more incapacitated. More recently, Ray and Street (39) have characterized family carers' experience as 'non-finite loss': the presence of continuing loss over the course of the illness. These include personal losses as the carer changes from, for example, wife and mother to caregiver and nurse, or from being socially active and integral to their community to being housebound and afraid to leave the person with MND at home on their own. They may gradually lose the sense of being loved by the person they are caring for, particularly as communication becomes more difficult or absent. Role change can be something that carers have to adapt to quite rapidly and can involve difficult decision-making; for example, when work and career come into conflict with the role of family carer (31). The relatively short prognosis in MND means that the carer has to not only consider the financial situation of giving up work, with the emotional issue of wanting to be with the person with MND, but also their own future after their relative's death, both financially and in terms of their career. This is particularly important if there are young children or other dependents to consider. Brown (31) illustrates this dilemma, quoting a family carer as saying 'I'd love to do my job and look after Liz but what do I do when Liz's gone and there's no job?' (31). Part-time working is often a compromise. Compounded with loss of income, often resulting directly from the person with MND's inability to work, financial difficulties can result, as these changes in income come just at the time when major home adaptations, aids and appliances, and additional carers may be needed. The degree to which these costs, and the costs associated with mechanical ventilation, are funded, vary between countries but they can cause families considerable financial strain (37). The extent to which these losses and changes in life are experienced as carer strain and, therefore, impact on health will, as always, depend on the coping strategies of the carer and the resources available to them, including social support (37).

A longitudinal study of carer distress found that, although initial distress was best predicted by the psychosocial impact of MND, how emotionally labile the person with MND was, and the number of dependents the carer had, over time the strongest predictors were their satisfaction with their social relationships and social support (40). Love et al. (41) have similarly reported that stress on carer social networks was the single best predictor of carer well-being in their study of family carers. It can become increasingly difficult for family carers to access social support, as the person with MND becomes more dependent on them: they become less able to participate in social activities (particularly if they are providing home care) and friends especially may visit less often (37). This may affect some families more than others: younger family carers in Australia were more likely than older carers to report declines in support and fluctuations in the strength of relationships, as the person with MND deteriorated and caregiving demands increased (42). Although wider social support networks may suffer, in their review, Mockford *et al.* conclude that negative impact on family relationships are not inevitable, with one study reporting that two-thirds of families reported that MND had brought them closer together, and several studies reported increased intimacy and improved relationships between partners (37).

Parkinson's disease

Parkinson's disease (PD) is the second most common neurodegenerative disorder after Alzheimer's disease (43). Diagnosis requires the presence of at least two of the symptoms: bradykinesia (slowness of movement), resting tremor, rigidity or postural imbalance. It is an age-related disease: few people under the age of 50 are affected, with prevalence increasing rapidly after the age of 60, with up to 4000 per 100 000 affected in those aged over 80, compared to an estimated prevalence of 300 per 100 000 in the total population and 1000 per 100 0000 in those aged over 60 (43). Standardized incidence rates of 8 to 18 per 100 000 have been reported. There is some evidence that it is more common in men than in women. People with PD have a reduced life-expectancy compared to the general population: this is estimated to be in the region of 9 years reduced life-expectancy for those with onset before age 40, compared to 3 years for those with onset at or above aged 65 (44). Decreased life-expectancy is probably largely due to the increased risk of dementia associated with PD: between a quarter and two-fifths are reported to eventually develop dementia, with the risk being between 1.7 and 5.9 times higher than for the general population (43). Other conditions most commonly confused with PD include vascular pseudo-Parkinsonism and the 'Parkinsons's plus syndromes', such as multiple systems atrophy (MSA) and progressive supranuclear palsy (PSP). These progress faster than PD with a life-expectancy of 7 to 9 years and include early falls, poor response to medication and autonomic failure.

In addition to movement disorders, such as bradykinesia, people with PD may also experience difficulty in speaking and in swallowing. Depression is also known to be more common in people with PD than in the general population, particularly at onset and in advanced disease, and to impact negatively on quality of life (45). Initially dopaminergic therapy may control symptoms, but over time response to these drugs may decline, balance problems become more evident and neuropsychiatric problems, such as hallucinations, psychosis and cognitive decline, emerge. These symptoms can cause particular problems for family carers who, the literature suggests, often continue in their caring role without complaint when the problems remain physical, even though these include falls, difficulties with mobility and with activities of daily living, but do seek help when patients develop confusion and/or hallucinations (46, 47). The impact of coping with falls may, however, have been underestimated: Schrag *et al.* (48) identify that falls, as well as neuropsychiatric symptoms, increase family carer burden, whilst a qualitative study (49) has highlighted the considerable consequences of caring for someone who falls repeatedly.

The usual late onset of PD means that many family carers are themselves older and may have their own health problems, particularly, given the long duration of the disease for many people, by the time the person with PD develops balance and neuropsychiatric problems. A UK survey (50) reported six out of ten of their carer respondents were aged 65 and over with almost a quarter aged over 75 years, who on average spent 9 years caring for a person with PD. As in MS and MND, family carers report experiencing negative impacts of caregiving on their physical and emotional health, on their sleep, on their social life and on their finances (48, 49, 51). Again, carer burden is associated with the person with PD's psychological status, the severity of PD and the associated level of disability, and with the carer's own psychological status (52, 48). The carer's satisfaction with their marital and sexual relationship has also been shown to be important (48).

Research into effective interventions for family carers is somewhat more advanced in PD than in MS and MND, in that a number of pilot and early-stage studies have recently been published, indicating a growing interest in this issue, in contrast to the dearth of studies in MS and MND. These provide preliminary evidence that cognitive behavioural therapy may be effective in reducing psychological morbidity, carer strain and subjective burden (53); and that psycho-educational interventions for patients and carers (54) may be beneficial in improving mood. In contrast, intensive multidisciplinary rehabilitation programmes for patients and carers have been shown to be associated with increased strain (55) for carers (as opposed to patients). A stronger evidence base will emerge as this research develops from preliminary to definitive studies.

Huntingdon's disease

Huntingdon's disease (HD) is a familial genetic, neurodegenerative disease, which is passed from parent to child and for which there is no treatment available to stop its progression. Onset is most typically between the ages of 35 and 45, although it can present at any age, as late as 80 years of age or as early as 2. It has a prevalence internationally of 1 per 10 000 in the total population (7). It is characterized by involuntary jerky movements called chorea, an abnormal gait, slurred speech and swallowing difficulties. Cognitive decline affects short-term memory and causes difficulties with problem-solving, leading to eventual dementia. Behavioural disturbance increase over time with personality changes, such as impulsiveness, disinhibition, depression, mood swings and agression (56). A study of over 2000 people with HD found that median duration of the disease was 21 years, and this ranged from 1 to 41 years, with those with disease onset when aged under 20 or in older age surviving for shorter periods than with onset between the ages of 20 and 49 (57).

HD has a significant impact on families for reasons similar to those discussed in relation to MS, MND and PD: as people with HD become progressively more dependent, they experience psychological and cognitive symptoms, already shown to be associated with high levels of carer strain and, as in MS, family carers may need to provide care for extended periods of time, whilst ageing themselves. The fact that HD is an inherited disease of (usually) mid-life onset puts it, however, in a class of its own in relation to family carers, as they live with the knowledge that they may well eventually develop the same symptoms and require the same care, and they may already have watched the impact of the disease in other family members. They are not, therefore, solely observers of another's suffering, a challenge for many in itself, as this book demonstrates, but are potentially also watching their own futures. Not surprisingly, the impact of HD is devastating for affected individuals, as well as for their families, not least because 'it is a disease with a long trajectory: many young people are aware that they may develop the illness for years before there are obvious symptoms' (56).

The situation for families with HD has become more complicated since 1993, with the discovery of the gene mutation for HD on chromosone 4. This means that genetic testing has been possible for people with a history of HD in their family. There are four categories of risk depending on the number of unstable trinucleotides in the IT15 gene (58), which range from an increasing chance of the disease to a certainty. People aware of HD in their families may chose to have predictive genetic testing to determine if they have the abnormal gene and thus potentially remove uncertainty, if not (depending on gene status) the need to live knowing that the future will include HD. Increasingly, research evidence demonstrates that the impact of genetic testing on HD families is complex and that it does not necessarily reduce the impact of HD on the family, not least because disclosing an individual's test results will also communicate information about the risk of their first-degree relatives, who may chose not to know. There is evidence that disclosing HD test results can lead to the loss of family support (59). One explanation given for this is that uncertainty influences the bond between family members and a person who chooses to be tested was perceived as not being strong enough to live with the uncertainty (60). Hamilton *et al.* (58) suggest that genetic testing is a 'family affair', affecting the dynamics of family relationships, involving obligations as well as the issue of how test results are communicated and to whom. Their qualitative research revealed that their participants engaged in three processes in disclosing genetic information: (1) they considered the effects on themselves and family members; (2) they selectively disclosed particular aspects of the information they had received; and (3) they planned the timing of the disclosure. People with HD have obvious sensitivity that this disease is not just theirs but a whole family issue, which explains why Quaid and Wesson (61) report increased focus on the effects of predictive testing in Huntington's disease on spouses and partners.

Perhaps because of the focus of attention on the dilemmas presented by genetic testing and the related hereditary aspects of HD, there has been very little research into the experiences of family carers in HD, or into effective interventions to support them. Skirton and Glendinning (62) identify that almost 20 per cent of carers suffer from a stress-related illness, and that their fears include fear of their loved ones' sudden death, to threats to their safety by violence or accident initiated by the person with HD. There has been some recent interest into the coping strategies family carers adopt (63) but this research is in its infancy.

Organ failure

Chronic heart failure

Chronic heart failure (CHF) has been defined as 'a syndrome with symptoms and signs caused by cardiac dysfunction, resulting in reduced longevity' (64). Symptoms include breathlessness, particularly at rest and at night, reduced exercise tolerance, fatigue, lethargy, orthopnoea, nocturnal cough, wheeze, loss of appetite and confusion or delirium, particularly in older people. These symptoms overlap with those of other conditions, so diagnosis of CHF is not straightforward: the European Society of Cardiology, therefore, requires there to be symptoms of CHF at rest or during exercise and objective evidence of cardiac dysfunction, preferably by echocardiography (64). The most common cause of CHF is ischaemic heart disease, and up to one-third of those surviving a heart attack will develop CHF within 10 years. The incidence of CHF is estimated to be 5 to 10 in 1000 persons per year, and the prevalence 1 or 2 per cent of the population. Both are, however, related to age, with a UK population-based study reporting incidence rates of 0.2/10 000 person years in those aged 45 to 55 years, rising to 12.4/1000 in those aged 85 years or over, and a similar study in the USA reporting prevalence to be 0.7 per cent in those aged 45 to 54 rising to 8.4 per cent in those aged 75 or above (64). CHF is more common in men, with an age-standardized ratio of 1.75. However, more women than men survive into older age and the increased incidence of CHF with age means that the total number of men and women living with heart failure is very similar.

People with CHF experience bouts of worsening symptoms and signs (decompensation of CHF), which may need hospitalization or more GP visits. Up to two-thirds of hospitalizations in CHF are thought to be preventable, with the primary reasons for them being poor compliance by people with CHF with pharmacological and non-pharmacological regimens and failure to seek help with worsening symptoms (65). They are encouraged (and expected) by health professionals to make sustained changes in their behaviour to help prevent these episodes, including fluid restriction, daily weighing to detect fluid retention (a sign of deterioration) early, dietary changes including salt restriction, and regular exercise, as well as managing complex medication regimes. CHF is, however, a progressive condition, with those with the most severe symptoms breathless at rest and, therefore, severely limited in their physical activities. There have been important pharmacological advances, including ACE inhibitors and B blockers, but CHF continues to have a signifi-cant impact on prognosis, with a recent Dutch study reporting 1-, 2- and 5-year survival rates in a study of newly diagnosed cases of 63 per cent, 51 per cent and 35 per cent, respectively (64). Predictors of prognosis in CHF are poorly understood (64): a substantial but unknown proportion are thought to die suddenly, and there is some evidence that people with relatively mild CHF are at the most risk of dying unexpectedly from arrhythmias and sudden car-diac deaths. Implantable cardioverter-defibrilliators (ICDs) and pacing devices are available to prevent this in those thought to be at risk of sudden death. Co-morbidities are common in CHF and have been shown to have a negative impact on survival: common co-morbidities include anaemia, cachexia, renal impairment, obstructive sleep apnoea, COPD, renal failure and diabetes.

There is, as indicated above, increasing recognition of the important role played by self-management in preventing deterioration in CHF and, associated with this, a growing number of interventions designed to support people with CHF on discharge from hospital in order to prevent future hospitalizations (66).

There is also increasing recognition of the substantial impact of CHF on health-related quality of life (67), with people with CHF reporting that they experience significant physical and social limitations, including reduced ability to perform activities of daily living and to fulfil family responsibilities, reduced mobility and ability to travel, disrupted social interaction with family and friends. Not surprisingly, they also have high levels of depression and anxiety (68). Despite this, there has been very little attention to the experiences or needs of family carers, with the authors of a recent review of the limited research evidence commenting that 'the available research evidence does not explicitly reflect the important role that carers may have in managing the illness' (69). Because of the levels of disability experienced by people with CHF, those with moderate and severe CHF are often dependent on family carers for help with shopping and household tasks, with those with severe CHF also needing help with activities of daily living. Family carers are, therefore, likely to play a key role in making and sustaining the necessary changes in life-style in prevent hospitalization and disease progression, and in managing medications. The lack of attention given to family carers in CHF is even more striking, given the emerging evidence of an association between social support and prognosis in CHF; for example, marital quality has been found to predict survival in CHF over an 8-year period, particularly in women (70), and a review has found evidence of a relationship between social support and both re-hospitalization and mortality (71).

Research evidence for the impact of caring on family carers in CHF is very limited. On the basis of their review of 16 papers, Molloy, Johnston and Witham (69) list the potential caregiving burden on family carers (specifically spouses or partners, although many are also relevant to other carers), as limitations in physical activities, fluctuating symptoms, dealing with complex medical and self-care regimes, mood changes, restricted social life, frequent hospitalizations, changes in social activities, worry associated with ICDs or other technological medical devices, and disturbed sleep patterns caused by CHF-related sleep apnoea and use of diuretics. They conclude that family carers in CHF appear to have at least moderately high levels of distress, and that there is some evidence that women carers seem to be more distressed than men. A recent study by Barnes et al. found carer strain to be associated with carer depression and with the severity of breathlessness and impairment patients were experiencing, whilst carer quality of life was associated with their own health, as well as with depression levels (72). Given the lack of interest until recently in family carers in CHF, it is not surprising that there is as yet no evidence of effective interventions to support them: one recent study is, however, encouraging in that it unusually considered the impact of an exercise intervention for frail older people with CHF on family carers, demonstrating that the intervention was associated with increased family burden (73). This demonstrates the importance of including the impact on family carers in future studies.

Chronic obstructive pulmonary disease

Chronic obstructive pulmonary disease (COPD) is characterized by a decline in lung function, which is not fully reversible, and encompasses chronic bronchitis, emphysema and chronic airway obstruction (74). There is little good prevalence and incidence data at present (74), with a pooled prevalence estimate from available studies of 7.6 per cent in the whole population, and about 9 to 10 per cent in those aged 40 years or above (74). Prevalence increases with age, particular in those who smoke. Smoking is the most important risk factor for COPD, with up to half of long-term smokers developing the disease (75). Other risk factors include occupational exposure, air pollution, airway hyper-responsiveness and asthma. Largely because of the associations with smoking and ageing, there is expected to be a substantial increase in the proportion of people dying from COPD in the 30 years from 1995 to 2025, with its projected rise from 6th to 3rd in the most common causes of death world-wide (76). Rates of death from COPD are higher amongst men than amongst women but, as in CHF, women live longer and are therefore more likely to develop COPD; as a consequence there are more deaths of women from COPD than of men (74).

COPD causes breathlessness, particularly on exertion, and fatigue. These lead to physical deconditioning and, as the disease progresses, to reductions in physical functioning and in the ability to carry out activities of daily living. Depression is common, with estimates of between 20 and 60 per cent, and impacts on ability to adhere to treatment plans, leading to increased loss of function, and may be related to worse outcomes during the acute exacerbations experienced by people with COPD (77). These periods of acute worsening affect quality of life and health, may result in hospital admission and eventually lead to death (78). During these periods, they experience increasing breathlessness, sputum purulence and volume, and may also have worsening exercise tolerance, fluid retention, increased fatigue, acute confusion and general malaise. If they are admitted to hospital, estimates of in-patient mortality range from 4 per cent to 30 per cent (78), with 14 per cent estimated to die within 3 months of discharge in the UK. Attention has been focused on improving functioning in COPD in order to prevent exacerbations and improve both quality of life and survival: a recent Cochrane Review concluded that pulmonary rehabilitation, exercise training for at least 4 weeks, with or without education and/or psychological support, is effective in reducing breathlessness and fatigue, and in improving emotional function and a sense of control over the condition (79). The impact of these interventions on family carers was not considered, despite the evidence that people with COPD become functionally impaired and experience psychological symptoms, both of which are likely to mean that they require support from family carers. Similarly, a systematic review of nurse-led management interventions in COPD concluded that there was no evidence for the effectiveness of these interventions on family carers (80). The need to consider the impact of interventions for people with COPD on family carers is given even greater impetus by the growing interest in the role of hospital-at-home, to prevent acute admissions in COPD (81).

The lack of evidence on the impact of COPD interventions on family carers is mirrored in the lack of knowledge about the experiences and needs of family carers in COPD. A qualitative study of the experiences of people with COPD, and their family carers, of living with severe COPD demonstrated that carers not only had to support the person with COPD in their experience of multiple losses (including loss of personal liberty and dignity, of previous expectations of the future, of ability to perform activities of daily living and of social life), but they experienced some of the same losses, with strain very apparent in the carers (82). In an interview study of bereaved relatives, respondents reported breathlessness as being the major symptom that had impaired the person with COPD's mobility and contributed to their being housebound, to high levels of anxiety and panic and to depression (83). They perceived oxygen therapy to have been helpful, but to have imposed considerable lifestyle restrictions on them both, due to increasing dependence upon it. Some had had very little support from health or social services beyond repeat prescriptions from family doctors and emergency hospital admissions. Other studies have also reported negative impacts of long-term oxygen therapy: Kanervisto *et al.* reported that it negatively impacts on family communication and roles (84), whilst Ibanez *et al.* (85) have reported negative impacts on both communication between spouses and on family carers, as well as for people with COPD. Breathlessness also impacted negatively on carers' lives: they experienced severe anxiety and helplessness as they watched their loved one suffering and were unable to help, and their lives were greatly affected by the restrictions imposed by this symptom (86). Little else is currently known about the experiences of family carers in COPD: it is not known, for example, whether particular carers experience more difficulties than others, or what enables some carers to be resilient and to find meaning in their experience. Given the lack of research in this area, it will come as no surprise to learn that there is no evidence for effective interventions to support family carers in COPD.

Discussion

This chapter has reviewed the evidence on the experiences of family carers of people with six disorders, which currently receive, at best, limited attention from hospices and specialist palliative care services. One, MND, is characterized by a relatively short prognosis, with two-thirds of those affected likely to die within 4 years, and a relentless progressive decline to paralysis and death. Given both the predictable prognosis and the only too evident 'total pain' of those with this condition, it is not perhaps surprising that some palliative care services have provided care for MND patients since the inception of the modern hospice movement, and many, but by no means all, do so today. CHF has received increasing attention from palliative care researchers and clinicians over the past 10 years, and emphasis is now turning from identifying and classifying palliative care needs in this patient group, to establishing effective interventions, particularly given continuing debates about prognostic uncertainty. Like MND, it is characterized by relatively poor survival, again with two-thirds expected to die within 5 years (although the high incidence of sudden deaths makes individual life-expectancy difficult to estimate). In contrast, MS, PD, HD and COPD are only just beginning to receive attention within palliative care, with very little research into the palliative care needs of those affected, or debate about the appropriate response of palliative care services. This may be because the time course of these conditions is either much longer than in MND or CHF (MS, PD and HD) or currently much less well understood (COPD). A lack of attention from palliative care does not necessarily indicate a lack of interest in the experiences of family carers, with the literature on family carers in MS and in PD being relatively well-developed in contrast to that in, for example, CHF. This provides evidence for the important point made earlier in this chapter, that palliative care is not alone in its interest and expertise in family carers. The question of whether palliative care has a role in supporting family carers in neurodegenerative conditions and in advanced organ failure will be returned to again later.

It is clear from the research reviewed in this chapter that caring for someone with a neurodegenerative disease or with advanced organ failure can impact negatively on the physical and emotional well-being of the family carer, their quality of life, their social life and their finances. Increased impact on family carers' well-being (quality of life, carer strain or carer burden) was associated with caring for more hours each day (MS and MND), with providing personal care (CHF), with increased severity of symptoms (MS, PD, CHF), with reduced functional status (MS, MND), with depression (MS, MND, CHF), and with cognitive impairment (MS, PD). In addition to these commonalities, it is important to recognize that each diagnostic group poses distinct caregiving challenges and disease-specific aspects of caregiving need, therefore, to be separated from general aspects. For example, family carers in MND and CHF have potentially to deal with complex medical technologies, which, in the case of MND involved ethical dilemmas about the commencement and withdrawal of artificial nutrition and ventilation, as well as complex care regimens, whilst ICDs in CHF bring different dilemmas. Carers in COPD often had to cope with the impact of long-term oxygen use. Because it is a genetic disorder, family carers in HD differ from other carers in having to provide care for a condition they themselves may get or for which they have already provided care for other family members. An unstable disease course has been found to be particularly stressful for family carers in MS, whilst a particularly rapid progression has been shown to be a cause of stress in MND. Family carers in COPD have to contend with the fact that COPD is often seen as a stigmatized condition because of its association with smoking. There is currently insufficient evidence to identify key disease-specific aspects of caregiving in HD, CHF and COPD, and limited evidence in MND and PD. Full understanding of the needs of family carers beyond cancer therefore requires further research into the experiences of those caring for people with these conditions.

This is particularly true when focus is shifted from negative to positive aspects of caring: with the exception of MS, little attention has been paid to how family carers in these conditions cope with the demands placed upon them or indeed, how they develop resilience or find meaning in their experience. Social support does, however, emerge as an important factor: it has been shown to have beneficial effects on health, family life and depression, and it is, therefore, of concern that family carers in MS, MND, PD and CHF all reported a negative impact of caring on their social lives. Satisfaction with social relationships and social support were found to be important predictors of carer distress in MND and PD, and, whilst the impact on carers is not known, social support is related to prognosis in CHF. Cognitive changes in MS, PD and HD may place family carers at particular risk of a lack of social support, both as a consequence of altered relationships with the person with the disorder and because of withdrawal by friends and relatives. The impact of breathlessness in CHF and COPD and long-term oxygen therapy in COPD on family communication and social support needs further exploration.

Not surprisingly, given the lack of research into family carers' experiences, there is a dearth of research into effective interventions for those providing care for people with these conditions. The evidence-base is most advanced in PD, but even here is restricted to pilot and early-stage studies, which suggest benefits of cognitive-behavioural and psycho-educational interventions. There is some evidence of increasing recognition of the importance of including carer outcomes in intervention studies for patients in these conditions, but few studies so far have done this. Palliative care may not be alone in recognizing the needs of family carers, but there is little evidence to date in neurodegenerative disorders or in advanced organ failure that others have fully grasped the task of understanding their experiences or of developing and testing effective interventions to support them in their caregiving roles.

Should hospices and specialist palliative care services extend their role to provide support for family carers in these conditions? In the light of the (albeit limited) research evidence presented above, it is not difficult to make a case that something should be done to support family carers, particularly given the reliance placed upon them by industrialized healthcare systems, which need to keep people at home to reduce healthcare costs. This has, of course, been recognized by Governments with, for example, the Government in England and Wales putting increasing emphasis on assessing and supporting carers. The rhetoric of palliative care goes beyond supporting family carers to enable them to continue to provide care by placing them alongside patients as the 'unit of care'. This is subject to debate, and the reality may differ from the rhetoric; but, at least in theory, palliative care has the potential to provide support for family carers, which addresses issues identified in this chapter, such as 'chronic loss', psychological distress and lack of social support, as well as meeting needs for practical support. One argument for the expansion of palliative care beyond cancer would suggest that to fail to provide this care outside of cancer is inequitable and cannot therefore be justified. It is important, however, to recognize that as yet there is no robust evidence for the benefits of palliative care for family carers outside of cancer and (perhaps) MND. Expertise developed within cancer-specific palliative care services may not translate well to other conditions, particularly given the disease-specific components of caring, which are currently poorly understood. Hospice and specialist palliative care services, therefore, need to develop interventions for specific groups of family carers beyond cancer, in conjunction with the family carers themselves and those who currently care for these patients. These interventions then need to be tested rigorously to see if they reduce distress and increase resilience in family carers. This will take time and resources. It may be a good thing that it will take time to develop an evidence-base for the involvement of palliative care in supporting family carers beyond cancer, given widespread concerns that moving beyond cancer will lead to services being swamped by referrals and by patients with uncertain prognoses (3): the need to develop an evidence-base will (if service development is evidence-based) provide time for services to be planned, growth controlled and important questions about, for example, funding to be addressed. Palliative care cannot fill all the gaps left by existing health and social services, despite the evident need amongst family carers: it needs to know what it has to offer family carers beyond cancer and why. Some of its contribution may (as in MND at present) be in direct service provision, underpinned by research, some in providing support for health and social care professionals delivering care, and some may involve campaigning to ensure that others too recognize that having a chronic or life-threatening condition is a family, not an individual, affair. Failing to recognize the needs of those caring for people with conditions other than cancer is not an option for palliative care, but neither is attempting to meet the needs of all family carers.

Key learning points

- Caring for someone with a neurodegenerative disease or with advanced organ failure can impact negatively on the physical and emotional well-being of the family carer, their quality of life, their social life and their finances. Although the research evidence is limited, it suggests that those family carers providing care for people who are depressed, who have cognitive problems, who have reduced functional status, who require personal care, who have severe symptoms and who require care for longer each day, are at increased risk of adverse consequences, as are carers who lack social support.

- In addition to these general points, each condition poses distinct caregiving challenges. It is therefore important to know enough about a specific condition to be able to anticipate the impact on family carers of, for example, its disease course, age of onset, pattern of symptoms and treatment requirements.

- Caring need not, however, be a negative experience. Although further research is needed to understand how family carers cope and find meaning in their experiences, it is clear that some do. Learning more about why some family carers cope better than others will inform the development of interventions to promote resilience in carers.

- There is an almost total lack of evidence about effective interventions to support family carers caring for those near the end of life with neurodegenerative disorders and advanced organ failure. This reflects the lack of attention given to date to family carers of people with these conditions.

◆ Whether, and to what extent, hospices and specialist palliative care services have a role in addressing the needs of family carers with neurodegenerative disorders and advanced organ failure is currently unknown. Given the growing evidence of the impact of caring, effective interventions need to be developed and tested. Robust evidence of benefit should be an essential prerequisite for palliative care involvement in meeting the needs of family carers.

Recommended reading and resources

Addington-Hall JM (2005). Extending palliative care to chronic conditions. *European Journal of Palliative Care* **12**(Supplement): 14–17.

Addington-Hall JM, Rogers A, McCoy A and Gibbs JSR (2003). Heart disease. In: Morrison RS and Meier D (ed.). *Geriatric Palliative Care*. New York: Oxford University Press, 110–122.

Field D and Addington-Hall JM (1999). Extending specialist palliative care to all? *Social Science and Medicine* **48**: 1271–1280.

Hudson PL, Toye C and Kristjanson LJ (2006). Would people with Parkinson's disease benefit from palliative care? *Palliative Medicine* **20**: 87–94.

Kumpfel T, Hoffman LA, Pollman W, Rieckmann P, Zetti UK, Kuhnbach R, Borasio GD and Voltz R (2007). Palliative care in patients with severe multiple sclerosis: two case reports and a survey among German MS neurologists. *Palliative Medicine* **21**: 109–114.

McKeown LP, Porter-Armstrong AP and Baxter GD (2003). The needs and experiences of caregivers of individuals with multiple sclerosis: a systematic review. *Clinical Rehabilitation* **17**: 234–248.

Mockford C, Jenkinson C and Fitzpatrick R (2006). A review: carers, MND and service provision. *Amyotrophic Lateral Sclerosis* **7**: 132–141.

Molloy GJ, Johnston DW and Witham MD (2005). Family caregiving and congestive heart failure. Review and analysis. *The European Journal of Heart Failure* **7**: 592–603.

Travers E, Jones K and Nichol J (2007). Palliative care provision in Huntington's disease. *International Journal of Palliative Nursing* **13**: 125–130.

Voltz R, Bernat JL, Borasio GD, Maddocks I, Oliver D and Portneoy R.eds (2004). *Palliative Care in Neurology*. Oxford: Oxford University Press.

References

1. National Council for Palliative Care (2006). *National Survey of Patient Activity Data for Specialist Palliative Care Services*. London: National Council for Palliative Care.

2. Addington-Hall JM (2005). Extending palliative care to chronic conditions. *European Journal of Palliative Care* **12**(Supplement): 14–17.

3. Field D and Addington-Hall JM (1999). Extending specialist palliative care to all? *Social Science and Medicine* **48**: 1271–1280.

4. Holmes T (2005). Motor neurone disease and the NSF for long-term neurological conditions. *Primary Health Care* **15**: 27–31.

5. Kumpfel T, Hoffman LA, Pollman W, Rieckmann P, Zetti UK, Kuhnbach R, Borasio GD and Voltz R (2007). Palliative care in patients with severe multiple sclerosis: two case reports and a survey among German MS neurologists. *Palliative Medicine* **21**: 109–114.

6. Hudson PL, Toye C and Kristjanson LJ (2006). Would people with Parkinson's disease benefit from palliative care? *Palliative Medicine* **20**: 87–94.

7. Travers E, Jones K and Nichol J (2007). Palliative care provision in Huntington's disease. *International Journal of Palliative Nursing* **13**: 125–130.

8. Pugliatti M, Rosati G, Carton H, Riise T, Drulovic J, Vecsei L and Milanov I (2006). The epidemiology of multiple sclerosis in Europe. *European Journal of Neurology* **13**: 700–722.

9. Gonzalez-Scarano F and Bima, B (1999). Infectious aetiology in multiple sclerosis: the debate continues. *Trends in Microbiology* **7**: 475–477.

10. Perkin GD and Wolinsky JS (2006). *Fast Facts: Multiple Sclerosis*. Abingdon: Health Press.

11. Chwastiak LA, Gibbons LE, Ehde DM, Sullivan M, Bowen JD, Bombardier CH and Kraft GH (2005). Fatigue and psychiatric illness in a large community sample of persons with multiple sclerosis. *Journal of Psychosomatic Research* **59**: 291–298.

12. Siegert RJ and Abernethy DA (2005). Depression in multiple sclerosis: a review. *Journal of Neurology, Neurosurgery and Psychiatry* **76**: 469–475.

13. Simioni S, Ruffieux C, Bruggimann L, Annoni JM and Schuep M (2007). Cognition, mood and fatigue in patients with the early stage of multiple sclerosis. *Swiss Medical Weekly* **137**: 496–501.

14. Johansson S, Ytterberg C, Claesson IM, Lindberg J, Hillert J, Andersson M, Widen Holmqvist L and von Koch L (2007). High concurrent presence of disability in multiple sclerosis. Associations with perceived health. *Journal of Neurology* **254**: 767–773.

15. Zorzon M, Zivadinov R, Monti Bragadin L, Moretti R, De Masi R, Nasuelli D and Cazzato G (2001). Sexual dysfunction in multiple sclerosis: a 2-year follow-up study. *Journal of the Neurological Sciences* **187**: 1–5.

16. Higginson IJ, Hart S, Silber E, Burman R and Edmonds P (2006). Symptom prevalence and severity in people severely affected by multiple sclerosis. *Journal of Palliative Care* **22**: 158–165.

17. McKeown LP, Porter-Armstrong AP and Baxter GD (2003). The needs and experiences of caregivers of individuals with multiple sclerosis: a systematic review. *Clinical Rehabilitation.* **17**: 234–248.

18. O'Brien MT (1993). Multiple sclerosis: health promoting behaviours of spousal caregivers. *Journal of Neurosciences Nursing* **25**: 105–112.

19. Figved N, Myhr K-M, Larsen J-P and Aarsland D (2007). Caregiver burden in multiple sclerosis: the impact of neuropsychiatric symptoms. *Journal of Neurology, Neurosurgery and Psychiatry* **78**: 1097–1102.

20. Aoun S (2004). *The Hardest Thing We Have Ever Done: the Social Impact of Caring for Terminally Ill People in Australia 2004.* Full report of the national inquiry into the social impact of caring for terminally ill people. Canberra, Australia, Palliative Care Australia.

21. Dawson S and Kristjanson LJ (2003). Mapping the journey: Family carers' perceptions of issues related to end stage care of individuals with muscular dystrophy or motor neurone disease. *Journal of Palliative Care* **19**: 36–42.

22. Good DM, Bower DA and Einsporn RL (1995). Social Support: gender differences in multiple sclerosis spousal caregivers. *Journal of Neurosciences Nursing* **27**: 305–311.

23. Hunt CK (2003). Concepts in caregiver research. *Journal of Nursing Scholarship* **35**: 27–32.

24. Neno R (2004). Spouse caregivers and the support they receive; a literature review. *Nursing Older People* **16**: 14–15.

25. Edmonds P, Vivat B, Burman R, Silber E and Higginson IJ (2007). 'Fighting for everything': service experiences of people severely affected by multiple sclerosis. *Multiple Sclerosis* **13**: 660–667.

26. Nolan M (2001). Positive aspects of caring. In: Payne S and Ellis-Hill C (ed.). *Chronic and Terminal Illness; New Perspectives on Caring and Carers*. Oxford: Oxford University Press, 22–44.

27. Pakenham KI (2005). The positive impact of multiple sclerosis on carers: associations between carer benefit finding and positive and negative adjustment domains. *Disability and Rehabilitation* **27**: 985–997.

28. Pakenham KI (2005). Benefit finding in multiple sclerosis and associations with positive and negative outcomes. *Health Psycholog.* **24**: 123–132.

29. Logroscino G, Traynor BJ, Chio A, Couratier P, Mitchell JD, Swingler RJ, Beghi E and for The pan-European ALS Register (EURALS) (2006). Descriptive epidemiology of amyotrophic lateral sclerosis: new evidence and unsolved issues. *Journal of Neurology, Neurosurgery and Psychiatry* **79**: 6–11.

30. Beresford S (1995). *Motor Neurone Disease*. London: Chapman & Hall.

31. Brown JB (2003). User, carer and professional experiences of care in motor neurone disease. *Primary Health Care Research and Development* **4**: 207–217.

32. Ringholz GM, Appel SH, Bradshaw M, Cooke NA, Mosnik DM and Schulz PE (2005). Prevalence and patterns of cognitive impairment in sporadic ALS. *Neurology* **65**: 586–590.

33. Kurt A, Nijboer F, Matuz T and Kubler A (2007). Depression and anxiety in individuals with amyotrophic lateral sclerosis: epidemiology and management. *CNS Drugs* **21**: 279–291.

34. Wicks P, Abrahams S, Masi D, Hejda-Forde S, Leigh PN and Goldstein LH (2007). Prevalence of depression in a 12-month consecutive sample of patients with ALS. *European Journal of Neurology* **14**: 993–1001.

35. Averill AJ, Kasarskis EJ and Segerstron SC (2007). Psychological health in patients with amyotrophic lateral sclerosis. *Amyotrophic Lateral Sclerosis* **8**: 243–254.

36. Ganzini L, Silveira MJ and Johnston WS (2002). Predictors and correlates of interest in assisted suicide in the final month of life among ALS patients in Oregon and Washington. *Journal of Pain and Symptom Management* **24**: 312–317.

37. Mockford C, Jenkinson C and Fitzpatrick R (2006). A review: carers, MND and service provision. *Amyotrophic Lateral Sclerosis* **7**: 132–141.

38. Krivickas LS, Shockley L and Mitsumoto H (1997). Home care of patients with amyotrophic lateral sclerosis (ALS). *Journal of Neurological Sciences* **152**(Supplement 1): S82–S89.

39. Ray R and Street A (2007). Non-finite loss and emotional labour: family caregivers' experiences of living with motor neurone disease. *Journal of Nursing and Healthcare of Chronic Illness* **16**: 35–43.

40. Goldstein LH, Atkins L, Landau S, Brown R and Leigh PN (2006). Predictors of psychological distress in carers with amyotrophic lateral sclerosis: a longitudinal study. *Psychological Medicine.* **36**: 865–875.

41. Love A, Street A, Harris R and Lowe R (2005). Social aspects of caring for people living with motor neurone disease: their relationships to carer well-being. *Palliative and Supportive Care* 3: 33–38.

42. Ray RA and Street AF (2005). Who's there and who cares: age as an indicator of social support networks for caregivers among people living with motor neurone disease. *Health and Social Care in the Community* 13: 542–552.

43. de Lau LML and Breteler MM (2006). Epidemiology of Parkinson's disease. *Lancet Neurology* 5: 525–535.

44. Ishihara LS, Cheesbrough A, Brayne C and Schrag A (2007). Estimated life-expectancy of Parkinson's patients compared with the UK population. *Journal of Neurology, Neurosurgery and Psychiatry* 78: 1304–1309.

45. Schrag A (2006). Quality of life and depression in Parkinson's disease. *Journal of the Neurological Sciences* 248: 151–157.

46. Thomas S and MacMahon D (2004). Parkinson's disease, palliative care and older people. *Nursing Older People* 16: 22–27.

47. Clough CG and Blockley A (2003). Parkinsons's disease and related disorders. In: Voltz R, Bernat A, Borasio G, Maddocks I, Oliver A and Portenoy R (ed.). *Palliative Care and Neurology*. Oxford: Oxford University Press, 48–58.

48. Schrag A, Hovis A, Morley D, Quinn N and Jahanshahi M (2006). Caregiver-burden in Parkinson's disease is closely associated with psychiatric symptoms, falls and disability. *Parkinsonism and related disorders* 12: 35–41.

49. Davey C, Wiles R, Ashburn A and Murphy C (2004). Falling in Parkinson's disease: the impact on informal caregivers. *Disability and Rehabilitation* 26: 1360–1366.

50. Parkinson's Disease Society/Policy Studies Institute (1999). *Survey of Members of the PDS*. London: PDS, 57–68.

51. Pal PK, Thennarasu K, Fleming J, Schulzer M, Brown T and Calne SM (2004). Nocturnal sleep disturbances and daytime dysfunction in patients with Parkinson's disease and in their caregivers. *Parkinsonism and Related Disorders* 10: 157–168.

52. Martinez-Martin P, Forjaz MJ, Frades-Payo B, Rusinol AB, Fernandez-Garcia JM, Benito-Leon J, Arillo VC, Barbera AM, Sordo MP and Catalan MJ (2007). Caregiver burden in Parkinson's disease. *Movement Disorders* 22: 924–931.

53. Secker DL and Brown RG (2005). Cognitive behavioural therapy for carers of patients with Parkinson's disease: a preliminary randomised controlled trial. *Journal of Neurology, Neurosurgery and Psychiatry* 76: 491–497.

54. Simons G, Thompson SB and Smith Pasqualini MC (2006). An innovative education programme for people with Parkinson's disease and their carers. *Parkinsonism and Related Disorders* 12: 478–485.

55. Wade DT, Gage H, Owen C, Trend P, Grossmith C and Kaye J (2003). Multidisciplinary rehabilitation for people with Parkinson's disease; a randomised control trial. *Journal of Neurology, Neurosurgery and Psychiatry* 74: 158–162.

56. Dawson S, Kristjanson LJ, Toye C and Flett P (2004). Living with Huntington's disease: need for supportive care. *Nursing and Health Sciences* 6: 123–130.

57. Foroud T, Gray J, Ivashina J and Conneally PM (1999). Differences in duration of Huntington's disease based on age at onset. *Journal of Neurology, Neurosurgery and Psychiatry* 66: 52–56.

58. Hamilton RJ, Bowers BJ and Williams JK (2005). Disclosing genetic test results to family members. *Journal of Nursing Scholarship* **37**: 18–24.

59. Sobel S and Cowen CB (2003). Ambiguous loss and disenfranchised grief: The impact of DNA predictive testing on the family as a system. *Family Process* **42**: 47–47.

60. Williams JK, Schutte DL, Evers C and Holkup PA (2000). Redefinition: Coping with normal results from predicitve genetic testing for neurodegenerstive disorders. *Research in Nursing & Health* **23**: 260–269.

61. Quaid KA and Wesson MK (1995). Exploration of the effects of predictive testing for Huntington's disease on intimate relationships. *American Journal of Medical Genetics* **57**: 46–51.

62. Skirton H and Gleninning N (1997). Using research to develop care for patients with Huntington's disease. *British Journal of Nursing* **6**: 83–90.

63. Helder DI, Kaptein AA, van Kempen GMJ, Weinman J, van Houwelingen JC and Roos RAC (2002). Living with Huntington's disease: illness perceptions, coping mechanisms, and spouses' quality of life. *International Journal of Behavioural Medicine* **9**: 37–52.

64. Mosterd A and Hoes AW (2007). Clinical epidemiology of heart failure. *Heart* **93**: 1137–1146.

65. Michalsen A, Konig G and Thimme W (1998). Preventable causative factors leading to hospital admissions with decompensated heart failure. *Heart* **80**: 437–441.

66. Riegel B, Carlson B, Kopp Z, LePetri B, Glaser D and Unger A (2002). Effect of a standardized nurse case-management telephone intervention on resource use in patients with chronic heart failure. *Archives of Internal Medicine* **162**: 705–712.

67. Johansson P, Dahlstrom U and Bromstrom A (2006). Factors and interventions influencing health-related quality of life in patients with heart failure: a review of the literature. *European Journal of Cardiovascular Nursing* **5**: 5–15.

68. Haworth JE, Moniz-Cook E, Clark AL, Wang M, Waddington R and Cleland JGF (2005). Prevalence and predictors of anxiety and depression in a sample of chronic heart failure patients with left ventricular systolic dysfunction. *European Journal of Heart Failure* **7**: 803–805.

69. Molloy GJ, Johnston DW and Witham MD (2005). Family caregiving and congestive heart failure. Review and analysis. *The European Journal of Heart Failure* **7**: 592–603.

70. Rohrbaugh MJ, Shoham V and Coyne JC (2006). Effect of marital quality on eight-year survival of patients with heart failure. *American Journal of Cardiology* **98**: 1069–1072.

71. Luttik ML, Jaarsma T, Moser D, Sanderman R and van Veldhuiden DJ (2005). The importance of social support on outcomes in patients with heart failure. *Journal of Cardiovascular Nursing* **20**: 162–169.

72. Barnes S, Gott M, Payne S, Parker C, Seamark D, Gariballa A and Small N (2006). Characteristics and views of family carers of older people with heart failure. *International Journal of Palliative Nursing* **12**: 380–388.

73. Molloy GJ, Johnston DW, Gao C, Witham MD, Gray JM, Argo IS, Struthers AD and McMurdo ME (2006). Effects of an exercise intervention for older heart failure patients on caregiver burden and emotional distress. *European Journal of Cardiovascular Prevention and Rehabilitation* **13**: 381–387.

74. Chapman KR, Mannino DM, Soriano JB, Vermeire PA, Buist AS, Thun MJ, Connell C, Jemai A, Lee TA, Miravitalies M, Aldington A and Beasley R (2006). Epidemiology and costs of chronic obstructive pulmonary disease. *European Respiratory Journal* **27**: 188–207.

75. Halbert RJ, Natoli JL, Gano A, Badamgarav E, Buist AS and Mannino DM (2006). Global burden of COPD: systematic review and meta-analysis. *European Respiratory Journal* **28**: 523–532.

76. Murray CJ and Lopez AD (1997). Alternative projections of mortality and disability by cause 1990–2020: Global Burden of Disease Study. *Lancet* **349**: 1498–1504.

77. Norwood R (2006). Prevalence and impact of depression in chronic obstructive pulmonary disease patients. *Current Opinion in Pulmonary Medicine* **12**: 113–117.

78. Donaldson GC and Wedzicha JA (2006). COPD exacerbations. 1: Epidemiology. *Thorax* **61**: 164–168.

79. Lacasse Y, Goldstein R, Lasserson TJ and Martin S (2006). Pulmonary rehabilitation of COPD. *Cochrane Database of Systematic Reviews* **18**: CD003793.

80. Taylor SJ, Candy B, Bryan RM, Ramsey J, Vrijhoej HF, Eszond G, Wedzicha JA and Griffiths CJ (2005). Effectiveness of innovations of nurse-led chronic disease management of patients with COPD: systematic review of evidence. *BMJ* **331**: 485–488.

81. Ram FS, Wedzicha JA, Wright J and Greenstom M (2004). Hospital at home for patients with acute exaceberations of COPD: systematic review of evidence. *BMJ* **329**: 315.

82. Seamark DA, Blake SD, Seamark CJ and Halpin DM (2004). Living with severe chronic obstructive pulmonary disease: perceptions of patients and their carers. An interpretative phenomenological analysis. *Palliative Medicine* **18**: 619–625.

83. Elkington H, White P, Addington-Hall J, Higgs R and Pettinari C (2004). The last year of life in COPD: a qualitative study of symptoms and services. *Respiratory Medicine* **98**: 439–445.

84. Ibanez M., Aguilar JJ, Maderal MA, Prats E, Farrero E, Font A and Escarrabill J (2001). Sexuality in chronic respiratory failure: coincidences and divergences between patient and primary caregiver. *Respiratory Medicine* **95**: 975–979.

85. Kanervisto M, Paavilainen E and Heikkila J (2007). Family dynamics in families of severe COPD patients. *Journal of Clinical Nursing* **16**: 1498–1595.

86. Booth S, Silvester S and Todd C (2003). Breathlessness in cancer and chronic obstructive pulmonary disease: using a qualitative approach to describe the experiences of patients and carers. *Palliative and Supportive Care* **1**: 337–344.

Chapter 14

Support for bereaved family carers

Sheila Payne and Liz Rolls

Introduction

Historically, bereavement support was regarded as the role of family and friends, and bereaved people found meaning in their experience through religious frameworks and spiritual guidance. Arguably, as many developed societies have become more secular and culturally diverse, these frameworks are no longer so widely accepted. In the context of palliative care services, the same people who become bereaved are those who have provided care and companionship throughout the final illness of the dying person. Yet this life transition is largely not reflected in the academic literature or in the organization and delivery of support services. Instead, there appears to be a disjunction between services for family carers during the life-time of the patient and following bereavement. The implications of this disjunction will be explored in this chapter.

This chapter will introduce different approaches to conceptualizing bereavement and loss, drawing upon international contemporary, competing accounts. It will provide an overview of three overarching theoretical perspectives that have come to dominate the way bereavement and loss is viewed in developed societies, especially in healthcare contexts; namely: accounts drawn from psychiatric and psychological perspectives; accounts based on models of stress and coping; and accounts derived from sociological, biographical and narrative frameworks. Each of these discourses contributes different ways to evoke the impact and meaning of bereavement and loss. It will be argued that the language used to represent bereavement and loss serves to both reflect and shape how these experiences are understood and enacted. We will also explore Walter's notion of 'clinical lore' with respect to the way that practitioners have interpreted these models as a linear process and then impose them as a template for mapping experience. This gives rise to notions of 'normal' and 'abnormal' (or complicated) grief, and raises broader issues about how practitioners use theory and research, and how theory and research are presented to them. The assumptions underpinning these discourses will be exposed and challenged and alternative accounts presented. Contemporary representations that emphasize resilience, well-being and coping with loss, will be examined. We will draw upon a number of research studies to consider the implications of loss and bereavement for family members both before and after the death of the patient. We will also highlight how loss impacts on healthcare workers and social care workers in hospices, hospitals and care homes for older people and in the community.

In the latter part of the chapter we will draw on recent research conducted by the authors examining the nature and purpose of bereavement support services provided by hospices and specialist palliative care services for adults and children in the UK. What functions do they have for bereaved family members, for the people who provide these services (both paid and unpaid), for health and social care workers who refer clients to them, and for the wider societies in which they are situated? Why do the majority of people decline to use these services? Do they somehow 'miss out' or are they making sensible decisions?

Bereavement, grief and mourning

It has been argued that there are no 'correct' or 'true' theories that explain the experience of loss or that fully account for the emotions, experiences and cultural practices that characterize grief and mourning (1, 2). Small (3) has argued that they are intimately linked to our theoretical understanding of loss. So the language we use to describe bereavement both reveals and shapes our understanding of this experience. Bereavement is usually associated with the experience of loss when a significant person is lost through death or when something that is important is lost (1). Grief is generally regarded as a normal emotional experience that follows the loss of a loved person. It is usually portrayed as intensely distressing, where the emotions of sadness, anger, guilt and anxiety predominate. It is, therefore, painful for the grieving person and vicariously painful for others to witness. Mourning refers to the social and culturally shaped behaviours through which individuals and communities express feelings of loss and grief. Within families, deaths of key members often precipitate beneficial and detrimental social transitions in status, power and access to resources; for example, with the transfer of family wealth between generations, ownership of the ancestral home and land or directorship of a family business, or with their loss. Transitions in relationships following death are formally socially sanctioned and acknowledged, such as spouse to widow or widower. Historically, and in many cultures, mourning behaviours have been the key way that people display their grief, rather than privileging emotional expression. Alternatively, a postmodernist position suggests that individual diversity is paramount, and that within broad cultural constraints each of us develops our own ways of *doing* and *expressing* bereavement (4).

Most major religions provide accounts of loss that enable shared meanings to be given for this experience. Religions also provide accounts of what happens in 'an afterlife'. They offer guidance on how bereaved people should respond after death and the nature of rituals and disposal practices, although these behaviours and practices may be modified over time and are sensitive to changes, such as migration and acculturation. For example, Firth (5) describes how British Hindus have had to adapt cremation and associated death rituals to the constraints of British crematoria. In the US, Chinese Americans have adapted ceremonial burial rituals, such as the traditional use of firecrackers and loud music to ward off evil spirits, to the contemporary inclusion of marching bands in the funeral possession to the cemetery (6). Cultural rituals that involve tending the grave and memorialization of family ancestors are found in many countries, such as Japan and China. In some countries including Mexico, Japan and Ireland, collective annual festivities are held to commemorate the dead on a specific day. For example, in Mexico the Day of the Dead is a very important cultural event marked by visiting the grave, socializing and sharing of foods in a cheerful, rather than morbid, occasion. In the UK, memorialization of significant deaths, such as soldiers in the First and Second World Wars, continues to be marked annually in more sombre mode. It is important to acknowledge that ideas derived from religious teaching have evolved and continue to do so. However, Britain has become an increasingly secular society and, arguably, religious teaching provides less guidance than in the past.

Distinctions between normal and abnormal grief are problematic, although one definition describes abnormal grief as 'a deviation from the (cultural) norm in the time course or intensity of specific or general symptoms of grief' (7). However, we would urge readers to critically reflect on the language of this definition, which conceptualizes grief in terms of symptomatology and highlights the burdensomeness of grief responses. For a review of the literature on complicated grief and recommendations for practice, see the Australian Department of Health and Ageing guidance (8). The following section examines common theoretical positions in more depth, in order to understand the different current discourses.

Loss and change: exploring models of grief and bereavement

Different models of bereavement have been developed and each offers various accounts of experience and 'outcomes'. There are a number of extensive reviews of the literature that provide more detailed examinations of the theoretical models than this chapter (9–11). We have grouped models conceptually into three categories: (1) psychoanalytic and attachment theories; (2) stress and coping; and (3) continuity theories.

Psychoanalytic and attachment theories

The first group of psychoanalytic and attachment theories constitute some of the most influential ways to conceptualize grief, loss and change. They are based on developmental notions of change and psychological growth. They make the assumption that bereavement is a *process* in which there is an *outcome*. Moreover, the successful resolution of grief involves psychic changes and offers the potential for psychological growth; for example, having successfully coped with previous losses, the individual learns how to cope more easily with subsequent bereavements. The idea of process is typically expressed as phases, stages or tasks to be accomplished over time. Notions of change and process are fundamental and failure to 'move on' or to 'progress' gives rise to potentially pathological positions of being 'stuck' in the midst of grieving. The theories have largely concentrated their attention on the intra-psychic domain—the inner workings of the mind. They have emphasized how people think and especially how they feel—their emotions, and that these can be accessed through talk. Moreover, they suggest that successful grieving requires effortful, but unconscious, mental processing called 'grief work' and that failure to do this is 'abnormal'. So where do these ideas come from?

A major contribution to theories of bereavement emerged from the psychoanalytic tradition, perhaps the most important being that of Freud (12). Freud contributed much to twentieth century thought and his ideas have been very influential in shaping our ways of understanding people. In 1917, Freud first pointed out the similarities and differences between grief and depression in his classic text *Mourning and Melancholia*. His paper offered one of the first descriptions of normal and pathological grief. The thoughts discussed in it underpin psychoanalytic theory of depression and provide the basis for many current theories of grief and its resolution. In the light of the impact of Freud's theory of grief on subsequent theoretical developments, it is surprising to acknowledge that grief, as a psychological process, was never Freud's main focus of interest. In the paper, he argued that people became attached to others who are important for the satisfaction of their needs and to whom emotional expression is directed. Love is conceptualized as the attachment of emotional energy to the psychological representation of the loved person. It is assumed that the more important the relationship, the greater the degree of attachment. According to Freudian theory, grieving represents a dilemma because there is a simultaneous need to relinquish the relationship, so that the person may regain the energy invested, and a wish to maintain the bond with the love object. The individual needs to accept the reality of the loss so that the emotional energy can be released and redirected. The process of withdrawing energy from the lost object is called 'grief work'. During this process the bereaved person is required to reconsider the past and dwell upon memories of the lost relationship (10). Freud regarded this intra-psychic processing as essential to the breaking of relationship bonds with the deceased, to allow the reinvestment of emotional energy and the formation of new relationships with others. Arguably, Freud's most important contributions to loss have been:

• developing psychoanalytic theory;

• introducing the 'grief work' hypothesis; and

• defining the difference between grief and depression.

Later psychoanalytic theorists have elaborated this theory of grief work. Klein (13) argues that bereavement results from the loss of a person's capacity to tolerate the ambivalence inherent in all human relations (a capacity Klein terms the 'depressive' position), through the re-activation of the early anxieties of what she called the 'paranoid-schizoid' position. In this early position, the infant oscillates between viewing objects in their world as either 'all good' or 'all bad'. When this position is re-activated as an adult as a result of bereavement, Klein likens the experience to a transitory manic-depressive state. It is the resolution, that is, the return of ambivalence, that is central to the bereavement process (14). Both Freud's and Klein's theories are based on notions of withdrawal and identification, although they are used in opposite ways. According to Littlewood, in Freud's theory, the withdrawal of libidinous attachment 'may be accomplished by the ego's *identification with* the lost object' (1992—our emphasis). In Klein's theory, the process of 'projective identification' is one in which we allow others to act for parts of ourselves, and it is this withdrawal, the *identification* we have lodged in the deceased person, from which we have to free ourselves (3). Nevertheless, Klein emphasizes that eventually the dead person is restored as a 'good object' within (13).

Based upon detailed observations of infants separated from their mothers, and his psychiatric clinical practise, Bowlby (15–17) proposed a complex theory to account for the formation of close human relationships, emphasizing those between mothers and their babies, and for what happened when separation occurred. He suggested that human evolution resulted in mothers and infants needing to be in close proximity for survival and that this was achieved through an interactional process involving reciprocal behaviours and emotions between mothers and infants, called attachment. Temporary separation was marked by characteristic behaviours and feelings such as distress, calling and searching. Permanent loss, such as bereavement, also triggered these feelings of intense distress and behavioural responses. The nature and quality of attachment bonds were used to predict vulnerability to adverse bereavement outcomes. Bowlby (17) drew upon psychoanalytic ideas to formulate a series of overlapping stages of grief involving: shock, yearning and protest, despair and recovery. Recent research has demonstrated that patterns of attachment in childhood profoundly influence the way people grieve (18). However, this study is based on analysis of questionnaire responses from patients attending a psychiatric clinic, which raises questions about their representativeness.

Bowlby's attachment theory was very influential in guiding health and social care services; for example, in encouraging early contact between mothers and babies after birth. Bowlby's attachment theory was also a key factor in the development of Parkes' theories of loss (19). Both Bowlby and Parkes were psychiatrists who were in contact with patients struggling to deal with complicated grieving and the impact of their bereavements. Parkes (20, 21) suggested that bereavement should be considered as a major psychosocial transition, which challenged the taken-for-granted world of the bereaved person. He argued that most people think of their world as relatively stable, in which they make assumptions of perceived control. Death, especially sudden death, challenges this, as people have to adapt to changes in relationships and social status (for example, from being a mother to being childless), and economic circumstances (for example, having less money). He, like Bowlby, proposed that people progress through a number of phases before resolving their bereavement; including numbness, pining and intense anxiety, disorganization and despair, and finally, reorganization.

Finally, there are two well-known models, which are widely recognized in palliative care. Kubler-Ross (22), a psychiatrist working in the USA who was heavily influenced by psychoanalytic theories, proposed a stage model of loss in relation to dying, which has been applied to bereavement. This model emphasized changing emotional expression throughout the final period of life. Worden (23, 24), working in the USA, based his therapeutic model on phases of grief and what he called 'tasks of mourning'. He emphasized the process of grieving and argued that people needed to work through their reactions to loss in order to achieve a final adjustment.

Over time, Parkes, Kubler-Ross and Worden have modified and developed their ideas and our simple account does not do justice to the complexity of their thinking. All these theories have been critiqued and challenged, especially in relation to notions of a linear progression through phases or stages and the necessity of 'grief work'; for example, see Wortman and Silver (25). In nursing and medical practice, they have gained the status of 'clinical lore' and their rigid application may arguably be disempowering and pathologizing for bereaved people (4). Furthermore, in some counselling models, there is also an assumption that people have some control over their feelings and thoughts. In addition, the emphasis on emotional expression does not take account of gender or cultural differences in expressiveness (26). Contemporary evidence suggests that bereaved people may be more resilient and less distressed than previously thought (27).

Stress and coping

An alternative theoretical position on loss has been derived from the psychological literature on cognitive processing and models of stress and coping. These ideas are based on an assumption that if certain things, called stressors, are present in sufficient amounts, they trigger a stress response (28). This response has both physical and psychological consequences. Stroebe and Schut (26), working in The Netherlands, drew upon a transactional model of stress and coping originally developed by Lazarus and Folkman (29). This model proposed that any event may be perceived as threatening by an individual, and cognitive appraisal is undertaken to estimate its degree of threat and to mobilize resources to cope with it. Coping may focus on dealing with the threat directly or may emphasize the emotional response. These are called 'problem focused' and 'emotion focused' coping. Stroebe and Schut, (26) applied this model within the context of bereavement. They proposed that stressors, following a death, can be categorized as to do with loss or restoration. They proposed that bereaved people oscillate between 'restoration focused' coping (for example, dealing with everyday life) and 'grief focused' coping (for example, by expressing their distress by yearning or crying). Both types of coping are taxing and anxiety provoking in the immediate aftermath of a loss. They suggest that people move between these two forms of coping with loss, although over time, coping responses become progressively more 'restoration focused'. However, there are no proscribed stages, and flexibility of oscillation between the different types of coping is emphasized. They called it 'the dual processing model'. From these ideas they have developed therapeutic interventions to help people address both types of coping to achieve a balance. This model can better account for gender and cultural differences in grieving but it continues to focus on psychological rather than social processes.

Continuity theories

Sociologists and anthropologists have challenged psychological theories, which suggest that successful resolution of grief involves 'moving on' and 'letting go' of the deceased person. They prioritize the social, cultural and interpersonal aspects of loss. They also remind us that in many places, such as in Chinese cultures (6), deceased ancestors continue to play an important part in the lives of the living. Therefore, bereavement outcomes that focus on disconnection and 'letting go' of the deceased are inappropriate. Instead, these theories are based on an assumption that people wish to maintain feelings of continuity across generations and that, even though physical relationships end at the time of death, these relationships become transformed but remain important within the memory of the individual and community. For example, memories of the large number of deaths that occurred during the First World War continue to haunt Britain, Germany, Russia and other countries, almost 100 years after the event (30). Rituals to mark these losses continue to occur frequently and some are even increasing in popularity and significance, yet no people remain alive who were present in the trenches and witnessed these events first-hand. Klass *et al.* (31), working in the USA, proposed that the goal of grieving is the transformation of relationships after death or other types of loss, and the creation of 'continuing bonds' with the deceased. Walter (32, 4), working in the UK, proposed a similar idea and illustrated this in relation to his own experiences of bereavement of his father and partner. He suggested that the purpose of grieving was the creation of a durable biography of the deceased, which allowed a bereaved person to integrate the memory of the deceased into their daily life. This biographical model of loss allowed bereaved people to create a narrative that describes both the person who has died and the part they play in their lives. He argues that these narratives are socially constructed. The elicitation of narratives (stories) is a common therapeutic device in counselling and is believed to help establish a lasting and tolerable memory of the deceased and how they died (33).

Supporting bereaved adults in palliative care contexts

The title of both this section and the chapter makes the assumption that bereaved adults either need, or could benefit from, 'support'. What is the evidence for this claim? Much of the palliative care literature makes the assumption that adults, either in the process of caring for their family members during their final illness and in bereavement, require additional support (34). Most bereavement services are based on an assumption that bereavement is a major stressful life event and that a minority of people experience substantial disruption to their physical, psychological and social functioning (19). Evidence from the first year after bereavement shows that physical and mental health is impaired for some people (35). Moreover, there are known to be increased mortality rates for men for a limited period of time after bereavement, especially in those with depression (36). Parkes (21) has argued that offering support to people who have adequate internal and external resources can be disempowering and can be detrimental to coping. Evidence suggests that bereavement support is of most benefit for individuals who recognize that they require support but there is little justification for providing proactive therapeutic intervention for bereaved people with no signs of poor bereavement outcome. Critical reviews of the literature have questioned the value of 'grief work', which challenges the basis of much of counselling with its focus on getting clients to talk about the loss and associated feelings (37).

Most adults, even when offered bereavement support, decline it. Bereaved people may be remarkably resilient, as they may draw upon personal resources, such as the experience of coping with previous bereavements, and social support, such as friendship and kinship networks. In the past, most health services have contributed little to bereavement support, with the exception of psychiatric treatment for those with complicated grief reactions and chaplaincy services at the time of the death. Proactive and reactive bereavement support has largely been delivered through religious and other community support networks or voluntary organizations, such as CRUSE (38). Hospices, as they have spread throughout the world, have recognized the continuing needs of bereaved relatives (39).

In this section we focus specifically upon a recent study that examined adult bereavement support services provided by hospices in the UK (for further information see 40–43), as an example of bereavement support services in palliative care. A survey was distributed to all 300 hospices and specialist palliative care units with adult bereavement services in the UK in 2003, and this was followed by detailed organizational case studies in five hospice bereavement services (44). The researchers collected information about the nature and role of bereavement support from the perspectives of service providers, including bereavement coordinators, professional bereavement workers and volunteers, and bereaved people who used services and those who declined. This study represents one of the first to investigate hospice bereavement support from multiple perspectives.

The postal survey identified 300 discrete bereavement services and 248 of them returned completed questionnaires. Of these, 80 per cent of services were located in England. Most had been in existence for at least 10 years and three-quarters of them were associated with in-patient hospice or specialist palliative care units (43). Staff involved in running the services were predominantly qualified nurses (56 per cent), social workers (46 per cent) and counsellors (46 per cent), with chaplains, psychologists and medical staff less commonly involved. The great majority of services employed paid staff. Typically hospice bereavement services usually involved two or three paid staff assisted by 11–12 volunteers; about a quarter of the services reported having insufficient staff to offer a full range of support. Nearly 80 per cent of the adult bereavement services were implementing or planning changes to their service, either in response to perceived difficulties and/or to expand existing services. Volunteers were reported to be involved in over two-thirds of the services, but seldom took sole responsibility for providing bereavement support activities. Volunteers may enhance the range of services offered and address the need to make services culturally appropriate by involving local people and those from different minority ethnic groups. However, there is controversy about the extent to which volunteer labour is valued and how the needs of volunteer workers are met (45). Volunteers require recruitment, selection, training and supervision. Relf (46) has pointed out that providing for the needs of volunteer workers in bereavement support is a demanding and skilled activity. Bereaved people appeared to value the input of trained volunteers, especially their approachability (43). A small but significant minority of services did not provide supervision for their bereavement staff. Formal audit and evaluation of adult bereavement services was uncommon. Less than half of the services had formal mechanisms for bereaved people to provide feedback about individual bereavement support.

One of the key findings from our research was the importance of pre-bereavement support offered by health and social care professionals associated with hospices (42, 43). Family members reported that the preparation for the loss was helpful, as was the sense that their family members were being cared for in a dignified and compassionate way. The pre-death care offered to patients influenced how bereaved people regarded their subsequent bereavement (43).

Following the death, services associated with in-patient units were more likely to use formal assessment tools to measure the need for bereavement support, but less than half (43 per cent) of UK hospice bereavement services reported using formal risk assessment, such as standardized questionnaires and checklists, to assess how likely it is that a bereaved person will have an adverse outcome (40). Half of the services reported that only informal assessment was used. The recognition of complicated (or abnormal) bereavement outcomes is important in identifying who might benefit from support services. While it is acknowledged that mental health problems, such as depression and anxiety, are relatively more common in bereaved people than others, there remains debate about definitions of complicated bereavement, as noted earlier. There are well-recognized attributes of the person such as age, gender, previous psychiatric history, their relationship with the deceased, such as the quality and intensity of the attachment, their social environment, such as availability of social support, religiosity, and the nature and place of the death, such as traumatic or unexpected deaths, which allow predictions to be made about which people are more likely to need help (47). For example, a person with previous mental health problems experiencing concurrent losses, such as their job or home, and witnessing a traumatic sudden death of their young child in a car accident, is likely to be more vulnerable than a person bereaved of their elderly grandmother after a chronic illness who was well-supported by hospice care. Although risk assessment measures are available, none are perfect. Previous research conducted in the UK in the early 1990s indicated that about 25 per cent of hospices used risk assessment to identify bereaved people in need of further support (48). Ten years later, the study showed little change in formal risk assessment and accounts of strong resistance from some bereavement workers to any form of selection or assessment. Instead, it was found that all services made unsolicited contact with bereaved relatives who had been in contact with the hospice, to offer them support; and it was left up to bereaved people to take up or decline services, as and when they required them.

The most commonly provided support activities were individual support, telephone support, written information, memorialization events and group support (40). Fewer services offered befriending and one-to-one counselling. It has been suggested that bereavement support can be conceptualized in three broad categories: social activities, such as memorial events, social evenings, information leaflets; supportive activities, such as drop-in centres, befriending; and therapeutic activities, such as counselling and group therapy (49). There may be considerable overlap in the aims and delivery of some of these activities. For example, a memorial event might enable a bereaved person to talk one-to-one with a bereavement worker, which may be perceived as therapeutic. Some services indicated they used social events to screen and assess bereaved people and they followed up those that they had concerns about.

Hospice bereavement support services need to be able to identify when clients present such difficult and complex problems that it exceeds their capacity to deal with them, and to have well-established mechanisms to refer on. Close and well-established links with other services, such as liaison psychiatric services, clinical psychology and specialist bereavement support services (e.g. suicide support groups), are needed but evidence from the five case studies indicated that these were either lacking or inadequate because of concerns about long waiting lists (43). Overall, evidence suggests that UK hospices were providing bereavement support that was well-regarded by bereaved people and fulfilled national recommendations (50). They provided information on the types of support available and the nature of grief, and provided a wide range of general support, but not necessarily access to specialist support. This was largely due to inadequate staffing and resources. Arguably this also meant that the skills developed in hospices were not available more generally in hospitals and the wider community to develop bereavement care (43).

Supporting bereaved children

Internationally, there is variation in the degree to which the deaths of infants and children have been publicly marked and mourned. Paradoxically, in developed countries where childhood deaths are less common there tends to be more attention to the loss of children. It is difficult to estimate the number of children who experience significant bereavements as many countries to not record this information. Winston's Wish (51) (a charity in the UK who offer childhood bereavement support) estimate that 3 per cent of 5–15-year-olds have experienced the death of a parent or sibling, equating to 510 000 children in the UK, whilst Easton (52) suggests that when the deaths of parents, siblings, grandparents and other significant people are taken into account, approximately 1 400 000 children are bereaved annually. Harrington and Harrison (53) argue that, based on reports on their experience of 'significant' loss, around 92 per cent of young people are bereaved of a significant relationship.

Initial developments in special childhood bereavement support occurred in the USA and these have now spread to Europe and Australia. In the UK, 14 per cent of childhood bereavement services are provided within freestanding organizations, but just under half (44 per cent) are provided in hospices and palliative care settings (54). What is the supportive role of these services and what is their justification? For this section, we will draw on a study undertaken between 2000 and 2003 that explored UK childhood bereavement services and the reasons why bereaved children and their parents had used a specialist service and the benefits they felt they drew from the experience.

The death of a parent is described as one of the most fundamental losses a child can face (55, 56), representing a profound psychological insult (57) and creating what Bertman (58) suggests is 'a new terror for a bereft child: the loss of one parent, and the symbolic or temporary loss—the unavailability—of the other [which] makes the actual loss of the lone surviving parent a threatening reality';

an experience that Riches and Dawson (59) term a 'double jeopardy'. The death of a sibling presents a different set of challenges for the bereaved child, who has been described as the 'forgotten mourner' (60), including negotiating the ambivalent feelings often found in sibling relationships, as well as feelings of guilt and self-reproach (55). Furthermore, when a child has died of a life-limiting illness, the well siblings will have already been living in what Bertman (58) calls 'houses of chronic sorrow' (58), citing Bluebond-Langner (61). However, the impact of bereavement on a child or young person is uncertain, and how a child experiences and responds to the death of a significant person, what happens afterwards and the accommodation, or 'timely reconstitution' (62), that a child is able to make, appears to be mediated by a number of factors. These include: who has died; the child's characteristics, such as age and stage of cognitive and emotional development; the circumstances surrounding the death, including how and what children are told, and what life is like afterwards; and relationships with peers and school (63). For this reason, Ribbens McCarthy (64) argues for a range of responses to be widely available to children who have been bereaved, particularly for those who are already vulnerable or living in disadvantaged circumstances. What is worthy of note here is that, whilst there are a range of bereavement theories that account for adult's experience, accounts of a child's bereavement experience are more problematic. There is no account conceptualized in their terms; rather, the issues are mainly conceptualized as to whether bereavement puts a child 'at risk' (64).

In the UK, services are offered to children in different ways: individually or in groups, with the child only, or with families; Fig. 14.1 shows this range of activity.

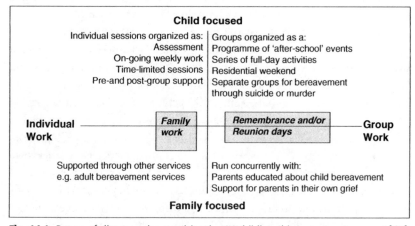

Fig. 14.1 Range of direct service provision in UK childhood bereavement support [63] Reproduced with permission from Taylor and Francis

The services used a wide range of techniques other than 'talk' with all age groups, including adults. Some services used bereavement-specific resources and workbooks, whereas others created their own activities. The activities included puppetry, making pictures, collages, 'memory boxes' and salt sculptures, as well as a range of experiential activities that contributed to naming feelings, thinking about the person who had died, about what had happened, and how users could help and support themselves in the future. Underlying these activities were a set of common objectives, which were to provide a secure place to enable them to create memory and story through an exploration of their experience of bereavement, accessing their unspoken and unconscious feelings, and helping them make sense of what had happened and how they felt. Services also help children manage these feelings, improve communication between family members, reduce feelings of isolation and hold the possibility of hope for their future.

Although children were not sure what to expect from a service, they had wanted something from the experience prior to attending. These included support and help to understand what was happening, and a place to 'get it off my chest'. However, not all children in each family used the service, the reasons for this varying from not wanting to attend, being unable to attend because of their age or because the non-attending child is seen as not needing to, as they either felt they were managing or were not displaying behavioural or emotional difficulties. Parents wanted support, either for themselves, for their own emotional needs or to support their capacity to parent; for their child, expressed in terms of their fear of the long-term effect of the loss, or recognizing the needs of a particular child that they were unable to meet; or for their family because the bereavement and its consequences were having a detrimental effect on the family unit, and they felt unable to restore it (65).

However, not all children or parents wanted to participate in the more structured interventions. Those who did, were able to describe the significant ways in which they found the experience helpful, and the ways in which this had an impact on both their internal (emotional) and external (social) worlds. Children were enabled to make sense of the experience of bereavement and to understand more, and it allayed their anxieties about what had happened to them, or to the dead person. It also helped them talk about their feelings, from which they experienced relief. Parents were supported, not just on their own account but also in their parenting. They found it very helpful to be with others; consoled that they were not alone, experiencing comfort in sharing their experiences, and in being with others who they felt were able to recognize and acknowledge their experiences. Although some parents had difficulties in attending group interventions, bereaved parents expressed their need for support and advice to help them provide appropriate care for their bereaved child (65).

Conclusion

Witnessing dying can be a profoundly disturbing event for some carers, while for others it is both a privilege and a relief. The death of the patient signals the transition into bereavement. This chapter has focused on that stage of the care-giving experience. We have provided an overview of the main theoretical perspectives and concluded that none fully explains the impact of loss. Internationally, death rituals and customs are derived from ethnic or religious groupings, and diversity is influenced by many factors, including social classes, urbanization and history (66). We have presented evidence drawn from a study of adult hospice bereavement services and a study of childhood bereavement services, both conducted in the UK. Support for adults may be delivered in a variety of forms but most rely on talking. Arguably, support for children has a different function to that for adults, in that it acts as both a support to children for their needs and support to parents in parenting a bereaved child. It also uses different approaches to those usually associated with 'counselling'—in that the work is more experiential rather than the traditional 'counselling' talk used with adults. Whatever the age group or needs of the bereaved person, they require compassionate, sensitive and sensible clinical practice.

Key learning points

- Bereavement is a life transition marked by the loss of a significant person.
- Grief refers to the expression of loss, while mourning refers to the behavioural response to loss and is typically shaped by social and cultural norms.
- Three types of theoretical perspectives provide competing accounts of bereavement and explain the experience of loss.
- Hospice bereavement support seeks to provide continuity of care for surviving family members.
- Childhood bereavement services seek to support children with their loss experience and to help parents deal with a bereaved child.

Recommended reading and resources

Christ G (2000). *Healing Children's Grief: Surviving a Parent's Death from Cancer.* Oxford: Oxford University Press.

Firth P, Luff G and Oliviere D (2005). *Loss, Change and Bereavement in Palliative Care.* Maidenhead: Open University Press.

Hockey J, Katz J and Small N (ed.) (2001). *Grief, Mourning and Death Ritual*. Buckingham: Open University Press.

Payne S, Horn S and Relf M (1999). *Loss and Bereavement*. Buckingham: Open University Press.

Riches G and Dawson P (2000). *An Intimate Loneliness: Supporting Bereaved Parents and Siblings*. Buckingham: Open University Press.

Stroebe MS, Hansson RO, Stroebe W and Schut H (2001). *Handbook of Bereavement Research. Consequences, Coping and Care*. Washington, DC: American Psychological Association.

Stokes J (2004). *Then, Now and Always: Supporting Children Through Grief: a Guide for Practitioners*.Cheltenham: Winston's Wish. http://www.winstonswish.org.uk/

Worden J (1996). *Children and Grief: When a Parent Dies*. New York: Guildford.

Walter T (1999). *On Bereavement*. Buckingham: Open University Press.

References

1. Payne S, Horn S and Relf M (1999). *Loss and Bereavement*. Buckingham: Open University Press.

2. Hockey J, Katz J and Small N (ed.) (2001). *Grief, Mourning and Death Ritual*. Buckingham: Open University Press.

3. Small N (2001). Theories of grief: a critical review. In: Hockey J, Katz J and Small N (ed.). *Grief, Mourning and Death Ritual*. Buckingham: Open University Press, 19–48.

4. Walter T (1999). *On Bereavement*. Buckingham: Open University Press.

5. Firth S (2001). Hindu death and mourning rituals: the impact of geographic mobility. In: Hockey J, Katz J and Small N (ed.). *Grief, Mourning and Death Ritual*. Buckingham: Open University Press, 237–46.

6. Chung SF and Wegars P (2005). *Chinese American Death Rituals: Respecting the Ancestors*. Lanham: Altamira Press.

7. Stroebe MS, Hansson RO, Stroebe W and Schut H (2001). *Handbook of Bereavement Research. Consequences, Coping and Care*. Washington, DC: American Psychological Association.

8. The Australian Department of Health and Ageing Guidance (2006). http://www. health. giv. au/internet/wcms/publishing. nsf/Contents/palliativecare-pubs-rsch-grief

9. Archer J (1999). *The Nature of Grief: the Evolution and Psychology of the Actions to Loss*. London: Routledge.

10. Stroebe MS and Schut H (2001). Models of coping with bereavement: a review. In Stroebe MS, Hansson RO, Stroebe W and Schut H (ed.). *Handbook of Bereavement Research. Consequences, Coping and Care*. Washington, DC: American Psychological Association.

11. Wimpenny P, Unwin R, Dempster P, Grundy M, Work F, Brown A and Silcock S (2006). *Literature review on Bereavement and Bereavement Care*. Joanna Briggs Collaborating Centre, School of Nursing and Midwifery, The Robert Gordon University, Aberdeen, Scotland.

12. Freud S (1917). *Mourning and Melancholia*. London: Hogarth Press.

13. Klein M (1940). Mourning and its relation to manic depressive states. In: Mitcheell J (ed.). *The Selected Melanie Klein*. London: Penguin, 146– 74.

14. Littlewood J (1992). *Aspects of Grief: Bereavement in Adult Life*. London: Routledge.

15. Bowlby J (1969). *Attachment and Loss, Vol. 1. Attachment*. London: The Hogarth Press.

16. Bowlby J (1973). *Attachment and Loss Vol. 2. Separation*. London: The Hogarth Press.

17. Bowlby J (1980). *Attachment and Loss Vol. 3. Loss: Sadness and Depression*. London: The Hogarth Press.

18. Parkes CM (2006). *Love and Loss. The Roots of Grief and its Complications*. Routledge: London.

19. Parkes CM (1996). *Bereavement* (3rd edn). London: Routledge.

20. Parkes CM (1971). Psychosocial transitions: a field for study. *Social Science and Medicine* 5(2): 101–14.

21. Parkes CM (1993). Bereavement as a psychosocial transition: processes of adaptation to change. In: Stroebe MS, Stroebe W and Hansson RO (ed.). *Handbook of Bereavement*. Cambridge: Cambridge University Press, 91– 101.

22. Kubler-Ross E (1969). *On Death and Dying*. New York, Macmillan.

23. Worden JW (1982). *Grief Counselling and Grief Therapy: a Handbook for the Mental Health Practitioner*. New York: Springer.

24. Worden JW (1991). *Grief Counselling and Grief Therapy* (2nd edn). New York: Springer Publishing.

25. Wortman CB and Silver RC (1989). The myths of coping with loss. *Journal of Consulting and Clinical Psychology* 57(3): 349–357.

26. Stroebe M and Schut H (1999). The dual process model of coping with bereavement: rationale and description. *Death Studies* 23: 197–224.

27. Bonanno GA (2004). Loss, trauma and human resilience: have we underestimated the human capacity to thrive after extremely aversive events? *American Psychologist* 59(1), 20–28.

28. Bartlett D (1998). *Stress*. Buckingham: Open University Press.

29. Lazarus RS and Folkman S (1984). *Stress, Appraisal and Coping*. New York: Springer–Verlag.

30. Hockey J (2001). Changing death rituals. In: Hockey J, Katz J and Small N (ed.). *Grief, Mourning and Death Ritual*. Buckingham: Open University Press, 185–211.

31. Klass D, Silverman PR and Nickman SL (1996). *Continuing Bonds*. Philadephia: Taylor and Francis.

32. Walter T (1996). A new model of grief: bereavement and biography. *Mortality* 1(1): 1–29.

33. Payne S, Jarrett N, Wiles R and Field D (2002). Counselling strategies for bereaved people offered in primary care. *Counselling Psychology Quarterly* 15(2): 161–177.

34. Harding R and Higginson I (2003). What is the best way to help caregivers in cancer and palliative care? A systematic literature review of interventions and their effectiveness. *Palliative Medicine* 17(1): 63–74.

35. Ringdal GI, Jordhoy MS, Ringdal K and Kaasa S (2001). The first year of grief and bereavement in close family members to individuals who have died of cancer. *Palliative Medicine* 15: 91–105.

36. Chen JH, Bierhals AJ, Prigerson HG, Kasl V, Mazure CM and Jacobs S (1999) Gender differences in the effects of bereavement–related psychological distress in health outcomes. *Psychological Medicine* 29: 367–380.

37. Stroebe W, Schut H and Stroebe M (2005). Grief work, disclosure and counselling: Do they help the bereaved? *Clinical Psychology Review* 25: 395–414.

38. Arnason A (2001). The skills we need: bereavement counselling and governmentality in England. In: Hockey J Katz and Small N (ed.). *Grief, Mourning and Death Ritual.* Buckingham: Open University Press.

39. Clark D and Seymour J (1999). *Reflections on Palliative Care.* Buckingham: Open University Press.

40. Field D, Reid D, Payne S and Relf M (2004). A national postal survey of adult bereavement support in hospice and specialist palliative care services in the UK. *International Journal of Palliative Nursing* 10(12): 569–576.

41. Field D, Reid D, Payne S and Relf M (2006). Evaluating adult bereavement support services provided by hospices: a comparative perspective on service provision. *International Journal of Palliative Nursing* 12(7): 320–327.

42. Reid D, Payne S, Field D and Relf M (2006). Adult bereavement support in five English hospices: research methods and methodological reflections. *International Journal of Palliative Nursing* 12(9): 430–437.

43. Field D, Payne S, Relf M and Reid D (2007). An overview of adult bereavement support in the United Kingdom: Issues for policy and practice. *Social Science and Medicine* 64(2): 428–438.

44. Payne S, Field D, Rolls L, Kerr C and Hawker S (2007). Evaluating case study methods research for use in end of life care practice: reflections on three studies. *Journal of Advanced Nursing* 58(3): 236–245.

45. Payne S (2001). The role of volunteers in hospice bereavement support in New Zealand. *Palliative Medicine* 15: 107–115.

46. Relf M (1998). Involving volunteers in bereavement counselling. *European Journal of Palliative Care* 5(2): 61–65.

47. Saunders CM (1993). Risk factors in bereavement outcome. In: Stroebe MS, Stroebe W and Hansson RO (ed.). *Handbook of Bereavement.* Cambridge: Cambridge University Press, 255–270.

48. Payne S and Relf M (1994). The assessment of need for bereavement follow–up in palliative and hospice care. *Palliative Medicine* 8: 291–297.

49. Payne S and Lloyd–Williams M (2003). Bereavement care. In: M Lloyd-Williams (ed). *Psychosocial Issues in Palliative Care.* Oxford: Oxford University Press.

50. National Institute for Clinical Excellence (2004). Services for families and carers, including bereavement care. In: *Improving Supportive and Palliative Care for Adults with Cancer. The Manual.* London: National Institute for Clinical Excellence, pp. 155–167.

51. Wiaston's Wish (2002). Key Facts – Children and Bereavement. Handout given at the Childhood Bereavement Network Conference, Birmingham, 28–29 June.

52. Easton C (2001). Child bereavement and children's rights. *Childright* 176: 15–16.

53. Harrington R and Harrison L (2001). Adolescents' bereavement experiences: prevalence, association with depressive symptoms, and use of services. *Journal of Adolescence* 24(2): 159–169.

54. Rolls L and Payne S (2003). Childhood bereavement services: a survey of UK provision. *Palliative Medicine* 17: 423–432.

55. Dyregrov A (1991). *Grief in Children: a Handbook for Adults.* London: Jessica Kingsley.

56. Worden JW (1996). *Children and Grief: When a Patient Dies* (3rd edn). New York: Guildford Publishing.

57. Raveis VH, Siegel K and Karus D (1999). Children's psychological distress following the death of a parent. *Journal of Youth and Adolescence* **28**(2): 165–180.

58. Bertman SI (1991). Children and death: Insights, hindsights and illuminations. In: Papadatou D and Papadatou C (ed.). *Children and Death*. New York: Hemisphere, 311–329.

59. Riches G and Dawson P (2000). *An Intimate Loneliness: Supporting Bereaved Parents and Siblings*. Buckingham: Open University Press.

60. Hindmarch C (1995). Secondary losses for siblings. *Child: Care, Health, and Development* **21**(6): 425–431.

61. Bluebond–Langner M (1989). Worlds of dying children and their well siblings. *Death Studies* **13**: 1–16.

62. Christ G (2000). *Healing Children's Grief: Surviving a Parent's Death from Cancer*. Oxford: Oxford University Press.

63. Rolls L and Payne S (2004). Childhood bereavement services: issues in UK provision. *Mortality* **9**: 4, 300–328.

64. Ribbens McCarthy J (2006). *Young People's Experience of Loss and Bereavement: Towards an Interdisciplinary Approach*. Maidenhead: Open University Press.

65. Rolls L and Payne S (2007). Children and young people's experience of UK childhood bereavement services. *Mortality* **12**(3): 281–303

66. Morgan J D and Laungani P (ed.).(2003). *Death and Bereavement Around the World, Volume 2: Death and Bereavement in the Americas*. Amityville, NY: Baywood Publishing Company.

Chapter 15

The future of family caregiving: research, social policy and clinical practice

Peter Hudson and Sheila Payne

Introduction

The World Health Organization (WHO) states explicitly that palliative care should not only improve the quality of life for patients but also for their families. Services should aim to enhance family members' coping during caregiving and through to bereavement (1). Accordingly, many countries have developed national standards for palliative care provision, which appear to endorse these recommendations (2–4). Some guidelines also advocate that family carers' needs are assessed and addressed separately from the patient's care plan (5).

It has been argued by others that health professionals' priority should be the patient and not family carers, and that health professionals do not have a therapeutic obligation to families (6). We maintain, however, that offering support for family carers should be an integral component of palliative care. This chapter begins by outlining why offering support to family carers is an imperative and introduces a pragmatic vision for the future of family carer support. We offer a conceptual framework to underpin this vision and then provide an overview of the priorities in relation to family carer research, psycho-social care, policy and clinical practice.

Our starting point is that family carers' experiences can only be understood in the context of their dynamic relationships with the ill person and other family members. The interplay of changing patterns of dependency, reciprocity, conflicts, rewards and challenges, love and affection, are both unique to each family and are universal of family life. While these features are rendered commonplace and 'known'—part of our common humanity—the way in which these relationships are played out in each family may be largely unknown to observers.

Why offering support for family carers is important

There are several key reasons why Governments (through policy and provision of resources) and health and social care agencies (through provision of services) should *offer* support to family carers. From the evidence available (7), we know that family carers in many circumstances:

- are profoundly affected by the life-threatening diagnosis of a close relative/friend;
- are responsible for numerous tasks (including symptom management);
- are prone to physical and psychological morbidity;
- are financially disadvantaged;
- have very limited first-hand exposure to death and dying;
- are pivotal to achieving 'successful' home care;
- are often excluded from information and care planning
- become socially isolated;
- commonly report unmet needs (typically aligned with lack of information about the carer role).

For these reasons we advocate the kind of support outlined by the WHO and the national standards of many countries. Illness, and indeed palliative care, is predominantly a family affair (8). Furthermore, the well-being of the patient may be significantly enhanced when their main family carer(s) is well supported (9). This alone makes a very convincing case for offering assistance to family carers.

Rhetoric versus reality

Even though there is a strong argument for supporting family carers in the context of palliative care, the reality does not always match the rhetoric. Palliative care standards, promoted on the websites and in the reports of numerous national palliative care organizations can give the impression that family carer needs are being assessed and evidence-based strategies implemented as normative practice. In the most part, however, there is a large gap between the 'theory' of so-called 'family support' and what actually occurs in every day practice.

Social and policy issues

Central to the philosophy of palliative care is the tenet that the patient and family form 'the unit of care'. It is often assumed, however, that family carers are a homogeneous group of willing contributors. In reality, many carers may not necessarily be undertaking the role by choice; others may not readily fit the ideal of a harmonious 'unit'. In this respect the commonly used term 'loved ones' is best avoided.

Caregiving, therefore, needs to be understood in the context of previous family history, relationships (including conflicts, guilt and dependency) and other social roles. A contemporary Western family structure commonly comprises two or less children nurtured in an adult heterosexual partnership. Increasing evidence suggests that family relationships are also characterized by serial transitions in adult partnerships, step-parenting and other relationship patterns. Health professionals need to be cognisant of the complex range of care provision, including the reciprocal relationships whereby patients provide care to their family members. It is also important to understand family caring within the broader public health approach to palliative care. This approach emphasizes that death is part of life; historically, and in many parts of the world, family members do not have access to formal end-of-life care, neither do they seek it.

While we endorse the practice of health professionals offering to assist family carers, we do not subscribe to the 'pathologization of the family carer role'. By this we mean the portrayal of family caregiving as an inherently burdensome experience predisposing carers to a variety of negative and distressing psychological and social outcomes. Unfortunately, the literature in many circumstances (sometimes based on less than optimal data sources) seems to support this view. Other research indicates that the overwhelming majority of family carers will not develop clinically significant depression, anxiety or traumatic grief. In fact, based on best available evidence, rates of these syndromes are not excessive (10). Attempting to identify those carers 'at risk' of negative outcomes and being able to offer them appropriate supports is, however, important (11).

While there has been an increase in policy initiatives related to family carers, the gap between theory and practice needs to be analysed more closely. As we have already highlighted (and will demonstrate further), it appears that services may not be equipped to meet carers' needs. They may lack the resources to undertake the assessment and the suitable strategies to respond. Furthermore, supports for family carers are inadequate and in many countries the rhetoric of 'choice' is being advocated while in reality there are often few desirable or equivalent options available. Many health and social care professionals are not adequately trained in palliative care, funding for services is limited and support for family carers may not be given high priority (12).

It would seem self-evident that policy for carers would include appropriate financial resources. In some developed countries, recent statutory policies have tended to promote home-based care near the end of life. Dying at home is being advocated, even where there have been marked declines in the home death rate for many decades, such as in the United Kingdom where home deaths account for approximately 20 per cent of all deaths. Clearly more needs to be done, as the financial burden placed on family carers who support a dying relative can be onerous (7, 13).

From a social and public health perspective, the family may not be viewed as a care recipient or healthcare consumer. There seems to be a paradox here; at another level family members are, in reality, construed as recipients of health and social care (e.g. via social policies mandating needs assessments) alongside 'the patient' or indeed as 'co-workers' alongside health professionals. Referring to family members as 'carers' (a term that family members themselves may not identify with) may then influence the way families of palliative care patients are viewed in day-to-day end-of-life care. We now examine this further as we focus on the reality and rhetoric of family caregiving in the clinical practice arena.

Clinical practice issues

The mantra of palliative care is that it is 'family centred' and the 'unit of care' is core to all its functions. Hence, perhaps by default, family carers (or family care-givers—the terms common to clinical parlance) are construed as part of the healthcare system, being regarded as care recipients. Some have argued that family carers have needs equal to, and/or greater than, the needs of patients, (see Monroe and Oliviere chapter in this volume). It is often assumed that family carers want their needs assessed and supportive interventions to be offered; however, this may not necessarily be the case. Unfortunately, for family carers who choose to have their needs assessed, the evidence barely supports the claim that palliative care services provide them with effective support (14).

Anecdotal evidence suggests it is not uncommon for patients who are dying at home, under the care of a 'specialist' palliative care service, to routinely not be visited when the death occurs. We are aware that some families may prefer to be alone during this time but a firm offer of a health professional visit should be made. We are also discouraged by stories of lack of resources (in countries with seemingly well-developed economies) to provide optimal 24-hour a day, 7 days a week access to specialist palliative care advice (13, 15, 16). As this is one of the hallmarks of palliative care, originating in the late 1960s, it is a major concern that this core function is so often lacking, with potentially very serious implications for vulnerable family carers.

An additional sobering fact is that in many countries with well-established palliative care networks and services, more than half of those expected to die will not be seen by specialist palliative care services and, typically, it is the minority cultural groups who miss out (17, 18). So, in reality much of the death and dying occurs in general medical/surgical wards in hospitals and in care homes for older people in the community. One wonders, therefore, whether or not this workforce is equipped to provide effective family-centred care. For example, in 2001, the British Government invested in a 3-year initiative to improve general palliative care education for community (district) nurses. An evaluation of the initiative indicated that one-third of all district nurses participated in additional education, and that local evaluations indicated increases in their knowledge (19) but overall there was no reduction in institutional deaths. Policy initiatives need to have a balance between a focus on specialist palliative care and general care to ensure maximum access to better end-of-life care (18).

Furthermore, while many definitions of palliative care espouse care from the time of diagnosis of a life-threatening illness, typically specialist care is only provided in the last phase of the patient's life and predominantly to those with cancer. There is, however, some evidence to show some changes in this area (see Chapters 10 and 13, in this volume). The question remains: how much support is actually provided to family carers from the outset, and who coordinates the care? Deficiencies in coordination of care are exemplified by this reflection from a family carer: 'The doctors and nurses don't seem to communicate properly to one another. I'm not sure who's in control of my wife's care' (20). Moreover, once in the 'specialist palliative care system', support for family carers is often crisis-driven and reactive, rather than following a comprehensive plan of care based on carefully assessed need. Once again the rhetoric versus reality gap is wide.

Family carers may also be viewed as 'co-workers' in the clinical setting. It is not uncommon for them to be referred to as 'part of the team' and to be given tasks that they sometimes may not be willing and/or equipped to undertake. In many situations this role may be quite appropriate; that is, family carers may welcome the opportunity to contribute to the direct care of their relative. However, it is not appropriate when carers neither have the desire or the skills to take on this role, as shown by the following comment: 'I was a bit surprised at the autonomy that was given to me by the nursing staff. To be responsible for the dosage of morphine and that sort of thing. I kept panicking and thinking about it.' (21).

Another commonplace scenario in the specialist palliative care clinical setting is that health professionals focus attention on the primary family carer and not the entire family. The reasons for this are pragmatic: many health and social care services may not be suitably resourced to try and meet the needs of the whole family. Furthermore, given the limited length of time that specialist palliative care is provided, even with comprehensive resources, it may simply be too difficult in some instances to coordinate a supportive care plan for the whole family. However, this may fail to adequately acknowledge the reality of difficult family dynamics; for example, where there are ex-partners, stepchildren or 'hidden' relationships. In such situations, a single named 'carer' is unlikely to adequately communicate information throughout the family or be in a position to 'represent' the collective view of the family.

In the reality of the clinical arena, family carers often want time alone (i.e. away from their dying relative/friend) with the health professional to discuss their issues and seek information. In the context of home-based palliative care these are referred to as 'letter box consultations', whereby the nurse (for example) conducts an assessment of needs in the home with the patient and family carer(s) together. Then, following farewells at the door, the family carer says something like: '… I'll just follow you out and check if the mail has arrived'. In the privacy of the outdoors (away from earshot of the patient) the family carer then proceeds to outline the concerns they did not feel comfortable raising in front of the patient. Typically, this discomfort arises from the carers' assumption that if the patient knows they are overwhelmed and burdened, then this will have a negative effect on the patient's well-being. In reality, therefore, the extra time required for family support can be significant and may increase substantially when more family carers are involved.

Healthcare professionals may not be sufficiently prepared for the complexities of family centred care. For example, nurses (the professional group typically with the most contact with palliative care families) report that 'family work' is often draining and challenging. Furthermore, they may lack the education and training (common to other disciplines such as psychology and social work) required to assess and respond to family needs. If palliative care is to have a family focus, then the professionals directly involved require appropriate training and resources (22, 23).

The rhetoric of family centred care is further called into question, as it is typically 'the patient' who is the focus of care. Parkes asserts that palliative care in recent years has perhaps focused too much on the patient's symptoms and suggests that this has detracted attention from Cicely Saunders' original intention—that the unit of care is not the patient but the family, which, of course, includes the patient (24). As Ashby and Mendelson have argued (in Chapter 6), supported by others such as Randall and Downie (6), in the eyes of the law and from a healthcare obligation perspective it is 'the patient' who is the priority and whose decisions should be adhered to. It is typically 'the patient' who consents to receive specialist palliative care and any associated interventions. This poses a dilemma for health and social care workers, particularly when the needs of the patient and family are incongruent (e.g. site of care decisions, discussions of prognosis). On the one hand, health professionals are to take a family centred approach, yet from a therapeutic and legal stance their primary obligation is to the patient.

Related to this issue is the lack of clarity about terms such as 'support' and 'quality of life', which are commonly seen as endpoints of effective care for family carers. The question remains, however, as to whether and how often these outcomes are evaluated in practice and whether they can, in fact, be accurately measured (6).

Research issues

Although family support has been advocated since the inception of the modern hospice movement, the reality is there are serious shortages in evidence-based strategies to assess and respond to family carer needs. Previous chapters in this volume (see Chapters 9, 12 and 13) have supported the findings of systematic reviews demonstrating significant gaps in evidence-based approaches to support family carers (25–27).

There are also considerable gaps in other areas related to family carer research. We outline these in more detail later in the chapter and recommend some strategies for overcoming key challenges. One issue that may not be readily rectified, however, is the limited funding for palliative care research. While on the one hand the rhetoric of 'evidenced-based palliative care' is dominant, the reality is palliative care research is significantly under-funded (17). The National Cancer Institute in the USA, for example, was reported to have spent less than 1 per cent of its budget on palliative care (28).

Toward a renewed vision of family carers and palliative care

A current evaluation of the global palliative care scene (29) reveals that:

- there is large variation in the provision of palliative care;
- it is not available to most patients who need it;
- it is not fully accepted by many medical professionals;
- it is not a core element of many national healthcare initiatives;
- the need for palliative care is increasing.

We have argued that there are significant social, policy and research gaps between the way family support is commonly portrayed and the everyday lived experience of families involved in end-of-life care. So what is the way forward? We advocate a vision of family carer support that is heavily informed by sociological perspectives in order to provide clinical services with a foundation, not only for their continued development but also for their involvement with policy and research. A better fit between healthcare policy in palliative care and family carers is needed (17). We believe it is worthless to promote an either/or approach, whereby a social model of family caregiving is advocated as more beneficial than a clinical/medical model or vice versa. Both approaches have their shortcomings, yet both are integral to shaping the way families are supported in palliative care.

The first step on the way forward is to provide a working definition of family carer. We define a palliative family carer (adapted from (23)) as:

> ... any relative, friend or partner who has a significant personal relationship and provides assistance (physical, social, and/or psychological) to a person with a life-threatening illness. These individuals may be primary or secondary carers and may or may not reside with the person receiving care.

What do we mean by family carer support? There are varying definitions and types of support; however, in the context of family carers and palliative care we define it thus:

> Support for family carers who are assisting a relative/friend requiring palliative care may incorporate practical, educational, psychological, spiritual, financial or social strategies (based on unmet needs and a desire by the caregiver(s) for assistance) with the intention of enhancing the caregiver's capacity to undertake their role, respond to its challenges and maintain their own health (including the bereavement period).

What then is the relationship between health and social care professionals and family carers in the context of palliative care? We believe health professionals have a clear responsibility toward family carers (who desire assistance) and that this should be a much more focused role than the notion of a 'professional friend' (6), which seems somewhat nebulous. Nor do we agree with the view of the family carer as 'co-worker' or 'part of the care team' (23).

We encourage an approach in clinical practice that views the patient and family carers as equals. We acknowledge, however, that in certain circumstances the patient has rights over and above family carers; for example, choices about treatments and about who receives medical information and who can make medical decisions on their behalf. If family carers' needs continue to be viewed as secondary to those of the patient, then resources, policy initiatives and research for family carers will be viewed as secondary and given a lower priority. This may also have implications for patients, based on the premise that lack of support for family may have negative implications for patients.

Realistic objectives are needed to support family carers. We concur with Randall and Downie (6) that it may indeed be quite untenable for health and social care professionals to improve family carers' quality of life (as promoted by the WHO). In addition, given the typically short time-frame that specialist palliative care professionals are directly involved with family carers, it would seem quite impracticable to set such unachievable goals.

In the context of clinical care, it is essential that care-planning decisions (e.g. discussions of prognosis, site of care options) are made in partnership with the family carer(s). Exceptions would pertain where the patient is unable or unwilling to make their own decisions or when, in extremely rare situations, the patient makes it quite evident that family members are not to be involved at all.

Where resources are not sufficient to support the needs of the entire family as well as the patient, care should be directed toward one or two persons who the patient perceives to be their most important lay support people. This could be a family member, partner or friend. This is not to say that others ought to be excluded; ideally, with the primary carer's permission, they could act as the information sharer with other members of the family and involve them in key decisions, as appropriate, taking on the role of family spokesperson.

We acknowledge that this may not work in all cases; for example, some families are disenfranchized and others experience significant conflict (30). In such cases palliative care services should do what they can to assist in matters related directly to end-of-life care. In our judgment it is not reasonable (unless suitable resources exist) to expect palliative care services to try and reconcile family differences, or to resolve conflict that may have existed for decades. This is not to ignore the need for referral to generic counselling services in some instances; however, unless there is a major injection of funding, therapeutically oriented general family counselling should not be the core function of palliative care services, whose priorities lie elsewhere.

Palliative care health professionals do, however, need to understand how caring behaviours are played out in the complex patterns of various kin and non-kin relationships. While research has investigated carers' experiences of burden, less research attention has been directed to patients' perception of themselves as 'burdensome' (31). Alertness is also needed for those situations where the dying experience causes conflict and where family carers may need referral to other services for specific therapeutic assistance.

However, in contrast to the view that many carers are unable to manage their role appropriately, it appears that the majority of carers, both during the carer experience and into bereavement, actually fulfil their role well. This is not to discount the fact that carers will need to know the role will be challenging and at times extremely difficult. Many will, however, identify some specific and positive consequences associated with the role (20). This does not mean that most carers do not need support. On the contrary, they should be offered support that is targeted in a way that will help sustain them in their role; provided, of course, the role is not becoming unduly onerous and they express a desire to continue.

A public health approach for families is also warranted so that death and dying can be viewed once again as a part of life (rather than, for example, as a medical failure) and the term palliative care be more widely understood. Increased public exposure about palliative care should then translate to increased confidence for families, so that when they are confronted with the impending death of a relative, and if they choose to access support, they will be familiar with the kind of resources available to them.

What follows is an overview of how this vision may be implemented. This incorporates a conceptual framework, followed by recommendations in the areas of social policy, research and clinical practice.

A conceptual framework for carer support

All strategic health and social care initiatives require a suitable framework. We acknowledge some tensions between social approaches and those that take a predominantly psychological perspective. There are merits and disadvantages in both. The transactional model of stress and coping (32) offers a potentially useful theoretical basis for understanding the carer experience and designing interventions. The applicability of this model for palliative care and family carers has been comprehensively described elsewhere (33). The model can be summarized thus:

> The diversity of responses related to end-of-life issues from patient and family carers can be understood from a psychological perspective based on a transactional model of coping in which carers make cognitive appraisals to determine the possible impact of a potentially stressful event (32, 33). The carer's perception of mastery or self-efficacy, or the greater the number of resources at their disposal to manage an event, the more likely the individual will demonstrate their ability to adapt to the situation. In this way, family caregiving need not necessarily be seen as stressful; it can vary, depending upon the person's internal cognitive appraisals and their resources for coping. Such resources include feelings of preparedness, competence, having sufficient social support, adequate information and focusing on positive aspects of the role. Indeed, the inclusion of the positive experiences, despite the often extraordinary challenges faced by carers of patients with life-threatening illness, was a major reason for reworking the original framework (34).

While the model has some shortcomings because it focuses primarily on individual coping and perhaps does not adequately address the social context in which caregiving is enacted, it continues to be endorsed (35). We believe it is a suitable theoretical framework to guide understanding of the carer experience and to assist in the development of strategies to enhance support.

A social agenda for family carers

An alternative approach to a psychological model has been advocated within the wider literature on family carers, and proposes a new social contract (36). Carers are seen as citizens with rights and responsibilities; this raises important challenges for public policy, the economy and the wider social fabric. Rather than concentrating on the individual carer's cognitions, 'coping' abilities (often task centred) or perceived vulnerabilities, this construal of caregiving sees interventions in terms of individual 'support needs'. These might be for additional education or information, or strategies, such as complementary therapies, to help them relax and deal with distress. While these interventions may have inherent value, we argue from a social perspective that (at least) three other considerations are needed.

First, carers need to be protected from health and social care systems that actually increase rather than lessen the burden of caregiving. For example, poor communication, lack of information, inflexible healthcare appointments (often at different hospital clinics and requiring repeated time off work), slow response to request for services, all add to the frustration of being a carer. To counteract some of these burdens, periods of respite might be found in physical rest, social interaction, education, recreation or employment outside the home (37).

Second, carers' economic and financial security is not always given the priority it deserves. Such security may be derived from flexible arrangements to continue work or to reduce work commitments and hours; together with protection of career progression and pension rights. Few researchers have investigated the impact of end-of-life care on carers' employment or incomes (38).

Third, carers' social inclusion requires increased attention. Evidence suggests that carers are often marginalized and social isolated. Their role within the home of a dying person can prevent their own particular voice being heard; for example, their opinion may be sought on service provision merely from the perspective of the patient's proxy. Increased policy recognition of carers' rights, and processes to involve them in major health and social care changes, are some of the means by which carers can make their contributions as citizens.

A research agenda for family carers

Challenges and strategies for improving family carer research

The challenges of palliative care research (including research with family carers) are well documented. However, there is also a significant amount of literature suggesting ways of overcoming some of these hurdles (39–49), and a number of books on strategies for palliative care research are emerging (50). While the debate about the place of evidence-based practice in palliative care continues (51), we maintain that more family carer studies are urgently required (ideally through a priority-based approach). The evidence base can be improved through rigorous research, despite the methodological challenges (many of which plague other areas of health and social care research). Rather than being dissuaded by a perception that 'research in palliative care is too difficult', we believe it is time to move forward. Palliative care research is not easy; however, it can be undertaken effectively through teamwork, modifying methods and the provision of adequate resources and funds. Nonetheless, there are some research issues that are specific to family carers within the context of palliative care. These issues are now outlined alongside recommendations for how these challenges might be met.

Recruiting family carers to research studies

Despite the notion of a family centred approach to palliative care, direct access to the primary family carer or next of kin is often compromised. It is not uncommon for ethics committees to demand that the patient is recruited to the study first and the patient's approval then sought for access to the carer. This can negatively influence the time taken for recruitment; it requires additional resources and in many instances the patient may be too unwell to consent. Furthermore, it lends credence to the commonly held view that, rather than being considered on equal terms, the carer is regarded as an appendage to the patient.

An approach we have used, with the approval of ethics committees, is to send a letter from the clinical director of the palliative care service to the primary family carer/next of kin (49). The letter outlines that the palliative care service is conducting an ethically approved study and that they (the carer) may be contacted by a researcher who would explain the study in more detail and potentially invite them to take part. The letter also emphasizes that the carer can choose not to be contacted or not to take part and this will not affect the care provided to them or their relative. This approach has not had any detrimental effects and very few carers have declined being approached by a researcher. Thus far, this strategy has aided recruitment but we acknowledge it is a long way from solving the problem.

Gate-keeping

A related issue that compromises recruitment is gate-keeping. Gate-keeping is the process by which people are inhibited by others in their capacity to be invited into a research project or make an informed decision regarding research participation (49). Health professionals who practice gate-keeping in relation to family carer recruitment often do so based upon a desire to 'protect' the family carer from becoming overburdened. The health professional may deliberately limit and/or influence a carer's opportunity to make an informed decision regarding research participation by either not advising them of the research project or suggesting that they are already too overburdened to consider participation.

Patients may also preclude a family member from making an informed choice about research participation for similar reasons. For example, the patient may deny the researcher access to a family member because they wish to protect the family member or be unwilling to impose further burden on them. The patient may also feel uncomfortable involving the family for other reasons; for example, the belief that the patient rather than the family should be the primary research focus (49).

Are palliative care recipients more vulnerable than other groups participating in research? While the debate continues, there is no legitimate argument precluding the application of standard ethical principles and guidelines in palliative care research (39, 52). Family carers of people with a life-threatening illness are self-directed individuals and, unless shown to the contrary, can decide for themselves whether or not they wish to participate in research (53). Furthermore, studying family issues in palliative care is a priority and excluding participants through paternalistic protectionism has had the paradoxical effect of limiting progress in evidence-based palliative care and intruding upon the rights of people to voluntarily contribute to research (52).

The impact of gate-keeping predominantly occurs in two key areas: restriction of autonomy and reduction of research quality (49). Restriction of autonomy arises when family carers are denied their right to informed choice regarding research participation (54, 55). Carers are, therefore, deprived of a valuable opportunity to reflect on their relative's illness, and a potential sense of satisfaction in their ability to add to the body of knowledge regarding their care (56). Research quality is reduced when gate-keeping causes selection bias, restricting the representativeness of the sample and therefore the generalizability of the findings (49). Several strategies for limiting gate-keeping are comprehensively outlined elsewhere (49).

Short intervention time

A priority area for inquiry related to family carers is intervention research. However, given the short length of time that people typically receive palliative care, intervention research is difficult. For example, the average length of stay in an Australian palliative care unit/hospice is approximately 2 to 3 weeks and in home-based care, approximately 14 weeks. This makes it extremely difficult to design studies that are applicable to practice, allow for recruitment, data collection and administration of the intervention. Despite these challenges, carefully designed studies (including randomised controlled trials) with carers can be undertaken (57, 58). We advocate the framework for complex interventions promoted by the United Kingdom's Medical Research Council (59).

Limited number of active family carer researchers and funding

The development of research networks to identify gaps in research areas, build capacity and translate the findings into day-to-day clinical practice, are considered to be a priority (60). Given the seemingly small number of researchers who are focusing on family carers, a recent collaborative initiative may prove a valuable model. The International Palliative Care Family Caregiver Research Collaboration (IPCFRC) was recently established with the aim of developing a more strategic approach to family carer research, production of resources and information sharing (61).

Bereavement research

The need for more bereavement research, specifically in palliative care contexts, is evident so that assessment of poor psychosocial outcomes is enhanced and the evidence base for strategies to lessen adverse outcomes are realized. It seems that, in order to accurately identify bereaved carers who are confronted with complicated grief, then at least 6 months should have passed since their relative's death (10). This means that tracking carers over time may be potentially difficult. For example, the carer may move house or may not have been residing with the patient in the first place.

We recommend recruiting family carers prior to the death of their relative/friend and, with their permission, taking their full contact details, including mobile phone and email address (if possible). Furthermore, prior to contacting the carer for the bereavement phase data collection (e.g. mail out questionnaire), we advocate phoning them to remind them of the study and to confirm their postal address.

Ethical obligations

Ethical issues can arise when administering psychological measurement instruments to family carers recruited to research studies (particularly in the home based setting). If carers score above the threshold on a self-report screening instrument for possible anxiety or depression in a bereavement study, for example, then what are the research team obliged to do? One could argue that they should contact the carer and advise them of this and suggest they contact their doctor to explore their psychological well-being in further detail. However, we contend that the benefit may outweigh the cost: screening instruments are not diagnostic and there is a significant chance of a false-positive; also the family carer may perceive this situation to be more than it actually is; that is, no matter how well explained, the carer may perceive that they have been assessed as being anxious and/or depressed. Alternatively, we suggest that at each data collection point the carer is advised verbally and in writing that, if they are feeling emotionally burdened, they should liaise with their health provider. This approach would of course need to be included in any ethics approval proposal.

Outcome measures

Another research issue related to family carers has been the limited number of psychometrically sound instruments available. It would seem that this situation is changing. The instruments outlined in Table 15.1, an extension of our earlier work (62), are a sample (not a definitive collection) of family carer measures, which have undergone some level of psychometric testing in palliative care populations. While there have been some collective validity and reliability reviews of family carer instruments (63, 64), it would be advantageous to have an overall critical review undertaken of family carer instruments used in palliative care and to make some recommendations to guide future work. It seems that there have been instruments developed to measure a variety of carer-related domains. If these instruments can be demonstrated to have adequate psychometric properties, perhaps there is not an urgency to develop new instruments. Further validation, particularly in different cultures and settings, would be valuable. However, what remains elusive is an instrument (or two) that can be readily used as primary outcome measures for family carers: in the same way that there are some commonly used primary outcome measures for patients. Having some consensus on primary instruments would allow for more meaningful comparisons between studies and perhaps internationally. There also needs to be more work done on identifying suitable instruments to screen family carers on entry to palliative care for risk of significant negative psychosocial well-being (11). This task is not easy given the need to specify (1) the degree of acceptable risk, and (2) negative psychosocial well-being.

Priority areas for family carer research

We concur with others that while there is still room for more 'needs-based' family carer research, intervention studies are a priority (25). It is encouraging that carer

Table 15.1 Examples of instruments used in palliative care family carer research

Instrument	References
Family inventory of needs scale	(65)
Preparedness for caregiving scale	(63, 66)
Caregiver competence scale	(63, 67)
Rewards of caregiving scale	(66)
Social support questionnaire	(63, 68)
Caregiver self-efficacy	(63, 69)
Caregiver reaction assessment	(63, 70)
Life orientation test	(63, 71)
Caregiver mutuality instrument	(63, 66)
FAMCARE-satisfaction	(72)
After death bereaved family interview	(73)
Inventory of traumatic grief	(74)
Modified Parkes'(1993)Bereavement Risk Index	(75)
Caregiving at life's End questionnaire	(76)
Quality of dying and death	(77)
Family strain questionnaire	(78)
Family assessment of treatment at end of life	(79)
Quality of Life in Life threatening illness- Family carer version	(80)
Brief assessment scale for caregivers of the medically ill	(81)
Family appraisal of caregiving questionnaire	(82)

The references listed refer to the author of the instrument and, where pertinent, an additional reference that reports additional reliability and validity data.

intervention studies are emerging, such as those targeting carer involvement in the reduction of patient symptoms (83) and patient depression (84); those aimed at reducing emotional distress in the carer (58); and increasing carers' comfort with their role (85). There also seems to be a strong foundation in psycho-educational studies focused on preparing family carers for their role (57, 86, 87).

However, there is still much to be done. The evidence base for some commonly used approaches to support family carers; for example, the use of family meetings and respite care, is lacking. Some interventions have been accepted as desirable for implementation in practice; however, they are commonly based on the findings of a single study and the applicability and cost of the intervention are often not measured. This does little to assist clinical services and policy advisors in implementing appropriate strategies. Ideally, in the near future, a suite of evidence-based interventions (whereby utility has also been checked) can be made available for those family carers who express a desire to access these types of services.

Based on the work presented in preceding chapters of this volume, together with recent literature reviews (14, 25), the following topics indicate areas that require further exploration in order to advance the body of knowledge related to family carers. We acknowledge that a more sophisticated and systematic approach to prioritize family carer research would be desirable.

- The experience of care giving.
  - Accounts of the psychosocial impact of caring.
  - Longitudinal studies (including studies conducted earlier in the patient's disease trajectory) of the caregiving experience.
  - The effect on family carers of the site/context of the patient's death (e.g. comparing negative/positive implications of death at home compared with death in hospital, hospice, aged care home, etc.).
  - The prevalence of family carers' wish for the patient's hastened death (e.g. in order to relieve their own, or the patient's suffering).
  - Reliable and valid means to assess family carers' satisfaction with service delivery.
  - The impact of migration and economic mobility.
  - The impact of 'fractured' families (e.g. by war, economic hardship, serial marriage, etc.).
  - Family 'resilience'.
- Specific groups of carers.
  - The impact and needs of younger and older carers.
  - The impact and needs of immigrant carers.
  - The impact and needs of carers not receiving 'specialist' palliative care.
- Development of assessment tools.
  - Validation of outcome measurement tools in palliative care setting.
  - Predictors of risk of poor psychological functioning.
  - Strategies to assess carer risk and need.
- Designing and evaluating interventions.
  - The efficacy of family meetings.
  - Meeting the needs of the entire family, or discerning who is 'worthy' of professionals' support.

- Intervention studies focused on preparing carers for their role.
- Strategies to reduce the negative psychosocial outcomes in those assessed as 'at risk'.
- Resources needed to support vulnerable population of carers e.g. older people.
- Supportive interventions for rural areas (e.g. telephone/video-conferencing based approaches).
- Cost-effectiveness of common family carer interventions.
- The efficacy of bereavement support programmes.
- Role of web-based educational and supportive interventions.
- Forecasting the role of Intelligent Technology.
- Identifying the educational initiatives required to teach health professionals how to support families.
- Care-planning strategies and their impact on carers and patient outcomes.
- Interventions that target the needs of patient and carer together.
- Impact of family carer policy on research and vice versa.
- Utility of interventions—accessibility, availability and affordability.
- Effective means of communication between carers and health professionals.
- Replication studies.

A clinical practice agenda for family carers

Carers have expressed their need for the following: education and information to prepare them for their role; guidance in terms of what to expect (for example, when their relative is approaching death); how to respond to the challenges (physical, social and psychological) of the role; and how to access resources (internal and external) to assist them to maintain optimal health (7, 88). These domains are commensurate with the 'good death' literature describing what most family carers seem to value in terms of an optimal end-of-life experience. Families expect that their relative's symptoms should be controlled, that they will receive emotional, social and spiritual support, that treatment decisions will be respected, that they will have access to respite care and bereavement support, and that preference for site of death will be upheld (89, 90).

We maintain, however, that this support should be targeted, time-limited, evaluated regularly and based upon best available evidence. For example, we agree that ongoing formal bereavement support may not be required by all family carers; rather, it must be based on need and justify prudent use of resources (6).

The common challenges for healthcare professionals providing family centred care have been comprehensively described elsewhere (22) and other issues have been identified earlier in this chapter. We now outline some recommendations and principles to guide health professionals in overcoming some of these challenges. We acknowledge that in circumstances where it is difficult to identify a family carer, or where there is conflict within families, then additional resources and strategies will need to be incorporated. Clinical practice guidelines for responding to conflict and incongruent needs between the patient and family have been addressed by others (91).

Recommendations for a family carer oriented approach to clinical practice

Setting up support for family carers

◆ Explain to the palliative care patient that the role of palliative care is to support the patient but also to offer support for family carers.

◆ Determine from the palliative care patient who they perceive to be their most important support person(s), i.e. their primary family carer (which could be family member, partner or friend). Complete a genogram as part of this process.

◆ Discuss with the patient their preferences for the involvement of the family carers in medical and care-planning discussions and note this in the medical record.

◆ Confirm with the primary family carer (PFC) that they understand their relative/friend has identified them for this role. Explain the meaning of 'family carer' (as some relatives/friends may not identify with this term).

◆ Explain to the PFC what services and resources (e.g. respite, financial support, practical support and information) can and cannot be provided, so that realistic expectations are established.

◆ Obtain permission from the PFC to be the key contact for the palliative care service and to assist where pertinent in care planning decisions.

◆ Seek willingness and capacity for the PFC to liaise (e.g. as spokesperson) with other family members (with the patient's permission) about updates on medical status and care planning matters.

Assessing need and establishing a plan of care

◆ Ascertain the PFC's understanding of the patient's prognosis and goals of care.

- Offer the PFC a needs assessment and screen for risk (including potential for complex/prolonged grief risk).
- Respond to needs using best available evidence-based approaches. Note and advise carer that it may not be possible to meet all needs due to limited resources and the longstanding nature of some issues.
- Offer to meet with the patient and PFC to discuss goals of care, site of care and other key care-planning matters, including process for regular review.
- If desired by the PFC, prepare them for the typical role of supporting a dying person, the potential impact of the role (including positive aspects) and strategies to optimise their own well being.
- Develop a care plan for the patient and PFG that is regularly reviewed in consultation with the patient and PFC'.

Bereavement support

- If death at home occurs (or is imminent) and resources permit, offer a home visit by the nurse (for example) to provide guidance and support.
- Contact the PFC within a few days of the patient's death to offer condolences and to check whether further advice and/or support are needed.
- Offer bereavement support in keeping with best available evidence and resources.

Conclusion

In this chapter, we have reflected on the social position of family carers, predominantly from a developed-world perspective. We have presented a potentially useful psychological model derived from the stress and coping literature. We have evaluated the role clinical services may play with family carers and established some research priorities. In addition, we have high-lighted the implications of a more socially inclusive perspective to understanding the position and needs of carers as citizens. No one position is adequate, instead we advocate that readers need to work at multiple levels to improve the welfare of carers; for example, by engaging with Governments, employers and politicians to highlight the 'hidden' work of carers, to mobilize resources within the community to establish in-home and institutional respite schemes, and to improve the flexibility of medical clinics to accommodate palliative care patients and their families. This may require new ways of working, an ability to engage with national and local policy makers, trade unions, industry chiefs and other stakeholders outside the normal comfort-zone of health and social care workers. The greatest benefit for carers might be from changes to fiscal policy, such as tax credits for caregiving or enhanced pension rights. Of course, most attention has been placed on direct 'support' services to carers, and we still have much to learn about what types of support are of most benefit to which carers and when. These are important research questions. We see the need for improved information, training and brokerage services for carers, so they are empowered to take greater control of their situation and utilize those services that are already available within their local communities, and to make effective choices about when, and if, to take up offers of help.

We have also used this chapter to refer to content elsewhere in this volume in order to support some of our claims. Finally, based on the contents of this and preceding chapters, we draw the conclusion that from the data available (albeit limited in several areas) similarities are emerging between the experiences of family carers across care settings and disease groups. This means that there may be ways of supporting carers that have generic application. We do not condone a prescriptive, 'one size fits all' approach: there will always be the need for individual variation. However, given the serious shortfall in family carer support, the development of research-based approaches that can be modified for specific carer groups or settings seems wise. The situation is urgent, without improvements in social policy, research and clinical service delivery 'family centred care' will remain merely perfunctory and therefore rendered irrelevant.

Key learning points

- Support for family carers is a core function of palliative care.
- Most family carers will be able to recognize positive aspects of their role; however, some family carers will experience poor psychological, financial and social outcomes.
- There is a large gap between the rhetoric of family centred palliative care and what actually occurs in practice: many family carers are unable to access suitable supports, social policies are commonly inadequate and limited research has been undertaken.
- There are some similarities between the experiences and needs of family carers between disease groups and across settings.
- In order to enhance family centred care, a combined approach that incorporates improved social policy, research and service delivery is required.

Recommended reading and resources

Advanced care planning initiative: www.respectingpatientchoices.org.au/

Clayton JM, Hancock KM, Butow PN, Tattersall MHN and Currow DC (2007). Clinical practice guidelines for communicating prognosis and end-of-life issues with adults in the advanced stages of a life-limiting illness, and their caregivers. *Medical Journal of Australia* 186(12): S77–S108.

Family Caregiver Alliance (2006). *Caregiver Assessment: Principles, Guidelines and Strategies for Change*. Report from a National Consensus Development Conference (Vol 1). San Francisco.

Girgis A, Johnson C, Currow D, Waller A, Kristjanson LJ, Mitchell G *et al.* (2006). *Palliative Care Needs Assessment Guidelines*. Newcastle, NSW: The Centre for Health Research & Psycho-oncology.

Instruments related to family carers. www.chcr.brown.edu/pcoc/toolkit.htm

International Palliative Care Family Caregiver Research Collaboration. http://www.ipcfrc.unimelb.edu.au/

Overview of evidence based interventions for family carers www.rosalyncarter.org/dynamic_grid/

References

1. World Health Organization (2002). *National Cancer Control Programmes: Policies and Managerial Guidelines* (2nd edn). Geneva: WHO.

2. Ferrell B, Connor SR, Cordes A, Dahlin CM, Fine PG, Hutton N, Leenay M, Lentz J, Person JL, Meir DE and Zuroski K (2007). The national agenda for quality palliative care: the National Consensus Project and the National Quality Forum. *Journal of Pain and Symptom Management* 33(6): 737–744.

3. National Institutes of Health (2004). *National Institutes of Health State-of-the-Science Conference Statement: Improving End of Life Care*. Conference report: http://consensus.nih.gov/2004/2004EndOflifeCare SOS 24main.htm(accessed 15 July 2008).

4. Palliative Care Australia (2005). *Standards for Providing Quality Palliative Care for all Australians*. Canberra, Australia: Palliative Care Australia.

5. National Institute for Clinical Excellence (2004). *Guidance on Cancer Services: Improving Supportive and Palliative Care for Adults with Cancer. The Manual*. London: National Institute for Clinical Excellence.

6. Randall F and Downie RS (2006). *Relatives. The Philosophy of Palliative Care—Critique and Reconstruction*. Oxford: Oxford University Press, 75–96.

7. Girgis A, Johnson C, Currow D, Waller A, Kristjanson LJ, Mitchell G, Yates P, Neil A, Kelly B, Tattersall M and Bowman D (2006). *Palliative Care Needs Assessment Guidelines*. Newcastle, NSW: The Centre for Health Research & Psycho-oncology.

8. Wright LM, Watson WL and Bell JM (1996). *Beliefs: the Heart of Healing in Families and Illness*. New York: Basic Books.

9. Mularski RA, Rosefeld K, Coons SJ, Dueck A, Cella D, Feuer DJ, Lipscomb J, Karpeh MS, Mosich T, Sloan JA and Krouse RS (2007). Measuring outcomes in randomized prospective trials in palliative care. *Journal of Pain and Symptom Management* 34(1S): S7–S19.

10. Zhang B, El-Jawahri A and Prigerson HG (2006). Update on bereavement research: evidence-based guidelines for the diagnosis and treatment of complicated bereavement. *Journal of Palliative Medicine* **9**(5): 1188–1203.

11. Hudson P, Hayman-White K, Aranda S and Kristjanson L (2006). Predicting family caregiver psychosocial functioning in palliative care: a pilot study. *Palliative Medicine* **20**(3): 266.

12. Help the Hospices (2007). *The End of Life Care Strategy for England: How the Government Could Change the Way We Die*. London: Help the Hospices.

13. McLaughlin D, Sullivan K and Hasson F (2007). Hospice at home service: the carer's perspective. *Supportive in Cancer Care* **15**(2): 163–170.

14. Harding R (2005). Carers: current research and developments. In: Firth P, Luff G and Oliviere D (ed.). *Facing Death: Loss, Change and Bereavement in Palliative Care* (1st edn). Berkshire: Open University Press, 150–166.

15. King N, Bell D and Thomas K (2004). Family carers/ experiences of out-of-hours community palliative care: a qualitative study. *International Journal of Palliative Nursing* **10**(2): 76–83.

16. Monroe B, Hansford P, Payne M and Sykes N (2007–08). St Christopher's and the future. *OMEGA Journal of Death and Dying* **56**(1): 63–75.

17. Lorenz KA, Lynn J, Dy S, Wilkinson A, Mularski RA, Shugarman LR, Hughes R, Asch S, Rolon C, Rastegar A and Shekelle PG (2006). Quality measures for symptoms and advanced care planning in cancer: a systemic review. *Journal of Clinical Oncology* **24**(30): 4933–4938.

18. Higginson IJ, Shipman C, Gysels M, White P, Barclay S, Forrest S, Worth A, Murray S, Shepherd J, Pale J, Dewar S, Peters M, White S, Richardson A, Hotopf M, Lorenz K and Koffman J (2007). *Scoping Exercise on Generalist Services for Adults at the End of Life: Research, Knowledge, Policy and Future Research Needs*. Report for the National Co-ordinating Centre for NHS Service Delivery and Organization R & D. London: NCCSCO.

19. Hughes P, Noble B, Payne S, Ingleton C and Parker C (2006). Evaluating an education programme in general palliative care for community nurses. *International Journal of Palliative Nursing* **12**(3): 121–131.

20. Hudson P (2004). Positive aspects and challenges associated with caring for a dying relative at home. *International Journal of Palliative Nursing* **10**(2): 58–66.

21. Hudson P, Aranda S and McMurray N (2002). Intervention development for enhanced lay palliative caregiver support—the use of focus groups. *European Journal of Cancer Care* **11**(4): 262–270.

22. Hudson PL, Aranda S and Kristjanson LJ (2004). Meeting the supportive needs of family caregivers in palliative care: Challenges for health professionals. *Journal of Palliative Medicine* **7**(1): 19–25.

23. Family Caregiver Alliance (2006). *Caregiver Assessment: Principles, Guidelines and Strategies for Change*. Report from a National Consensus Development Conference (Vol 1). San Francisco. Family Caregiver Alliance: National Centre on Caregiving; California USA.

24. Parkes CM (2007–08). Introduction. *OMEGA Journal of Death and Dying* **56**(1): 1–5.

25. Hudson P (2004). A critical review of supportive interventions for family caregivers of patients with palliative-stage cancer. *Journal of Psychosocial Oncology* **22**(4): 77–92.

26. Harding R and Higginson I (2003). What is the best way to help caregivers in cancer and palliative care? A systematic literature review of interventions and their effectiveness. *Palliative Medicine* **17**(1): 63–74.

27. McMillan SC (2005). Interventions to facilitate family caregiving at the end of life. *Journal of Palliative Medicine* **8**(1): S132–S139.

28. Foley KM and Gelband H (ed.) (2001). *Improving Palliative Care for Cancer.* (www.nap.edu/books/0309074029/html): Institute of Medicine.

29. Twycross R (2007–08). Patient care: Past, present and future. *OMEGA Journal of Death and Dying* **56**(1): 7–19.

30. Kramer BJ, Boelk AZ and Auer C (2006). Family conflict at the end of life: lessons learned in a model program for vulnerable older adults. *Journal of Palliative Medicine* **9**(3): 791–801.

31. McPherson CJ, Wilson KG, Lobchuk MM and Brajtman S (2007). Self-perceived burden to others: patient and family caregiver correlates. *Journal of Palliative Medicine* **23**(3): 135–142.

32. Lazarus R and Folkman S (1984). *Stress, Appraisal, and Coping.* NY, USA: Springer Publishing Co.

33. Hudson P (2003). A conceptual model and key variables for guiding supportive interventions for family caregivers of people receiving palliative care. *Palliative and Supportive Care* **1**(4): 353–365.

34. Folkman S (1997). Positive psychological states and coping with severe stress. *Social Science and Medicine* **45**(8): 1207–1221.

35. Hebert RS, Arnold RM and Schulz R (2007). Improving well-being in caregivers of terminally ill patients. Making the case for patient suffering as a focus for intervention research. *Journal of Pain and Symptom Management* **34**(5): 539–546.

36. Yeandle S and Buckner L (2007). *Carers, Employment and Services: Time for a New Social Contract?* Leeds, UK: Carers UK: University of Leeds.

37. Ingleton C, Payne S, Nolan M and Carey I (2003). Respite in palliative care: a review and discussion of the literature. *Palliative Medicine* **17**(7): 567–575.

38. Smith P, Payne S and Ramcharan P (2006). *Carers of the Terminally Ill and Employment Issues: a Comprehensive Literature Review.* Help the Hospice London.

39. Casarett D and Karlawish J (2000). Are special guidelines needed for palliative care research? *Journal of Pain and Symptom Management* **20**(2): 130–139.

40. Dean RA and McClement SE (2002). Palliative care research: methodological ethical challenges. *International Journal of Palliative Nursing* **8**(8): 376–380.

41. Ferrell B (2004). Palliative care research: the need to construct paradigms. *Journal of Palliative Medicine* **7**(3): 408–410.

42. Penrod JD and Morrison RS (2004). Challenges for palliative care research. *Journal of Palliative Medicine* **7**(3): 398–402.

43. Hopkinson JB, Wright DNM and Corner JL (2005). Seeking new methodology for palliative care research: challenging assumptions about studying people who are approaching the end of life. *Palliative Medicine* **19**(7): 532–537.

44. Addington-Hall J (2005). Palliative care research in practice. *Canadian Journal of Nursing Research Special Issue: Palliative Nursing and End-of-Life Care* **37**(2): 85–93.

45. Christakis NA (2006). Advances in palliative care research methodology. *Palliative Medicine* **20**(8): 725–726.

46. Kaasa S, Jenson Hjermstad M and Havard Loge J (2006). Methodological and structural challenges in palliative care research: how have we fared in the last decades? *Palliative Medicine* **20**(8): 727–734.

47. Fielding S, Fayers PM, Loge JH, Jordhoy MS and Kaasa S (2006). Methods for handling missing data in palliative care research. *Palliative Medicine* **20**(8): 791–798.

48. Hudson P (2003). Focus group interviews: a guide for palliative care researchers and clinicians. *International Journal of Palliative Nursing* **9**(5): 202–207.

49. Hudson P, Aranda S, Kristjanson L and Quinn K (2005). Minimising gate-keeping in palliative care research. *European Journal of Pallaitive Care* **12**(4): 165–169.

50. Addington-Hall J, Bruera E, Higginson I and Payne S (ed.) (2007). *Research Methods in Palliative Care*. New York: Oxford University Press.

51. Hallenbeck J (2008). Evidence-based medicine and palliative care. *Journal of Palliative Medicine* **11**(1): 2–4.

52. Fine PG (2003). Maximising benefits and minimizing risks in palliative care research that involves patients near the end of life. *Journal of Pain and Symptom Management* **25**(4): S53–S62.

53. Addington-Hall J (2002). Research sensitivities to palliative care patients. *European Journal of Cancer Care* **11**: 220–224.

54. Raudonis B (1992). Ethical considerations in qualitative research with hospice patients. *Qualitative Health Research* **2**(2): 238–249.

55. Stevens T, Wilde D, Paz S, Ahmedzai S, Rawson A and Wragg D (2003). Palliative care research protocols: a special case for ethical review? *Palliative Medicine* **17**(6): 482–490.

56. Lee S and Kristjanson L (2003). Human Research Ethics Committees: issues in palliative care research. *International Journal of Palliative Nursing* **9**(1): 13–18.

57. Hudson PL, Aranda S and Hayman-White K (2005). A psycho-educational intervention for family caregivers of patients receiving palliative care: a randomised controlled trial. *Journal of Pain and Symptom Management* **30**(4): 329–341.

58. Walsh K, Jones L, Tookman A, Mason C, McLoughlin J, Blizard R and King M (2007). Reducing emotional distress in people caring for patients receiving specialist palliative care. *British Journal of Psychiatry* **190**: 142–7.

59. Medical Research Council (2000). *A Framework For Development And Evaluation Of Rcts For Complex Interventions To Improve Health*. MRC. London.

60. Abernethy AP, Hanson LC, Main DS and Kutner JS (2007). Palliative care clinical research networks, a requirement for evidence-based palliative care: time for coordinated action. *Journal of Palliative Medicine* **10**(4): 845–850.

61. Hudson P and Payne S (2006). An international collaboration for family carer research. *European Journal of Palliative Care* **13**(4): 135.

62. Payne S and Hudson P (In press). Assessing the family and caregivers. In: Walsh D (ed.). *Palliative Medicine*. Philadelphia: Elsevier.

63. Hudson PL and Hayman-White K (2006). Measuring the psychosocial characteristics of family caregivers of palliative care patients: psychometric properties of nine self-report instruments. *Journal of Pain and Symptom Managment* **31**(3): 215–228.

64. Deeken JF, Taylor KL, Mangan P, Yabroff KR and Ingham JM (2003). Care for the caregivers: A review of self-report instruments developed to measure the burden, needs, and quality of life of informal caregivers. *Journal of Pain and Symptom Management* **26**(4): 922–953.

65. Kristjanson LJ, Atwood J and Degner LF (1995). Validity and reliability of the Family Inventory of Needs (FIN): measuring the care needs of families of advanced cancer patients. *Journal of Nursing Measurement* **3**(2): 109–126.

66. Archbold P and Stewart B (1996). *Family Caregiving Inventory*. Portland: Oregon Health Sciences University.

67. Pearlin L, Mullan S, Semple S and Skuff M (199). Caregiving and the stress process: an overview of concepts and their measures. *The Gerontologist* **30**(5): 583–593.

68. Saranson I, Saranson B, Shearin E and Pierce G (1987). A brief measure of social support: practical and theoretical implications. *Journal of Social and Personal Relationships* **4**: 497–410.

69. Zeiss A, Gallagher-Thompson D, Lovett S, Rose J and McKibbin C (1999). Self-efficacy as a mediator of caregiver coping: development and testing of an assessment model. *Journal of Clinical Geropsychology* **5**(3): 221–230.

70. Given C, Given B, Stommel M, Collins C, King S and Franklin S (1992). The caregiver reaction assessment (CRA) for caregivers to persons with chronic physical and mental impairments. *Research in Nursing and Health* **15**: 271–283.

71. Scheir M and Carver C (1985). Optimism, coping, and health: assessment implications of generalized outcome expectancies. *Health Psychology* **4**(3): 219–247.

72. Kristjanson L, Sloan JA, Dudgeon D and Adaskin E (1996). Family members' perceptions of palliative cancer care: Perdictors of family functioning and family members' health. *Journal of Palliative Care* **12**(4): 10–20.

73. Teno JM, Clarridge B, Casey V, Edgman-Levitan S and Fowler J (2001). Validation of toolkit after-death bereaved family member interview. *Journal of Pain and Symptom Management* **22**(3): 752–758.

74. Prigerson H and Jacobs S (2001). Traumatic grief as a distinct disorder: a rationale, consensus criteria, and preliminary empirical test. In: Stroebe M, Hanson R, Stroebe W and Schut R (ed.). *Handbook of Bereavement: Consequences, Coping and Care*. New York: APA, 613–647.

75. Kristjanson LJ, Cousins K, Smith J and Lewin G (2005). Evaluation of the Bereavement Risk Index (BRI): a community hospice care protocol. *International Journal of Palliative Nursing* **11**(12): 610–618.

76. Salmon JR, Kwak J, Acquaviva KD, Egan KA and Brandt K. Validation of the caregiving at life's end questionnarie. *American Journal of Hospice & Palliative Medicine* **22**(3): 188–194.

77. Curtis JR, Patrick DL, Engelberg RA, Norris K, Asp C and Byock I (2002). A measure of the quality of dying and death: initial validation using after-death interviews with family members. *Journal of Pain and Symptom Management* **24**(1): 17–31.

78. Ferrario SR, Baiardi P and Zotti AM (2004). Update on the family strain questionnaire: A tool for the general screening of caregiving-related problems. *Quality of Life Research* **13**: 1425–1434.

79. Casarett D, Pickard A, Bailey FA, Ritchie CS, Furman CD, Rosenfeld K, Shreve S and Shea J (2008). A nationwide VA palliative care quality measure: the family assessment of treatment of the end of life. *Journal of Palliative Medicine* **11**(1): 68–75.

80. Cohen R, Leis AM, Kuhl D, Charbonneau C, Ritvo P and Ashbury FD (2006). QOLLTI-F: measuring family caregiver quality of life. *Palliative Medicine* **20**(8): 755–767.

81. Glajchen M, Kornblith A, Homel P, Fraidin L, Mauskop A and Portenoy RK (2005). Development of a brief assessment scale for caregivers of the medically ill. *Journal of Pain and Symptom Management* **29**(3): 245–254.

82. Cooper B, Kinsella GJ and Picton C (2006). Development and initial validation of a family appraisal of caregiving questionnaire for palliative care. *Psycho-Oncology* **15**(7): 613–622.

83. McMillan SC and Small BJ (2007). Using the COPE intervention for family caregivers to improve symptoms of hospice homecare patients: a clinical trial. *Oncology Nursing Forum* **34**(2): 313–321.

84. Kurtz ME, Kurtz Jc, Given CW and Given B (2005). A randomized, controlled trial of a patient/caregiver symptom control intervention: effects on depressive symptomatology of caregivers of cancer patients. *Journal of Pain and Symptom Management* **30**(2): 112–122.

85. Kwak J, Salmon JR, Acquaviva KD, Brandt K and Egan KA (2007). Benefits of training family caregivers on experiences of closure during end-of-life care. *Journal of Pain and Symptom Management* **33**(4): 434–445.

86. Hudson PL, Quinn K, Kristjanson LJ, Thomas T, Braithwaite M, Fisher J and Cockayne M (2008). Evalution of a psycho-educational group programme for family caregivers in home-based palliative care. *Palliative Medicine*, **22**(3): 270–280.

87. Hebert RS, Dang Q and Schulz R (2006). Preparedness for the death of a loved one and mental health in bereaved caregivers of patients with dementia: findings from the REACH Study. *Journal of Palliative Medicine* **9**(3): 683–693.

88. Hudson P, Aranda S and Kristjanson L (2004). Information provision for palliative care families. *European Journal of Palliative Care* **11**(4): 153–157.

89. Howell D and Brazil K (2005). Reaching common ground: a patient-family-based conceptual framework of quality EOL care. *Journal of Palliative Care* **21**(1): 19–26.

90. Steinhauser KE, Christakis NA, Clipp EC, McNeilly M, Grambow S, Parker J and Tulsky JA (2001). Preparing for the end of life: preferences of patients, families, physicians, and other care providers. *Journal of Pain and Symptom Management* **22**(3): 727–737.

91. Clayton JM, Hancock KM, Butow PN, Tattersall MHN and Currow DC (2007). Clinical practice guidelines for communicating prognosis and end-of-life issues with adults in the advanced stages of a life-limiting illness, and their caregivers. *Medical Journal of Australia* **186**(12): S77–S108.

Index